Nonparametric Statistical Tests

Test Name (Statistic)	Purpose	Measurement Level*		
		IV	DV	
Chi-square goodness-of-fit test (χ^2)	To test the predicted value of a proportion for a population	—	N	Nonparametric Tests → Chi Square
Chi-square test of independence (χ^2)	To test the difference in proportions in 2+ independent groups	N	N	Descriptive Statistics → Crosstabs
Fisher's exact test	To test the difference in proportions (2 × 2 table) when expected frequency for a cell < 5	N	N	Descriptive Statistics → Crosstabs
McNemar test (χ^2)	To test the difference in proportions for 2 dependent groups (2 × 2 design)	N	N	Descriptive Statistics → Crosstabs
Cochran's Q test (Q)	To test the difference in proportions for 3+ dependent groups	N	N	Descriptive Statistics → Crosstabs
Mann-Whitney U test (U)	To test the difference in the ranks of scores of 2 independent groups	N	O	Nonparametric Tests → 2 Independent Samples
Kruskal-Wallis test (H)	To test the difference in the ranks of scores of 3+ independent groups	N	O	Nonparametric Tests → K Independent Samples
Wilcoxon signed ranks test (T or z)	To test the difference in the ranks of scores of 2 dependent groups	N	O	Nonparametric Tests → 2 Related Samples
Friedman test (χ^2)	To test the difference in the ranks of scores of 3+ dependent groups	N	O	Nonparametric Tests → K Related Samples
Spearman's rank order correlation (r_S)	To test the existence of a relationship/correlation between two variables	O	O	Correlate → Bivariate
Kendall's tau (τ)	To test the existence of a relationship/correlation between two variables	O	O	Correlate → Bivariate

*Measurement level of the independent variable (IV) and dependent variable (DV):

N = nominal

O = ordinal

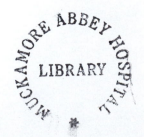

Second Edition

STATISTICS AND DATA ANALYSIS FOR NURSING RESEARCH

Denise F. Polit, PhD

*Humanalysis, Inc., Saratoga Springs, New York
and School of Nursing, Griffith University, Gold Coast, Australia*

Pearson

Boston Columbus Indianapolis New York San Francisco Upper Saddle River
Amsterdam Cape Town Dubai London Madrid Milan Munich Paris Montreal Toronto
Delhi Mexico City Sao Paulo Sydney Hong Kong Seoul Singapore Taipei Tokyo

Library of Congress Cataloging-in-Publication Data

Polit, Denise F.

    Statistics and data analysis for nursing research/Denise Polit.—2nd ed.

      p. ; cm.

    Rev. ed. of: Data analysis & statistics for nursing research/Denise F. Polit. c1996.

    Includes bibliographical references and indexes.

    ISBN-13: 978-0-13-508507-3

    ISBN-10: 0-13-508507-1

    1. Nursing—Research. 2. Nursing—Research—Statistical methods. I. Polit, Denise F. Statistics & data analysis for nursing research. II. Title.

    [DNLM: 1. Nursing Research—methods. 2. Statistics as Topic. W 20.5 P769s 2010]

    RT81.5.P62 2010

    610.72'7—dc22

                                          2009009967

Publisher: Julie Levin Alexander
Assistant to Publisher: Regina Bruno
Editor-in-Chief: Maura Connor
Assistant to Editor-in-Chief: Marion Gottlieb
Executive Editor: Pamela Fuller
Editorial Assistant: Jennifer Aranda/Lisa Pierce
Director of Marketing: Karen Allman
Marketing Specialist: Michael Sirinides
Marketing Assistant: Crystal Gonzalez
Senior Managing Editor: Patrick Walsh
Project Manager: Heather Willison, S4Carlisle Publishing Services
Senior Operations Supervisor: Ilene Sanford
Cover Art Director: Jayne Conte
Cover Designer: Bruce Kenselaar
Lead Media Project Manager: Rachel Collett
Full-Service Project Management: S4Carlisle Publishing Services
Composition: S4Carlisle Publishing Services
Printer/Binder: Edwards Brothers
Cover Printer: Lehigh Phoenix

This book was set in 10/12 Times by S4Carlisle Publishing Services. It was printed and bound by Edwards Brothers.

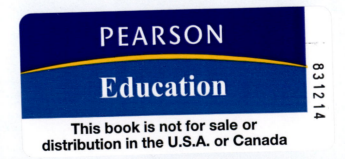

PEARSON Education

This book is not for sale or distribution in the U.S.A. or Canada

831214

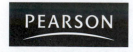

www.pearsonhighered.com

10 9 8 7 6 5 4 3 2
ISBN-10:   0-13-508507-1
ISBN-13: 978-0-13-508507-3

To the Memory of David P. Carroll

*Whose encouragement and support motivated me
to write the first edition of this book,
and whose ongoing friendship I sorely miss*

CONTENTS

CONTENTS

PREFACE

RATIONALE FOR THE SECOND EDITION

So very much has changed since the first edition of this book was published in 1996! The advances in statistical procedures and statistical software over the past 15 years have been substantial, and these advances alone would have warranted a second edition. A primary impetus for the revision, however, reflects the push for evidence-based practice (EBP) in nursing and health care. EBP has resulted in major changes in thinking about statistical analysis as a tool for generating, evaluating, and using evidence in clinical decisions. I hope that the excitement I experienced in revising this book is contagious.

Another impetus for this edition has come from students and faculty who have beseeched me to write a new edition. These advocates have consistently praised the accessibility, clarity, and user-friendliness of the book, features that are especially valuable on a topic that can be intimidating and frustrating. The style and practical emphasis of the first edition have been retained in this new edition, but important innovations have also been introduced, hopefully making it even easier to embark on a professional pathway that includes statistical analysis.

OVERVIEW OF THE BOOK

A fundamental belief underlying this book was that most students using it would have little interest in mathematics, probability, or statistical theory. For most of us, the primary reason for learning about statistics is to understand *how to analyze data*. This edition, like the first, is based on the premise that learning about data analysis is the ultimate goal of a statistics course in healthcare fields like nursing. Although this book *does* present statistical techniques, it does so within a broad data analytic framework. For example, each chapter explains not only *how* to perform a statistical analysis, but *why* and *when* in the analytic process it should be done. Each chapter has a section on the practical applications of the material covered, and also includes a section on how to report statistical information in a research article or dissertation.

Statistics and Data Analysis for Nursing Research (2nd ed.) is designed as a textbook for a one-semester course on statistics and data analysis, primarily for nursing students. It covers descriptive statistics, bivariate inferential statistics, and many widely used multivariate statistics. It assumes virtually no prior knowledge of statistics, and advanced mathematical grounding (e.g., calculus, matrix algebra) is not required. The book is written in a nontechnical manner, and the emphasis is on understanding how to use, understand, and interpret statistics, not on how to calculate them. Indeed, widely available software for statistical analysis has made hand calculations virtually obsolete. In writing and revising this book, I made a deliberate effort to present concepts in an incremental fashion, introducing complex topics only after first developing a firm foundation. My sincere hope is that the book will succeed in making a course on statistics less formidable than is often anticipated, and more practical than it often is.

NEW TO THIS EDITION

Emphasis on Evidence-Based Practice

I have made several changes to emphasize the importance of statistics as a tool in the evidence-building process. The first chapter provides a framework for understanding the types of EBP questions that can be addressed through statistical analysis. The book's focus is no longer exclusively on a traditional hypothesis-testing framework, which the medical community has all but abandoned. Virtually every chapter in this edition offers content on evaluating the *reliability* of statistical results (as communicated through *p* values), the *precision* of statistical results (as communicated through confidence intervals), and the *magnitude* of results (as communicated through effect size indexes). Information on effect size is especially important, given its crucial role in meta-analysis. This edition also describes various *risk indexes*, such as relative risk, absolute risk, odds ratios, and number needed to treat. These statistical indexes are routinely discussed in textbooks on EBP, but have not been adequately described in statistical textbooks for nurses.

SPSS Version 16.0

Computer output from statistical analyses is presented throughout the book, together with guidance on how to read the printouts. The Statistical Package for the Social Sciences (SPSS) is the most widely used statistical software by nurse researchers, and SPSS version 16.0 was used to generate the output for the book. Each chapter has exercises for students that involve using SPSS files. Three SPSS datasets are offered with the book on the book's Web site. The exercises have step-by-step instructions on how to run the analyses, and the answers to the exercises are provided in Word files, also on the book's Web site.

Missing Values

Almost all data analysts face the problem of missing values, and yet this topic is given scant attention in most statistics books. The final chapter of the book covers strategies for detecting patterns of missing values, and approaches to dealing with ensuing problems. State-of-the-art imputation techniques are discussed.

Scale Development

Most quantitative nurse researchers use composite scales in their studies, and often have to develop them from scratch. In this edition, the chapter on factor analysis has been expanded, and a new section on evaluating internal consistency reliability has been added. Even researchers using a preexisting scale routinely compute coefficient alpha, so this addition to the text is highly practical.

Power Analysis

Approaches for doing a power analysis to estimate sample size needs have been expanded and greatly simplified in this edition. Web sites with free power analysis software are noted, when appropriate.

ORGANIZATION OF THE TEXT

The content of this edition is organized into 14 chapters. Chapter 1 offers an introduction to statistical analysis, its role in research, and its importance to evidence-based nursing practice. The next three chapters cover descriptive statistics: Chapter 2 discusses data organization and frequency distributions; Chapter 3 describes indexes of central tendency, variability, and location; and Chapter 4 covers bivariate descriptive indexes, including the various risk indexes.

Chapter 5 offers an introduction to the complex topic of statistical inference. Care was taken in this chapter to provide a solid foundation for understanding the logic of inferential statistics, using fairly simple examples and analogies. Chapters 6 through 9 cover bivariate statistical tests, such as *t* tests (Chapter 6), analysis of variance (Chapter 7), chi-square tests and other nonparametric tests (Chapter 8), and correlation and simple regression (Chapter 9).

The next four chapters introduce students to important and widely used multivariate tools. The chapter on multiple regression (Chapter 10) is especially detailed, because several topics have relevance for other multivariate techniques (e.g., the concept of *residuals*, problems such as *multicollinearity*). Chapter 11 describes several multivariate techniques within the general linear model (GLM), such as analysis of covariance, multivariate analysis of variance, and repeated measures analysis of variance. Two less widely used analytic options, discriminant analysis and canonical analysis, are briefly reviewed. Chapter 12 offers a greatly expanded description of logistic regression, a widely used type of analysis in nursing research. Chapter 13 covers factor analysis and internal consistency reliability analysis.

The final chapter (Chapter 14) discusses the important topic of missing values. Although researchers typically address missing values problems early in the data analysis process, we postponed this chapter until the end because several innovative methods of analyzing missing values are fairly sophisticated and needed to be grounded in material covered earlier in the book.

KEY FEATURES

This textbook was designed to be helpful to those who are learning how to undertake research and analyze research data. Many of the features successfully used in the previous edition have been retained in this edition. Among the basic principles that helped to shape this book are (1) a conviction that the development of research and statistical skills is critical to the nursing profession; (2) a firm belief that research is an intellectually and professionally rewarding enterprise, and that data analysis is part of that enterprise; and (3) a view, based on personal experience, that learning about statistics need not be intimidating. Consistent with these principles, I have tried to present the fundamentals of statistics and data analysis in a manner that both facilitates comprehension and arouses interest. Key features of my approach include the following:

- *Research Examples.* Each chapter concludes with the description of an actual study that features the analyses described in the chapter. In addition, many research examples are used to illustrate key points in the text and to stimulate students' thinking about research questions and analytic options.
- *Clear, "user friendly" style.* The writing style used in this book was designed to make the content digestible and nonintimidating. Concepts are introduced carefully and systematically, difficult ideas are presented clearly, and readers are assumed to have no prior exposure to technical terms.
- *Specific practical tips on performing analyses.* The book is filled with practical guidance on how to translate the abstract notions of statistical methods into realistic strategies for analyzing data. Every chapter includes several tips for applying the chapter's lessons to real-life situations.
- *Guidance on presenting statistical results.* Each chapter offers advice on how to report the statistical results for statistics covered in the chapter. The guidance indicates what information to report in the text versus in tables and figures, and includes exemplary tables that can be used as templates for many statistical analyses.
- *Exercises.* Student exercises are included at the end of every chapter. The exercises are in two parts. Part A exercises ask students to apply their newly acquired knowledge, but do not require actual data analysis. Answers to Part A questions are in Appendix C at the back of the book. Part B exercises *do* require students to run analyses using the datasets provided with this book. The data are from a large and interesting study of low income women, and offer opportunities to test new skills using SPSS. Answers to the Part B exercises are included on the book's Web site.
- *PowerPoint slides.* PowerPoint slides have been prepared for each chapter of the book. These slides offer a more dynamic and colorful way to review textbook content, and also provide explicit guidance for undertaking SPSS analyses.
- *Further aids to student learning.* Several additional features are used to reinforce learning and to focus the student's attention, including the following: bolded terms when new concepts are introduced; succinct, bulleted summaries at the end of each chapter; and tables and figures that provide examples and graphic materials in support of the text discussion. A glossary of key terms is included at the end of the book for easy reference.
- *Online applications manual for* Statistics and Data Analysis for Nursing Research 2nd Edition. This online resource provides three complete datasets, compatible with SPSS, that students will use to complete the Part B exercises. Part B exercises are presented in an interactive form on the site, so students can submit their answers for instant feedback. Answers to Part A exercises are also available here, as well as links to additional Web sites for further study. *www.pearsonhighered.com/polit*

It is my hope that the content, style, and organization of this book will meet the needs of a broad spectrum of nursing students whose career paths will involve research. I also hope that the book will help to foster interest and enthusiasm for the kinds of discoveries that research and data analysis can produce, and for the knowledge that will help support an evidence-based nursing practice.

DENISE F. POLIT, PhD
President, Humanalysis, Inc., Saratoga Springs, NY
and Adjunct Professor, Griffith University School of Nursing, Gold Coast Australia
(WWW.DENISEPOLIT.COM)

ACKNOWLEDGMENTS

This second edition of *Statistics and Data Analysis for Nursing Research* (2nd ed.) relied on the contribution of many individuals. I would like to thank the numerous faculty and students who used the earlier edition and who made valuable suggestions for its improvement. In addition, several individuals deserve special mention.

I would like to acknowledge the comments of several anonymous reviewers of the previous edition, whose feedback influenced the revisions. Faculty at Griffith University in Australia made important suggestions, and also inspired the inclusion of some new content. Dr. Eileen Lake of the University of Pennsylvania was a strong supporter of this project and offered useful advice. Nathan O'Hara (my son) provided excellent technical expertise on many fronts.

We also extend our thanks to those who helped to turn the manuscript into a finished product. The staffs at Pearson Education and S4Carlisle Publishing Services have been of great assistance in seeing this project through. We are indebted to Pamela Fuller, Jennifer Aranda, Patrick Walsh, and Heather Willison, and all the others behind the scenes for their fine contributions.

Finally, I need to thank my family and friends, who provided critical support throughout the preparation of this book. I am grateful to my husband Alan and my son Nate, who did not complain when I worked long into the night, over weekends, and during holidays (including all day Christmas Eve and New Years Eve 2008) to get this edition finished.

FOREWORD

for *Statistics and Data Analysis for Nursing Research*

I am delighted to welcome you to this book. While I happen to be a nurse who is passionate about statistics, I know well that many nursing students are mystified or frightened by them. This book is the answer for all of us: This is the most clearly written, illustrative, and relevant statistics and data analysis textbook available.

Over my 20+ year research career, I have been fortunate to witness the development of a sizable amount of empirical evidence for nursing practice. When research questions emerge from our clinical experiences, the proper selection and use of statistics permits researchers to generate valuable answers, and thereby, ultimately, serve nurses and patients. Achieving the best match between a research question and an empirical answer, however, requires specialized knowledge. This knowledge is essential to prepare today's nurses to evaluate research critically, to integrate evidence into practice, and to participate in research.

As an associate professor of nursing at a research-intensive university, I set a high standard that my students will become avid, competent consumers of and advocates for nursing research. For over a decade I have been using Denise Polit's textbooks to teach required statistics and research methods to undergraduate nursing students. I teach large classes in which the textbook is the cornerstone to building complex, distinctive knowledge in a single semester. I have consistently used the first edition of this book, published in 1996, to teach statistics, and Polit and Beck's *Nursing Research* text (8th edition published in 2008) to teach research methods. What appealed to me about the first edition of the statistics book was its clarity, logical presentation, and comprehensive coverage of statistics and data analysis, illustrated by examples of contemporary nursing research.

You will learn how data are analyzed and it will not feel like a daunting prospect, because Dr. Polit presents technical material in plain language. This may seem to be an obvious expectation of a statistics textbook, but other textbooks do not actually walk you through examples with data. Although this book presents statistics and data analysis in a simple and straightforward style, do not be concerned that it is written for dummies. The coverage of statistics, including detailed equations, tests of significance, and underlying assumptions, is thorough.

Many other attractive features increase the book's practical value and distinguish it from other texts. Each chapter shows multiple research applications of the topic, provides computer printouts of the analytic results (using the widely used software called SPSS), gives tips on presenting the statistics in reports, and contains clinically relevant exercises to test yourself on the fundamental concepts as well as to answer research questions with a real dataset. Each chapter summarizes a published nursing research example. These examples are presented in a common format (purpose, methods, analysis, and results), demonstrating by consistent example how to think about a research study. Collectively, the book's features foster critical thinking, skill development, and an appreciation for research.

A hallmark of this textbook is the integration of an evidence-based practice perspective. I see firsthand many nursing students who struggle with statistics and are reluctant to engage in the research literature. Nursing students tell me that practicing nurses who precept them in clinical settings offer limited role models for evidence-based practice. My students understand the imperative of evidence-based practice, but need guidance to implement it fully. Dr. Polit provides the essential guidance in an accessible fashion.

I know that Dr. Polit felt an obligation to update the highly regarded first edition for the benefit of our newest nurse researchers. I applaud her for preparing a volume that builds substantially on the success of the earlier edition. This book is a useful companion for all nurses to understand the meaning and use of statistics and data analysis in research. By fostering a research foundation in student nurses, we can begin to close the gap between researchers and clinicians, and to enable nurses to use research evidence to improve patient care. Enjoy this "how to" guide on your path to evidence-based practice.

Eileen Lake, PhD, RN, FAAN
University of Pennsylvania School of Nursing

ABOUT THE AUTHOR

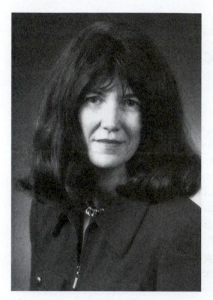

Dr. Denise F. Polit graduated from Wellesley College in 1969, and went on to obtain her Master's and Ph.D. degrees from Boston College. While in graduate school, where she obtained her doctoral degree in Research Methods and Statistics, she taught research methods courses at the Boston College School of Nursing. In 1978, she published *Nursing Research: Principles & Methods*, which quickly became a leading research methods textbook for nurses worldwide. (The 8th edition of this classic was released in 2008, under the new title *Nursing Research: Generating and Assessing Evidence for Nursing Practice*. This edition won the AJN Book-of-the-Year Award for research). In 1985, Dr. Polit published the award-winning undergraduate textbook, *Essentials of Nursing Research*. The 7th edition, published in early 2009, has a new title: *Essentials of Nursing Research: Appraising Evidence for Nursing Practice*. Two editions of a Canadian adaptation of this book have been released, and a third is underway. In 2009, the long-awaited second edition of *Statistics and Data Analysis for Nursing Research,* which was first published in 1996, was released. Her books have been translated into many languages.

Dr. Polit has established a strong track record as a researcher, with most of her research focusing on health-related issues among low-income women. She was a research scientist for 4 years at the American Institutes for Research in Cambridge, MA and Washington, DC, before starting her own research and consulting firm, Humanalysis, Inc., in 1983. She has received several grants from the National Institutes of Health (NIH), and has served on several study sections of NIH, including the National Institute of Nursing Research.

Dr. Polit has lectured and offered consulting services throughout the United States and in several countries. Several lectures were filmed and are offered as part of online nursing research courses by Walden University. She is a permanent adjunct professor at the Griffith University School of Nursing (at the Research Centre for Clinical and Community Practice Innovation) on the Gold Coast, Australia, where she works with faculty and students during yearly visits. She has published in numerous top-tier nursing journals, including *Nursing Research, Research in Nursing & Health, International Journal of Nursing Studies, Journal of Advanced Nursing,* and *Journal of Nursing Scholarship*.

Denise and her husband, Alan Janosy, live in Saratoga Springs, NY. Denise has a son (Nathan, a U.S. Marine), and 3 stepdaughters. Denise and Alan have a dog (a bearded collie) and 2 cats. Denise is an active volunteer for numerous nonprofit organizations in Saratoga Springs, including Saratoga Hospital.

Introduction to Data Analysis in an Evidence-Based Practice Environment

DATA ANALYSIS AND NURSING RESEARCH

Throughout the world, nursing is experiencing dramatic changes. Nurses are now being called on to base their professional practice on sound *evidence* that their actions and decisions will be effective—that is, to adopt an **evidence-based practice (EBP).** The EBP culture change means that nurses are increasingly expected to understand and critique research so that they can assess the quality of new evidence, and to conduct their own research so that they can contribute to the evidence base. This book is designed to teach some of the important skills needed to achieve these goals.

Research and Evidence-Based Practice

EBP is broadly defined as the use of the best clinical evidence in making patient care decisions. Evidence for EBP comes from a variety of sources, but most people concur that research findings from rigorous studies provide particularly strong evidence for informing nursing practice. Nursing leaders acknowledge the desirability for nurses to base specific clinical actions on evidence indicating that the actions are appropriate, cost effective, and efficacious for client outcomes.

Developing an evidence-based practice means learning skills for finding relevant evidence and evaluating its worth. For individual nurses, typical steps in EBP include: (1) asking clinical questions; (2) searching for research evidence that addresses the question; (3) appraising the evidence; and then (4) integrating the evidence with one's own clinical expertise and information about patient preferences (Polit & Beck, 2008; DiCenso, Guyatt, & Ciliska, 2005; Melnyk & Fineout-Overholt, 2005).

Example of a clinical question:

Among patients with cancer cachexia, is a fish oil–enhanced supplement better than other dietary supplements in stabilizing weight?

After posing a clinical question, the next steps are to locate and then critically appraise studies that address this question. Appraisals of research evidence involve a scrutiny of all aspects of a relevant study—how the sample of participants was selected, how confounding variables were controlled, how concepts were measured, how the research information was gathered, and how the information was analyzed. The appraisal process usually involves understanding and interpreting statistical evidence—hence the need for some proficiency in statistics even among nurses who will never actually conduct a study.

Statistical know-how is needed to address several key EBP questions for appraising research evidence (Box 1.1). These questions—especially the first three—can be addressed using statistical techniques described in this textbook.

The Analysis of Research Data

Just as with an EBP inquiry, a study begins with a question. **Research questions** are the queries that researchers pose with regard to a *research problem,* which is a perplexing or troubling condition (e.g., a high rate of patient falls). Research questions involve **concepts** (sometimes called *constructs),* which are abstractions inferred from observing behaviors or characteristics. For example, pain, stress, and body temperature are all concepts.

Researchers seek to answer their research questions by collecting information about the concepts of interest from people who serve as the *study participants* (or *subjects*). In the context of a study, the information collected is called **data**. Data can be gathered in a number of different ways—by asking people questions,

BOX 1.1
Key Evidence-Based Practice Questions

1. How reliable is the evidence?
2. What is the magnitude of effects?
3. How precise is the estimate of effects?
4. Is there evidence of side effects (or side benefits)?
5. What is the financial cost of using (or not using) the evidence in practice?
6. Is this evidence, if reliable and of sufficient magnitude, relevant in my particular clinical situation?

by observing their behavior, or by taking biophysiologic measurements, to name the most typical methods. Whatever the data collection method or research design, the data gathered by the researchers enables them to answer their research questions.

TIP: *A datum (singular for data) is a single measurement or observation, and is sometimes called a* score, raw score, *or* data value.

Research data can be either qualitative or quantitative. **Qualitative data** consist of verbal, narrative pieces of information. For example, Box 1.2 presents some fictitious qualitative data provided by two people in response to the question: Have you felt sad or depressed at all lately, or have you generally been in good spirits? Here the data are narrative descriptions that provide details about the respondents' emotional state.

Quantitative data consist of information in numerical form. Box 1.3 presents quantitative data from two study participants responding to the question: Thinking about the past week, how depressed would you say you have been on a scale from 0 to 10, where 0 means "not at all" and 10 means "the most possible"? The participants have provided a number indicating their degree of depression: 9 for Person 1, suggesting a high level of depression; and 0 for Person 2, indicating no depression.

In a study, researchers would ask many different people the research questions. These people, as a group, constitute the research sample. The responses of the sample members would, collectively, comprise the data for the study. By themselves, however, the data do not answer research questions. The data must be organized, synthesized, and interpreted through the process of **data analysis**.

BOX 1.2

Example of Qualitative Data

Question

Have you felt sad or depressed at all lately, or have you generally been in good spirits?

Data (Participant 1)

Well, I probably shouldn't burden you with this, but I've been in really rough shape this past month or so, to tell you the truth. I mean, I, like, just can't seem to shake the blues. When I think about the future, like, even just tomorrow, I just don't, um, I can't see anything to feel hopeful about. There are days when I just feel like, "What's the use of it all? What's the point of going on?"

Data (Participant 2)

Honestly, I feel great! I was thinking just yesterday how incredibly fortunate I am. It's like, I must be just about the happiest person in the world. About 3—no, it was 4—months ago I started a great new job that's interesting and has good benefits. The people at work are super, um, super friendly and fun to be around. And I've lost, like, 20 pounds and feel so much healthier. I can't remember when I've been happier.

BOX 1.3
Example of Quantitative Data

Question

Thinking about the past week, how depressed would you say you have been on a scale from 0 to 10, where 0 means "not at all" and 10 means "the most possible"?

Data (Participant 1)

9

Data (Participant 2)

0

The analysis of qualitative data is a complex, labor-intensive process. Those interested in learning about methods of qualitative data analysis should consult such references as Grbich (2007) or Miles and Huberman (1994).

Quantitative data are subjected to **statistical analysis**. The term *statistics*, in its broadest sense, refers to a collection of mathematical methods for organizing, summarizing, analyzing, and drawing conclusions based on data gathered in a study. This textbook focuses on methods of analyzing data through statistics. Statistical skills help to describe data, explore relationships, test hypotheses, predict outcomes, and, more broadly, answer research questions.

RESEARCH VARIABLES

In quantitative studies, the concepts in which researchers are interested are called variables. In our example in Box 1.3, the variable is depression. A **variable** is something that varies or takes on different values. Weight, *sex*, blood pressure, and heart rate are all examples of characteristics that vary from one person to the next. (If they did not vary, they would be **constants.**) Variation is at the root of much scientific inquiry.

Researchers are interested in explaining and understanding variation—for example, why do some hospitalized patients fall while others avoid falls? Research questions communicate information about the study variables and about the study *population*—the broad group of people who are the focus of the inquiry. In quantitative studies, many research questions take this form: In (population), what is the relationship between (variable X) and (variable Y)? As an example, here is a research question: Among women who are victims of partner violence during pregnancy (the population), is a nursing case management intervention (variable X) effective in reducing pregnancy complications (variable Y)? The "X" and the "Y" variables have distinct names in a research context, as discussed next.

Independent and Dependent Variables

Variables can be characterized in several different ways. One important distinction concerns the role that the variable plays in an analysis—the distinction between independent and dependent variables. The **independent variable** ("X") is the hypothesized cause of, or influence on, the **dependent variable** or "Y" (sometimes called the **outcome variable**). In the research question, "Does a low-cholesterol diet reduce the risk of heart disease among middle-aged men?" the independent variable is the amount of dietary cholesterol, and the dependent variable is heart disease; the population is middle-aged men. Cholesterol level is a variable, because people consume different amounts of it, and heart disease is a variable because not everyone has this disease. The research question is whether variation in the independent variable is related to, or causes variation in, the dependent variable.

Example of independent and dependent variables:

Research question: What is the effect of an educational program on fluid compliance among patients with end-stage renal disease undergoing hemodialysis? (Barnett, Li-Yoong, Pinikahana, & Si-Yen, 2008).

> *Independent variable*: Exposure or nonexposure to a special educational program
>
> *Dependent variable*: Compliance with fluid restrictions

TIP: *Although the concept of* **causality** *is controversial, many research questions are about causes and effects (e.g., does aromatherapy* cause *reductions in nausea among ambulatory surgical patients?). Statistical analysis in and of itself does not shed light on whether an independent variable* caused *or affected the dependent variable. Statistical analysis is used to assess how likely it is that variables are truly interrelated, not whether one caused the other, or vice versa (except in certain types of complex causal modeling analyses not described in this book). Inferences about causality are influenced more by features of the research design than by statistical analysis per se.*

Operationalizing Variables

In a quantitative study, the abstract concepts of interest must be captured in a way that they result in numerical data. Researchers begin by clarifying the theoretical or conceptual meaning of their concepts by developing *conceptual definitions*. They must then figure out a way to *operationalize* the concepts, by selecting or inventing methods to translate their abstractions into data. An **operational definition** identifies the precise set of operations or procedures that will be used to measure research variables. It is important to understand that the operational definition *defines* the underlying abstract concept in terms of the resulting measurements, and so researchers must strive for excellent operational definitions.

A key issue in developing operational definitions is to have sound conceptual definitions. Another is to understand the underlying nature of the variable in question. One useful distinction that has relevance for statistical analysis concerns discrete and continuous variables. A **discrete variable** consists of separate, indivisible categories, with a finite number of values between any two points. For example, if people were asked how many times they had been hospitalized, they might answer 0, 1, 2, 3, or more times. The variable for number of times hospitalized is discrete, because a number such as 1.2 is not a meaningful value: Between the values 1 and 3, the only possible value for number of hospitalizations is 2. A **continuous variable** is one that, at least in theory, can assume an infinite number of values between any two points. Weight is an example of a continuous variable. Between 1 and 2 pounds (or kilograms), there is an unlimited number of possible values: 1.01, 1.245, 1.379, and so on. In practice, however, many variables that are theoretically continuous are captured as discrete values. For example, we measure weight in whole pounds or kilos (or perhaps to one decimal place), even though there is theoretically an infinite number of values between any two weights. Thus, discrete variables offer greater possibility for *exact* measurement, whereas the measurement of continuous variables is always an approximation.

> **TIP:** *The Internet has dozens of resources that can supplement material included in this textbook. For example, if you search in Google or Yahoo! for a term like "continuous variable," you will find many sites that expand on our discussion of continuous versus discrete variables.*

LEVELS OF MEASUREMENT

Operational definitions guide the measurement of research variables. For every variable, researchers must devise methods of assigning values, typically numerical values that differentiate people appropriately. **Measurement** involves assigning numbers to qualities of people or objects to designate the quantity of the attribute, according to a set of rules. No attribute *inherently* has a numerical value. Humans invent the rules to quantitatively measure abstract concepts.

For some variables, measurement is straightforward. There are widely accepted rules for measuring such variables as height, weight, and blood pressure, for example. For other variables, researchers must often develop new rules of measurement. Sometimes the rules are complex—for example, when researchers measure psychological concepts such as stress, health beliefs, and so on, complex rules may be required. In other cases, the rules involve the assignment of an arbitrary **code**—for example, when the researcher designates a code of 1 for females and a code of 2 for males, for the variable *sex*.

Thus, there are different types of measurement rules, and the system for describing these differences concerns the **level of measurement** of a variable. There are four different levels of measurement: nominal, ordinal, interval, and ratio. This classification system is important because the type of analysis that researchers can undertake depends on the measurement level of the variables.

Nominal Measurement

Nominal measurement, the lowest form of measurement, involves using numbers (or, less frequently, alphabetical codes) simply as labels to name attributes and classify them into categories. In fact, variables measured on the nominal scale are sometimes called **categorical variables**. Many characteristics can be measured on a nominal scale: a person's race, marital status, and blood type, for instance. Some examples of nominal-level variables and possible codes are shown in Box 1.4. In nominal measurement, the numbers are arbitrary and have no inherent quantitative meaning: It would be just as appropriate to code males as 1 and females as 0 as vice versa. Because the numbers are arbitrary, they cannot be treated mathematically. For example, it is not meaningful to compute the average *sex* of a sample, although we could compute the percentage of males and females.

BOX 1.4

Examples of Nominal-Level Variables

VARIABLE	CODE			
Sex	1=Female	0=Male		
Group	1=Experimental	2=Control		
Blood Type	1=Type A	2=Type B	3=Type AB	4=Type O

TIP: *In nominal measurement, any coding scheme is, in theory, just as good as any other because the codes are just labels. However, for reasons that will not become apparent for many chapters, when a nominal-level variable is dichotomous (has only two values), such as the variable* sex, *researchers sometimes prefer using codes of 1 and 0, rather than codes of 1 and 2. This coding makes certain statistical analyses more straightforward.*

Ordinal Measurement

Ordinal measurement involves using numbers to designate *ordering* on an attribute. Ordinal measurement allows researchers to classify people and to indicate their relative standing on a dimension of interest. The numbers are no longer arbitrary, but rather convey some information about the *amount* of an attribute. Sometimes an ordinal scale is a series of ranks, like the rank ordering of students in a class (1st, 2nd, etc.). In other situations, ordinal measurement represents categories that may have verbal labels, such as *small*, *medium*, and *large* or *never, sometimes,* and *always.* Yet, unlike nominal measures, these categories are in a specific order indicating the amount of a variable, and the corresponding numerical codes (such as 1, 2, and 3) could not be rearranged. Some additional examples are presented in Box 1.5. The codes for pressure sore stages, for example, indicate incremental levels of damage, from Stage 1 (redness and edema) to Stage 4 (necrosis and muscle deterioration). Ordinal measurement does not, however, tell us anything about the distance between categories—that is, about absolute amounts. The difference between Stage 1 and Stage 2 is not equivalent to the difference between Stage 3 and Stage 4: The ordinal codes provide no clue about the relative magnitude of the differences. As with nominal-level measures, it is not generally meaningful to compute an average with variables measured on an ordinal scale.

Interval Measurement

Interval measurement involves assigning numbers that indicate both the ordering on an attribute, and the distance between score values on the attribute. Temperature on the Fahrenheit scale is an example of interval-level measurement. Equal distances on the Fahrenheit scale represent equal distances in temperature. That is, the difference between 100° F and 101° F is equivalent to the difference between 101° F and 102° F. Thus, interval-level measures provide information about not only rank ordering but also about the magnitude of difference between different numeric values. There are many analytic options for variables measured on the interval scale. For example, it is perfectly reasonable to compute averages

BOX 1.5

Examples of Ordinal-Level Variables

VARIABLE	CODE	
Pressure Ulcer Stage	1 = Stage 1, skin stays red for 5 minutes after removal of pressure	
	2 = Stage 2, breaks appear in the skin and discoloration may occur	
	3 = Stage 3, a hole may develop that oozes foul-smelling fluid	
	4 = Stage 4, the sore destroys tissue and necrosis extends through fat layers	
Educational Attainment	1 = High school diploma	3 = College degree
	2 = Some college, no degree	4 = Graduate degree
Cancer stage	1 = Stage 0	5 = Stage IIIB
	2 = Stage I	6 = Stage IV
	3 = Stage II	7 = Stage V
	4 = Stage IIIA	

for interval-level variables (e.g., the average body temperature of a sample of patients). Psychosocial scales that measure attributes of interest to nurse researchers (e.g., self-efficacy, spirituality, depression) are typically treated as interval-level measurements.

Ratio Measurement

Ratio measurements are similar to interval-level measurements, with one additional characteristic: the presence of a natural, meaningful zero point. Because of this feature, variables measured on the ratio scale provide information about the absolute amount of the attribute being measured. If we were measuring the amount of pain medication administered to a patient, 0 milliliters would be a legitimate value, indicating the absence of pain medication. Interval measures, by contrast, do not have a rational zero point. A temperature of 0° F does not indicate the total absence of heat. Because ratio-level measurements have an absolute zero, all mathematical operations are possible. It is possible to add, subtract, multiply, and divide values on a ratio scale. Thus, it is possible to say that 80 meters is twice as long as 40 meters (meters are on a ratio scale), although it is not meaningful to say that 80° F is twice as hot as 40° F.

Example of different measurement levels:

Kowalski and Bondmass (2008) studied physiological and psychological symptoms of grief in a sample of 173 widows. Ethnicity and type of health insurance were measured as nominal-level variables. In this study, annual income was measured as an ordinal variable in five income categories, coded from 1 (under $25,000) to 5 (>$100,000). Widows' grief was measured on an interval-level scale using the Revised Grief Experience Inventory. Age and number of months widowed were ratio-level variables.

Measurement Scale Considerations

The four levels of measurement can be thought of as a hierarchy, with nominal measurements at the base and ratio measurements at the pinnacle. Researchers usually strive to have variables measured on the highest level of measurement possible. There are several advantages to using higher levels of measurement: greater analytic flexibility, more powerful statistical options, and a greater amount of information than at lower levels.

As we move from ratio measures to interval, ordinal, and nominal measures, there is a successive loss of information. We can demonstrate this information loss with a fictitious example. Table 1.1 presents data on the amount of sodium intake for six people, measured on the four measurement scales. Column 1 shows the actual amount of sodium consumed, in milligrams. These ratio measures give us information regarding the absolute amount of sodium each person consumed, and the absolute differences among them. The next column shows interval measures that represent the amount of sodium over a specified criterion, which we have set at 2,500 mg. Chris has a value of 0 (2,500–2,500), while Nathan has a value of 5,000 (7,500–2,500) on this admittedly contrived measure. These interval-level values provide no clue about the absolute amount of sodium consumed, but the distances between the values are still meaningful. For example, the difference in sodium consumption between Mike and Daniel is the same as the difference between Daniel and Nathan (i.e., 2,000 mg). In column 3, the data have been reduced to an ordinal scale by rank ordering participants' sodium intake. Chris is ranked Number 1 because his sodium intake was lowest, Mike is ranked second, and so forth. These numbers no longer tell us how much more sodium was consumed by one person than the next. The amount separating Chris and Mike might be 1 mg or 5,000 mg. Finally, the last column presents nominal-level measures; here, the participants are simply classified as being high or not high on sodium intake, using 5,000 mg or greater as the cutoff value for the "high" category. Within each category, there is no information regarding who consumed more sodium than whom: Alan, Chris, and Mike are considered equivalent with regard to sodium intake.

It usually is preferable to use the highest possible level of measurement so that the fullest information available can be exploited. There are important exceptions. For example, some health variables may have cutoff values that are clinically important and that suggest different actions. For example, the distinction between low versus normal birth weight may be more important than ratio-level values such as 2,499 grams versus 2,501 grams.

TABLE 1.1 Fictitious Data Showing Four Measurement Levels for Daily Amount of Sodium Intake

Participant	(1) Ratio (Actual mg)	(2) Interval (Values above 2,500 mg)	(3) Ordinal (Rank order)	(4) Nominal (1 = not high, 2 = high)
Alan	4,000	1,500	3	1
Nathan	7,500	5,000	6	2
Chris	2,500	0	1	1
Mike	3,500	1,000	2	1
Vadim	6,000	3,500	5	2
Daniel	5,500	3,000	4	2

TIP: *It is best to* measure *a variable at the highest possible level, because it is always possible to collapse the information to a lower level during an analysis. For example, in Table 1.1, it was possible to convert ratio information to nominal information, but the reverse is not true. If we began by measuring sodium intake on a nominal high/not high scale, we would never be able to reconstruct ratio-level milligram values.*

For the most part, the measurement level of variables is fairly easy to determine. Yet, there is some controversy regarding the measurement level of scales that measure psychosocial attributes. Such scales typically have been treated in statistical analyses as interval-level measures, but some people argue that they are really ordinal measures. Although many psychosocial scales do yield measures that are (strictly speaking) ordinal, methodological studies have suggested that treating them as interval measures is not likely to result in distortions if the scales approximate interval characteristics.

TIP: *Variables are sometimes categorized into two basic measurement groups. Variables on the nominal level are* **qualitative variables** *because the numbers associated with the variables convey no quantitative information. The categories could as easily be designated with words or letters as with numerical codes. Variables measured on the ordinal, interval, or ratio scale—all of which convey information about the* amount *of an attribute—are* **quantitative variables.**

TYPES OF STATISTICAL ANALYSIS

Once research variables have been measured, the resulting quantitative data can be analyzed in various ways. The analyses can serve many different purposes, as discussed in this section.

Computerized and Manual Statistical Analysis

In the not-so-distant past, statistical analysis involved calculations performed using simple aids such as calculators. Even today, people sometimes quickly compute percentages or averages in this fashion. In research applications, however, virtually everyone uses specialized computer software for statistical analysis. Indeed, for many widely used analyses, manual calculations are out of the question.

There are dozens of statistical programs available, and some are even available for free over the Internet. One of the most widely used statistical software packages by nurse researchers is called Statistical Package for the Social Sciences, or SPSS®. This software is widely available on college and university campuses, and is the software we used to create examples of computer printouts for this book, using version 16.0. It is also the software that is the basis for assignments and exercises linked to the datasets that are available on the book's Web site. These datasets have data on over 100 variables for 1,000 low-income women who were randomly sampled in four U.S. cities.

Analyses for Description Versus Inference

A basic distinction in statistical analysis is the difference between descriptive statistics and inferential statistics.

DESCRIPTIVE STATISTICS   Researchers want to *describe* their data in a convenient and informative manner. Figure 1.1 presents an array of data that is sometimes referred to as a **data matrix**. The 15 rows in this matrix correspond to 15 study participants, and the columns correspond to data for 16 variables—the first 16 variables for the first 15 people in one of the datasets (Polit2SetA) on the book's Web site. Looking at the numbers in Figure 1.1, it is clearly impossible to make any sense of the data. Entering data into a statistical software data file is the first step in organizing data. Figure 1.2 shows a portion of an SPSS data file for the first seven variables in the Polit2SetA dataset. SPSS data files are in spreadsheet-type arrays, with a row for a study participant, and a column for each variable.

Descriptive statistics, which are used to describe and summarize data, help to make data even more comprehensible. A variety of descriptive statistics is available to researchers. Averages and percentages are examples of descriptive statistics. With regard to the variables in Figure 1.2, we could answer the following questions through descriptive statistics:

1. What percentage of the sample is Hispanic?
2. What is the average age of the participants in the sample?
3. What is the age range of study participants?
4. Are White participants older, on average, than African-American participants?
5. Is there a relationship between highest grade completed and age at first birth in this sample?

As these illustrative questions suggest, descriptive statistics allow researchers to *describe* (questions 1 through 3); to *compare* (question 4); and to *characterize a relationship* (question 5). Descriptive statistics can involve a single variable at a time (e.g., question 1 involves the variable race/ethnicity) or two variables simultaneously (for example, question 4 involves the variables race/ethnicity and age). Descriptive statistics are straightforward computationally.

Descriptive statistics can be communicated in three ways: in a narrative fashion, in a graph, or in a table. We could describe a sample in a narrative fashion as being 55% female and 45% male. We could display this same information graphically, as shown in Figure 1.3. A table could be used to characterize the sample in terms of

```
1200130.14822.81121414053204000
1200230.723  .  11110  .520.6000
1200330.18915.7812804  .87070000
1200426.67917.69121414053225000
1200639.33425.48111114053296000
1200736.39720.21121314554366000
1200927.51015.8312120  .56546000
1201131.81414.6811100  .55215600
1201225.01620.83121214053211000
1201538.03815.53121114058759000
1201738.01119.7531100  .58614110
1202125.42516.4911110  .65050000
1202328.88217.9411101 575050000
1202423.72318.47111112454155000
1202527.32323.31121012552145000
```

FIGURE 1.1   A matrix of data for 16 variables for 15 study participants.

id	age	age1bir	racethn	educatn	higrade	worknow
12001	30.148	22.81	1	2	14	1
12002	30.723	.	1	1	11	0
12003	30.189	15.78	1	2	8	0
12004	26.679	17.69	1	2	14	1
12006	39.334	25.48	1	1	11	1
12007	36.397	20.21	1	2	13	1
12009	27.510	15.83	1	2	12	0
12011	31.814	14.68	1	1	10	0
12012	25.016	20.83	1	2	12	1
12015	38.038	15.53	1	2	11	1
12017	38.011	19.75	3	1	10	0
12021	25.425	16.49	1	1	10	1
12023	28.882	17.94	1	1	11	1
12024	23.723	18.47	1	2	10	1
12025	27.323	23.31	1	2	1	0

FIGURE 1.2   Portion of an SPSS data file for 7 variables and 15 participants.

sex, race/ethnicity, marital status, and other traits. Throughout this book, we offer suggestions for when graphs or tables can be used effectively to supplement narrative presentations.

INFERENTIAL STATISTICS   Researchers typically derive their data by obtaining measurements from a **sample**, that is, from a subset of people with characteristics that are relevant to the research question. Yet researchers are almost always interested in answering research questions about a **population**—the entire group of people with the relevant characteristics—rather than about the particular people who are sampled from the population. Indeed, descriptive indexes computed for a population, such as an average value, are called **parameters**, whereas descriptive indexes for a sample are **statistics**.

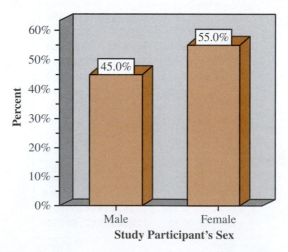

FIGURE 1.3   Graphic presentation of descriptive statistics (SPSS printout).

When researchers use data from a sample to make inferences or draw conclusions about a population, they use **inferential statistics**. Inferential statistics use *laws of probability* to help researchers draw objective conclusions about population characteristics, based on information from samples. Inferential statistics are widely used to generate research evidence about populations and concepts of interest to healthcare professionals.

Inferential statistics are sometimes used to draw conclusions about a single population value. For example, a researcher might want to know the average birth weight of infants born with AIDS. Without data from all babies born with AIDS, the researcher would estimate the value based on data from a sample of such babies. Inferential statistics would allow the researcher to infer how accurate the estimate was.

More frequently, inferential statistics are used to test **hypotheses** (predictions) about relationships between variables in the population. A **relationship** is a bond or association between variables. For example, the researcher might want to test the hypothesis that the average birth weight of babies with AIDS is *lower than* the birth weight of other babies. The relationship in question concerns birth weight (the dependent variable) in relation to AIDS status (the independent variable) in a population of infants.

Inferential statistics can be used to address several questions about relationships:

1. *Existence*   Is there a relationship between variable X and variable Y in the population?
2. *Magnitude*   How strong is the relationship between variable X and variable Y in the population?
3. *Precision*   How precise is the estimate about the existence and strength of the relationship?

Sometimes a single statistic can be computed to address several of these questions, but often separate statistics are needed for different questions. Statistics for all three types of question are described in this book. Note that these questions are consistent with the first three EBP appraisal questions shown in Box 1.1.

TIP: *Inference is an integral part of the research process. Inference is the attempt to generalize or draw conclusions based on limited information, using logical reasoning processes. Inference is essential because researchers use proxies that are meant to "stand in" for the things that are of fundamental interest.* A sample *of participants is a proxy for an entire* population. *An operational definition provides proxy (approximate) information about an abstract concept. A control group that does not receive an intervention is a proxy for what would happen to the same people if they simultaneously received* and *did not receive the intervention. Inferential statistics are thus a critical tool in allowing some types of inference to be made in an objective fashion.*

Univariate, Bivariate, and Multivariate Statistics

Another dimension along which statistical methods can be described concerns the number of variables in the analysis. **Univariate statistics** involve one variable at a time. Examples include the percentage of men and women in the sample, or the average heart rate of the sample members. **Bivariate statistics** involve two variables examined simultaneously. If the researcher compared the average heart rate of men versus women, bivariate statistical procedures would be used because there are two variables: *heart rate* and *sex*. When three or more variables are included in the same analysis, **multivariate statistics** are needed. For example, a researcher might use *sex*, weight, and amount of exercise (three independent variables) to better understand variations in heart rate (the dependent variable). Multivariate statistics are computationally formidable, but the widespread availability of computers has made these complex procedures accessible to most researchers.

THE DATA ANALYSIS PLAN

Researchers do not move directly from data collection to data analysis. Before addressing research questions and testing hypotheses, researchers typically undertake many preliminary steps with their **dataset** (i.e., the total collection of data for all sample members), as shown in the flow chart in Figure 1.4.

Preanalytic tasks include coding the data and entering data into a computer file. In developing a coding plan, researchers decide what codes to use for legitimate values (e.g., assigning a code of 1 for females and 0 for males, for the variable *sex*), and also what codes to use for missing information. **Missing values** represent the absence of substantive data for a variable, as a result of data collection errors, refusals, and so on.

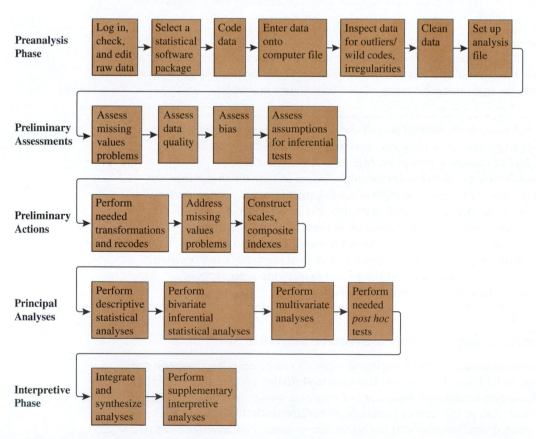

FIGURE 1.4 Flow of tasks in analyzing quantitative data.

TIP: *Missing values are sometimes assigned codes—codes that the researcher uses to designate a refusal or a "don't know" response. These codes must be numbers that are not used for legitimate values. Sometimes, however, missing data occur when information is totally absent—for example, when a question is skipped because it was not relevant for a particular participant (e.g., number of times pregnant for males). These missing values are often designated with a blank or (in SPSS) a period, and are called* **system missing.** *For example, in Figure 1.2, we can see that there is missing information about age at first birth (age1bir) for the second participant.*

There are many ways to enter the **raw data** (the actual information provided by study participants) into a file. In SPSS, data can be entered directly into a data editor, which, as previously noted, looks like a spreadsheet. The SPSS data editor allows you to give abbreviated **variable names** to each variable. Variable names must (in some versions of SPSS) be no longer than eight characters, and must be unique, with no duplication of names. In the data editor, these variable names are shown as column headers. For example, in Figure 1.2, the first four variable names are: *id* (a unique identification number for each participant), *age* (the participant's age), *age1bir* (age at first birth), and *racethn* (race/ethnicity). The SPSS data editor also allows you to provide all kinds of information about each variable, such as whether it is nominal, ordinal, or scale (interval and ratio levels combined); what the extended name of the variable is; what the numerical codes mean; how many decimal places are needed (if any); and what codes were used for missing values. A final pre-analytic step is to make sure that the data are "clean," i.e., error free. Data entry is an error-prone activity, so it is imperative to correct mistakes before undertaking actual analyses. Some data-cleaning steps are described in the next chapter.

Statistical analyses that we describe in this book are also used to make preliminary assessments of the data (Row 2 of Figure 1.4) and to take some preliminary actions (Row 3). Statistical procedures are used to deal with such issues as:

- assessing whether the data meet certain assumptions for advanced analyses;
- addressing the problem of missing values;
- assessing whether there are any **biases** in the dataset (e.g., it might be important to compare the characteristics of people who agreed to participate in the study with those of people who declined, to determine if they are different);
- evaluating the reliability and overall quality of **composite scales** (scales whose scores represent the aggregation of responses to several related questions);
- manipulating raw data to create new variables (e.g., converting infants' actual birth weights to an ordinal variable indicating normal, low, or very low birth weight); and
- understanding the characteristics of a sample.

Finally, researchers proceed to their principal analyses (Row 4 of Figure 1.4) and may follow these with further analyses designed to aid in interpreting results (Row 5). Prudent researchers develop a realistic **data analysis plan** that takes into account the need for the varied preliminary steps and guides progress toward the goal of answering the research questions and interpreting the results. Not all of the steps in Figure 1.4 are necessary in all studies, and in some cases the ordering of the steps might be different. The figure is intended not as an explicit guide, but rather to show that careful planning of analytic activities is critical. Throughout this textbook we describe statistical techniques that are appropriate for many of the steps in this flow of analytic activity.

TIP: *We did not order the material in this book in a sequence that corresponds with the order of activities in the flow chart in Figure 1.4. For example, we include information about addressing missing data problems (an early task in the flow of analytic activities) in the last chapter of this book. This is because some of the best methods of addressing missing data problems are fairly sophisticated and would be difficult to understand at the outset.*

Research Example

The following example describes the key variables in a study by a prominent team of nurse researchers.

Study: "A telephone-only motivational intervention to increase physical activity in rural adults" (Bennett, Young, Nail, Winters-Stone, & Hanson, 2008).

Study Purpose: The purpose of this research was to test whether an intervention—a telephone-only motivational interviewing intervention—would increase physical activity among physically inactive adults living in rural communities.

Research Design: A sample of 86 participants was assigned at random to an intervention group or a control group. Those in the intervention group received a pedometer and monthly motivational calls from a physical activity counselor over a 6-month period. Those in the control group had monthly phone calls, but without the motivational content. Data were collected via questionnaires administered at baseline (prior to the intervention) and then 6 months later.

Key Variables: The independent variable (IV) in this study was whether or not study participants received the special intervention. This IV is a dichotomous nominal level variable: Participants either received the intervention or they did not. One dependent variable was a ratio-level variable, caloric expenditure per week in all activities. Another dependent variable was self-efficacy for exercise, an interval-level variable measured on a six-item scale with scores ranging from 6 to 30. Stage of change for exercise, another key outcome, was measured on a five-category ordinal scale (precontemplation, contemplation, preparation, action, and maintenance). The researchers also gathered a variety of descriptive data about participants—for example, their age (ratio level); *sex*, race/ethnicity, and marital status (nominal-level); and illness/comorbidity (as measured in this study, an ordinal-level variable with three categories of illness severity).

Key Findings: The results suggested that the intervention increased participants' self-efficacy for exercise, but did not increase levels of physical activity compared to controls. Both groups changed their average stage of change for exercise over the 6-month study period.

Summary Points

- In a nursing environment in which **evidence-based practice (EBP)** is valued, skills in understanding and undertaking statistical analysis have become increasingly important.
- **Statistical analysis** involves a collection of mathematical methods for summarizing, analyzing, and drawing conclusions about quantitative data. **Quantitative data** are pieces of information that are in numerical form which, when analyzed and interpreted, contribute evidence to nursing practice.
- In a quantitative study, the abstract concepts of interest are called **variables**. Research often involves an **independent variable** (the presumed cause, influence, or antecedent) and a **dependent variable** (the presumed effect or **outcome**).

- **Research questions** are typically queries about the **relationship** between the independent and dependent variables within a **population** (the entire set of individuals or objects with characteristics of interest). **Hypotheses** are predictions about relationships among variables.
- Researchers first develop *conceptual definitions* of the study variables, and then formulate **operational definitions**, which specify the set of operations or procedures required to measure them.
- Some variables are **discrete** (take on a finite number of values), while others are **continuous** (capable of assuming an infinite number of values between two points).
- **Measurement** of variables involves assigning numbers to qualities of objects to designate quantitative information, according to a set of rules.
- There are four **levels of measurement** for research variables: (1) **nominal measurement**—classification into mutually exclusive categories; (2) **ordinal measurement**—the ordering or ranking of people based on their relative standing on an attribute; (3) **interval measurement**—indicating not only rank but the amount of distance between people on an attribute; and (4) **ratio measurement**—distinguished from interval measurement by having a rational zero point. The measurement level of variables often determines the type of analysis that is appropriate.
- **Descriptive statistics** are used to summarize and describe quantitative information. **Inferential statistics** are used to make inferences in an objective fashion about values for a population based on information from a **sample** (the subset of people selected for the study from the population).
- Statistical procedures vary in terms of the number of variables in the analysis (**univariate**, **bivariate**, and **multivariate statistics**).
- Statistical analyses can be used for many purposes in a study. Given the many uses and types of statistical analysis, prudent researchers develop a **data analysis plan** to guide the analytic activities. After coding and entering data into a data file, early steps in an analysis include cleaning the **raw data** and determining the extent of **missing values**—information that is absent from the dataset because of refusals and errors.

Exercises

In this and in following chapters, there are two types of exercises. Exercises in Part A are designed to reinforce your understanding of new concepts, and can be done on the basis of textbook content. Exercises in Part B are for those who wish to practice and hone their statistical skills by undertaking actual analyses with datasets we provide with this book, available on the book's Web site. Answers to most Part A exercises (as indicated with a dagger) are included in Appendix C of this book. Answers to the Part B exercises are provided on the Web site.

PART A EXERCISES

† **A1.** For each of the following, indicate which item is a variable and which item is a constant:
   (a) The number of minutes in an hour
   (b) Patients' diastolic blood pressure
   (c) Pi (π)—e.g., for finding the circumference of a circle
   (d) Level of anxiety among patients with cancer

† **A2.** For each of the following research questions, identify the independent variable and the dependent variable:
   (a) Is a person's age related to his/her psychosocial adjustment following a burn injury?
   (b) How do physically handicapped children differ from nonhandicapped children with respect to health self-concepts?
   (c) Do patients who administer their own pain medication have lower pain ratings than patients whose pain medication is administered by nurses?
   (d) Is the intracranial pressure of comatose patients affected by the presence of conversing visitors?
   (e) How does a bonnet compare to a stockinette in preventing heat loss in newborns?

† **A3.** For each of the variables listed below, indicate which variable is discrete and which variable is continuous:
   (a) Number of beds in a hospital
   (b) Height in inches or centimeters
   (c) Number of pregnancies a woman has had
   (d) Amount of time spent sleeping
   (e) Body temperature measured in Fahrenheit/Celsius degrees

† **A4.** For each of the variables listed below, indicate whether the measurement is nominal, ordinal, interval, or ratio:
   (a) Degrees on the Celsius scale
   (b) Runners' ranking in a race (1st, 2nd, etc.)
   (c) Number of cigarettes smoked per day
   (d) Scores on a 100-point scale measuring nurses' empathy
   (e) Adherence versus nonadherence to a treatment regimen
   (f) Academic rank (professor, associate professor, etc.)
   (g) Type of delivery (vaginal vs. cesarean)
   (h) White blood cell count

PART B EXERCISES

The book's Web site includes three real data files with, collectively, over 100 variables for 1,000 study participants—in this case, low-income women from four major U.S. cities facing various health challenges. We have created three separate data files, Polit2SetA.sav, Polit2SetB.sav, and Polit2SetC.sav. We created three files, with some redundant variables, because the student version of SPSS accommodates no more than 50 variables. The files were created in SPSS, Version 16.0, but are compatible with earlier versions of SPSS. Students can download the files and use the data to practice statistical analyses in SPSS for Windows. (For faculty preferring different statistical software, the file will need to be converted, and variable information such as value labels may need to be re-input.) We suggest several possible assignments related to these datasets in each chapter of this book.

The datasets can be downloaded on the book's Web site (please see the Preface or the back cover for the URL). The Web site also includes two Microsoft Word files to help you understand the datasets. The file "Dataset_Description.doc" provides an overview of the variables in the datasets, and a brief description of the study that generated these data. SPSS codebooks (data dictionaries) for the datasets are also available in a Word file on the Web site, "Codebooks_for_Datasets.doc." This codebook file[1] shows detailed information about each variable—for example, for the variable Race/ethnicity, the codebook shows that the code of 1 signifies *Black, not Hispanic*, and so on. It also provides information about the missing value codes that were assigned when legitimate values were not available, either because the participant refused to answer a question or the participant could not answer the question and gave a "don't know" response. Note that these missing values are the *assigned codes* that were specifically entered into the data file to designate a particular type of missing value. System-missing codes are not shown in the codebook. Thus, if a variable has no missing values information, it does not mean that there are no missing values, only that there are no separate user-missing values.

Complete one or more of the following exercises to begin to familiarize yourself with the dataset.

† **B1.** Open the data file Polit2SetA.sav in SPSS. The file should open in "Data View," which shows the spreadsheet of data values. (If not, click on the tab in the lower left of the screen that says "Data View.") You should be viewing information that looks like what we presented in Figure 1.2. Navigate down the rows of the spreadsheet to see the extensiveness of the file in terms of number of cases; each row corresponds to a study participant, each of whom was assigned a unique identification number (ID). What is the ID number for case 1,000—i.e., the last case in the file?

† **B2.** Now navigate across the spreadsheet to quickly peruse the variable names in the dataset. What is the eight-character variable name for the last variable in this dataset?

† **B3.** Look at the intersection of the variable *age1bir* and case number 10 (ID 12015) in the spreadsheet. How old was this woman when she first gave birth?

† **B4.** Click on the "Variable View" tab in the lower left of the screen. This view presents information about all variables, in the order they appear in the file. Find the fourth variable in the file, *racethn*. Click in the rectangle for *Values* for this variable, which will bring up a box with information about how this variable was coded. What code was used for Hispanic participants? What does the code of 7 mean? What codes were used to designate missing information for *racethn*? Now, keeping the codes for this variable in mind, go back to "Data View." What is the race/ethnicity of the first case (ID 12001)?

† **B5.** Now, open (and perhaps print) the Word file called "Codebooks_for_Datasets." What is the variable name (and extended variable description) for the variable that is the seventh variable in this file? If a person had a code of 1 for this variable, what would that mean? If a person had a code of 7, what would that mean? What is the level of measurement of this variable?

B6. Glance through the codebook and the other Word file, "Dataset Description." Find variables in the dataset that you think would be (a) a nominal variable; (b) an ordinal variable; (c) an interval-level variable; and (d) a ratio-level variable. Justify your selection.

B7. Find variables within any of the three dataset files that *you* might be interested in learning more about, and ask a research question. For example, suppose you choose as your variable "Frequency of being highly stressed"*(stressed),* in the file Polit2SetB.sav. You might ask: In a sample of low-income women, what percentage is highly stressed? Or, your research questions might involve two variables. For example, suppose you choose as your variables "Currently employed"*(worknow)* and "Frequency of being highly stressed*" (stressed).* You might ask: In a sample of low-income women, are those who are working less highly stressed or more highly stressed than those who are not working?

---

[1] Codebook information is available in a different format within each of the three SPSS files if you are using SPSS 16.0. Use the File → Display Data File Information command to see a matrix-style display of variable information.

2

Frequency Distributions: Tabulating and Displaying Data

Researchers use a variety of descriptive statistics to describe data from a research sample. This chapter presents methods of calculating, organizing, and displaying some descriptive statistics.

FREQUENCY DISTRIBUTIONS

Researchers begin their data analyses by imposing some order on their data. A simple listing of the raw data for a variable rarely conveys much information, unless the sample is very small. Take, for example, the data shown in Table 2.1, which represent fictitious resting heart rate values (in beats per minute or bpm) for 100 patients. It is difficult to understand these data simply by looking at the numbers: We cannot readily see what the highest and lowest values are, nor can we see where the heart rate values tend to cluster.

Ungrouped Frequency Distributions for Quantitative Variables

One of the first things that researchers typically do with data is to construct frequency distributions. A **frequency distribution** is a systematic arrangement of data values—from lowest to highest or vice versa—together with a count of how many times each value was observed in the dataset. Table 2.2 presents a frequency distribution for

TABLE 2.1 Fictitious Data on Heart Rate for 100 Patients, in Beats Per Minute

60	65	63	57	64	65	56	64	71	67
70	72	68	64	62	66	59	67	61	66
56	69	67	73	68	63	69	70	72	68
60	66	61	60	65	67	74	66	65	66
65	72	66	58	62	60	73	64	59	72
65	68	61	59	68	71	67	65	63	70
67	59	66	69	61	70	58	62	66	63
74	69	68	57	63	65	71	67	62	66
55	70	69	62	66	67	62	72	64	68
64	58	64	66	63	69	71	64	67	57

the heart rate data. Now we can tell at a glance that the lowest value is 55, the highest value is 74, and the value with the highest frequency (11 people) is 66.

> **TIP:** *Statistical software provides options for ordering variables in ascending or descending order. We show ascending order in our examples, but researchers preparing tables for journal articles may use reverse ordering for conceptual or theoretical reasons.*

TABLE 2.2 Frequency Distribution of Heart Rate Values

Score (X)	Tallies	Frequency (f)	Percent (%)
55	I	1	1.0
56	II	2	2.0
57	III	3	3.0
58	III	3	3.0
59	IIII	4	4.0
60	IIII	4	4.0
61	IIII	4	4.0
62	IIII I	6	6.0
63	IIII I	6	6.0
64	IIII III	8	8.0
65	IIII III	8	8.0
66	IIII IIII I	11	11.0
67	IIII IIII	9	9.0
68	IIII II	7	7.0
69	IIII I	6	6.0
70	IIII	5	5.0
71	IIII	4	4.0
72	IIII	5	5.0
73	II	2	2.0
74	II	2	2.0
		$N = 100 = \Sigma f$	$100.0 = \Sigma\%$

Researchers constructing a frequency distribution manually list the data values (the Xs) in a column in the desired order, and then keep a tally next to each value for each occurrence of that value. In Table 2.2, the tallies are shown in the second column, using the familiar system of four vertical bars and then a slash for the fifth case. The tallies can then be totaled, yielding the frequency (f) or count of the number of cases for each data value.

In constructing a frequency distribution, researchers must make sure that the list of data values is mutually exclusive and collectively exhaustive. The sum of the frequencies must equal the number of cases in the sample. We can express this with some notation that will appear again in this textbook:

$$\Sigma f = N$$

where $\Sigma =$ the sum of
$\quad\quad f =$ the frequencies
$\quad\quad N =$ the sample size

This equation simply states that the sum of (symbolized by the Greek letter sigma, Σ) all the frequencies of score values (f) equals the total number of study participants (N).

A frequency count of data values usually communicates little information in and of itself. In Table 2.2, the fact that five patients had a heart rate of 70 bpm is not very informative without knowing how many patients there were in total, or how many patients had lower or higher heart rates. Because of this fact, frequency distributions almost always show not only **absolute frequencies** (i.e., the count of cases), but also **relative frequencies**, which indicate the percentage of times a given value occurs. The far right column of Table 2.2 indicates that 5% of the sample had a heart rate of 70. Percentages are useful descriptive statistics that appear in the majority of research reports. A percentage can be calculated easily, using the following simple formula:

$$\% = (f \div N) \times 100$$

That is, the **percentage** for a given value or score is the frequency for that value, divided by the number of people, times 100. The sum of all percentages must equal 100% (i.e., $\Sigma\% = 100\%$). You will probably recall that a **proportion** is the same as a percentage, before multiplying by 100 (i.e., proportion $= f \div N$).

Of course, researchers rarely use a tally system or manually compute percentages with their dataset. In SPSS and other statistical software packages, once the data have been entered and variable information has been input, you can proceed to run analyses by using pull-down menus that allow you to select which type of analysis you want to run. For the analyses described in this chapter, you would click on Analyze in the top toolbar, then select Descriptive Statistics from the pull-down menu, then Frequencies.

Another commonly used descriptive statistic is **cumulative relative frequency**, which combines the percentage for the given score value with percentages for all values that preceded it in the distribution. To illustrate, the heart rate data have been analyzed on a computer using SPSS, and the resulting computer printout is presented in Figure 2.1. (The SPSS commands that produced the printout in Figure 2.1 are Analyze → Descriptive Statistics → Frequencies → *hartrate*.)

TIP: *Throughout this book, we present SPSS printouts to illustrate statistical analyses, and we point out the commands we used to create the output within SPSS 16.0. Note, however, that different versions of SPSS—including the Student Version—may involve slightly different commands, and a few analytic options might not be available in other versions.*

Frequencies

Heart Rate in Beats per Minute

		Frequency	Percent	Valid Percent	Cumulative Percent
Valid	55	1	1.0	1.0	1.0
	56	2	2.0	2.0	3.0
	57	3	3.0	3.0	6.0
	58	3	3.0	3.0	9.0
	59	4	4.0	4.0	13.0
	60	4	4.0	4.0	17.0
	61	4	4.0	4.0	21.0
	62	6	6.0	6.0	27.0
	63	6	6.0	6.0	33.0
	64	8	8.0	8.0	41.0
	65	8	8.0	8.0	49.0
	66	11	11.0	11.0	60.0
	67	9	9.0	9.0	69.0
	68	7	7.0	7.0	76.0
	69	6	6.0	6.0	82.0
	70	5	5.0	5.0	87.0
	71	4	4.0	4.0	91.0
	72	5	5.0	5.0	96.0
	73	2	2.0	2.0	98.0
	74	2	2.0	2.0	100.0
	Total	100	100.0	100.0	

FIGURE 2.1   SPSS printout of a frequency distribution.

In Figure 2.1, cumulative relative frequencies are shown in the last column, labeled *Cumulative Percent*. The advantage of these statistics is that they allow you to see at a glance the percentage of cases that are equal to or less than a specified value. For example, we can see that 87.0% of the patients had heart rates of 70 bpm or lower. This figure also has a column labeled *Valid Percent*. In this example, the values in this column are identical to the values in the preceding column (*Percent*) because there are no missing data—heart rate information is available for all 100 patients. It is common, however, to have missing data in actual studies. The percentages in the column *Valid Percent* are computed after removing any missing cases. Thus, if heart rate data were missing for ten sample members, the valid percent for the value of 55 would be 1.1% ([1 ÷ 90] × 100) rather than 1.0%.

Grouped Frequency Distributions

The values in the heart rate example ranged from a low of 55 to a high of 74, for a total of 20 different values. For some variables, the range of values is much greater. For example, in a sample of 100 infants, it would be possible to obtain 100 different values for the variable birth weight measured in grams. An ordinary frequency table to examine the birth weight data would not be very informative, because each value would have a frequency of 1. When a variable has many possible values, researchers sometimes construct a **grouped frequency distribution**. Such a distribution involves grouping together values into sets, called **class intervals**, and then tabulating the frequency of cases within the class intervals. For example, for infants' birth weights, we might establish the following class intervals:

- 1,500 or fewer grams
- 1,501–2,000 grams
- 2,001–2,500 grams
- 2,501–3,000 grams
- 3,001 or more grams

In grouping together data values, it is useful to strike a balance between insufficient detail when too few groups are used, and lack of clarity when too many groups are created. For example, if infants' birth weight was grouped in clusters of 10 grams (e.g., 1,001 to 1,010; 1,011 to 1,020, and so on), there would be dozens of groups. On the other hand, for some purposes it might be inadequate to cluster the birth weight data into only two groups (e.g., $<2,000$ grams and $\geq 2,000$ grams). As a rule of thumb, a good balance can usually be achieved using between four and 10 class intervals.

Once you have a general idea about the desired number of intervals, you can determine the size of the interval. By subtracting the lowest data value in the dataset from the highest data value and then dividing by the desired number of groups, an approximate interval size can be determined. However, you should also strive for intervals that are psychologically appealing. Interval sizes of two and multiples of five (e.g., 10, 100, 500) often work best. All class interval sizes in a grouped frequency distribution should be the same.

Given that the heart rate data resulted in a total of 20 different values, it might be useful to construct a grouped frequency distribution. Clustering five values in a class interval, for example, we would have four intervals. The printout for this grouped frequency distribution is shown in Figure 2.2.[1] In this distribution, we can readily see that, for example, there were relatively few cases at either the low end or high end of the distribution, and that there is a substantial clustering of values in the 65 to 69 interval. On the other hand, there is also an information loss: For example, we cannot determine from this distribution what percentage of cases is 70 or below, as we could with the original ungrouped distribution. Decisions on whether to use an ungrouped or grouped distribution depend, in part, on the reason for constructing the distribution.

Frequency Distributions for Categorical Variables

When a variable is categorical or qualitative (i.e., measured on the nominal scale), you can also construct a frequency distribution. As with quantitative variables, the variable categories are listed in the first column, followed by frequencies and/or relative frequencies in succeeding columns. A fictitious example of a frequency distribution for the nominal variable marital status is shown in Table 2.3.

With categorical variables, it is usually not meaningful to display cumulative relative frequencies because there is no natural ordering of categories along any dimension. In Table 2.3, for example, the ordering of the categories could be changed without affecting the information (e.g., the category "Single, never married" could come first). Several strategies can be used to order the categories in tables prepared

---

[1] For producing the frequency distribution in Figure 2.2, we created a new variable (we called it *grouphr*) by using the Transform → Compute commands. For example, we instructed the computer to set *grouphr* to 1 if *hartrate* >54 and *hartrate* <60. A procedure in SPSS called "Visual Binning" (within the "Transform" set of commands) can also be used.

Frequencies

Grouped Heart Rate

		Frequency	Percent	Valid Percent	Cumulative Percent
Valid	55-59 bpm	13	13.0	13.0	13.0
	60-64 bpm	28	28.0	28.0	41.0
	65-69 bpm	39	39.0	39.0	80.0
	70-74 bpm	20	20.0	20.0	100.0
	Total	100	100.0	100.0	

FIGURE 2.2   SPSS printout of a grouped frequency distribution.

for research reports. Two common approaches are ascending or descending order of the frequencies, and alphabetical order of the categories. We ordered the categories in Table 2.3 in descending order of frequency.

GRAPHIC DISPLAY OF FREQUENCY DISTRIBUTIONS

Frequency distributions can be presented either in a table, as in Tables 2.2 and 2.3, or graphically. Graphs have the advantage of communicating information quickly, but are not common in journal articles because of space constraints. By contrast, graphs are excellent means of communicating information in oral and poster presentations at conferences. They can also be useful to researchers themselves early in the analysis process when they are trying to understand their data.

Bar Graphs and Pie Charts

When a variable is measured on a nominal scale, or on an ordinal scale with a small number of values, researchers can construct a **bar graph** to display frequency information. An example of a bar graph for the marital status data from Table 2.3 is presented in Figure 2.3. A bar graph consists of two dimensions: a horizontal dimension (the *X* **axis**) and a vertical dimension (the *Y* **axis**). In a bar graph, the categories are typically listed along the horizontal *X* axis, and the frequencies or percentages are displayed on the vertical *Y* axis. The bars above each category are drawn to the height that indicates the frequency or relative frequency for that category. In a bar graph for categorical data, the bars for adjacent categories should be drawn not touching each other; each bar width and the distance between bars should be equal. Researchers sometimes indicate exact percentages at the top of the bars, as shown in Figure 2.3.

TABLE 2.3 Frequency Distribution of a Nominal-Level Variable: Patients' Marital Status

Marital Status	Frequency (*f*)	Percent (%)
Married	124	49.6
Single, Never Married	55	22.0
Divorced	49	19.6
Widowed	22	8.8
Total	*N* = 250	100.0%

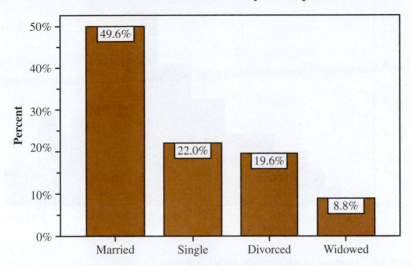

FIGURE 2.3 Example of an SPSS bar graph for a nominal-level variable.

An alternative to a bar graph is a **pie chart** (sometimes called a *circle graph*), which is a circle divided into pie-shaped wedges corresponding to the percentages. Figure 2.4 presents an SPSS-generated pie chart for the marital status data. All the pieces of the pie must add up to 100%. The pie wedges are generally ordered from highest to lowest frequency, with the largest segment beginning at "12 o'clock."[2]

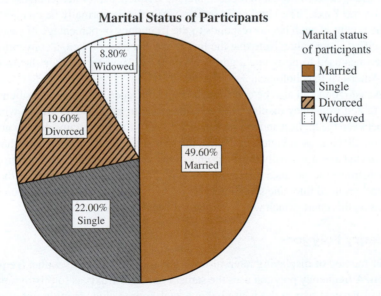

FIGURE 2.4 Example of an SPSS pie chart for a nominal-level variable.

---

[2] To produce Figures 2.3 and 2.4, we used the SPSS commands Analyze ➔ Descriptive Statistics ➔ Frequencies ➔ Charts for the variable *marstat,* opting for the Bar Chart option first and the Pie Chart option next. We could also have used the commands Graphs ➔ Legacy Dialogs ➔ Bar (or Pie).

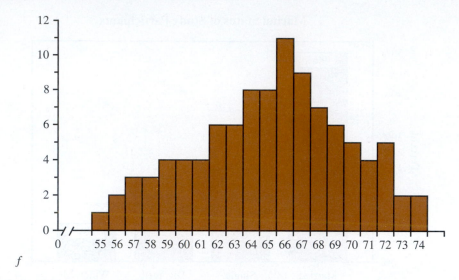

FIGURE 2.5   Example of a histogram: Heart rate data.

Histograms

Frequency information for interval-level and ratio-level data can be displayed in a **histogram**, which is a graphic display similar to a bar graph. In a histogram, however, the bars touch one another because adjacent values are not distinct categories, but rather contiguous scores on an ordered dimension.

An example of a histogram is shown in Figure 2.5, which is a graphic presentation of the heart rate data from Table 2.2. Data values are typically indicated on the X axis, arranged from lowest to highest, and the frequencies (or percentages) are presented on the Y axis. The numbering on this vertical axis normally begins with 0, or 0%. The height of each bar corresponds to the frequency or percentage of cases with the specified score value. Note that the line of the X axis is broken, a convention that is sometimes used to designate a gap between 0 and the first number shown on the scale (American Psychological Association, 2001).

A histogram can also be constructed from a grouped frequency distribution. As with a tabled frequency display, it is advantageous to group score values when the range between the highest and lowest scores is great. Most histograms display no more than about 20 bars, as in Figure 2.5. When the scores are grouped, the values shown on the horizontal axis are usually the midpoints of the score intervals. Computer programs can be instructed to produce histograms. Figure 2.6 presents a histogram of the heart rate data,[3] grouped into nine score intervals. Note the curved line that has been superimposed on this chart, which will be explained later in this chapter.

Frequency Polygons

Another method of displaying interval-level and ratio-level data is with a **frequency polygon**. A frequency polygon uses the same X axis and Y axis as for histograms, but instead of vertical bars, a dot is used above each score value (or midpoint of a class interval) to designate the appropriate frequency. The dots are then connected by a solid line. Figure 2.7, created within SPSS, displays the heart rate data from Table 2.2

---

[3] To produce the histogram in Figure 2.6, we used the Graphs ➔ Legacy Dialog ➔ Histogram commands in SPSS for the variable *hartrate*. We could also have used the Analyze ➔ Descriptive Statistics ➔ Frequencies ➔ Charts commands.

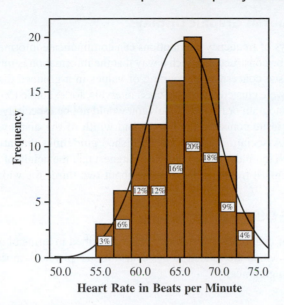

FIGURE 2.6   Example of an SPSS histogram with grouped data.

in a frequency polygon. Frequency polygons typically show one score value below the lowest obtained value and one score value above the highest obtained value. Sometimes the line connecting the dots is brought down to the horizontal axis to show a frequency of 0 for these two out-of-range values.

TIP: *There are no rules about whether a histogram or a frequency polygon should be used to display data. By convention, histograms are often the preferred method of displaying data for discrete variables, while frequency polygons are more likely to be used with continuous variables. From a visual perspective, a frequency polygon is more likely than histograms to emphasize the* shape *of a distribution, and highlights the notion of a continuum.*

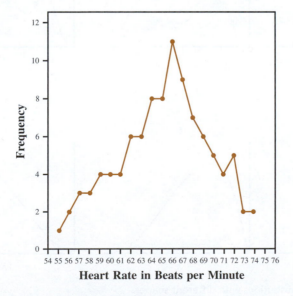

FIGURE 2.7   Example of an SPSS frequency polygon.

General Issues in Graphic Displays

Graphic displays of frequency distributions can communicate information at a glance, but graphs can be constructed in such a way that the information is misleading or ineffective. One issue concerns the grouping of values in a grouped distribution. If the heart rate data were clustered into two class intervals, for example (55–64 and 65–74), the resulting histogram or frequency polygon would not be especially informative.

Another issue concerns the height and width of the display. The American Psychological Association (2001) has published guidelines that are used by many nursing research journals. These guidelines suggest that the height of a graph (i.e., the height at the highest frequency) should be about two thirds the width of the X axis.

SHAPES OF DISTRIBUTIONS

Distributions of quantitative variables can be described in terms of a number of features, many of which are related to the distributions' physical appearance or shape when presented graphically.

Modality

The **modality** of a distribution concerns how many peaks or high points there are. A distribution with a single peak—that is, one value with a high frequency—is a **unimodal distribution**. The distribution of heart rate data (Figure 2.7) is unimodal, with a single peak at the value of 66.

Multimodal distributions have two or more peaks, and when there are exactly two peaks, the distribution is **bimodal**. Figure 2.8 presents six distributions with different shapes. In this figure, the distributions labeled A, E, and F are unimodal,

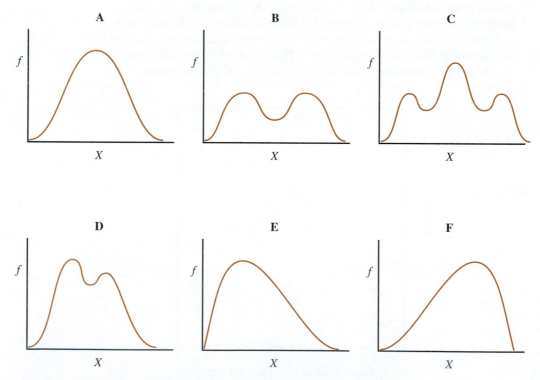

FIGURE 2.8 Examples of distributions with different shapes.

while B, C, and D are multimodal. Distributions B and D have two peaks, and thus can also be described as bimodal.

Symmetry and Skewness

Another aspect of a distribution's shape concerns symmetry. A distribution is **symmetric** if the distribution could be split down the middle to form two halves that are mirror images of one another. In Figure 2.8, distributions A through C are symmetric, while D through F are not.

Distributions of actual study data are rarely as perfectly symmetric as those shown in Figure 2.8. For example, the distribution of heart rate values in Figure 2.7 is roughly symmetric, and researchers would likely characterize the data as symmetrically distributed. Minor departures from perfect symmetry are usually ignored when describing the shapes of data distributions.

In **asymmetric distributions**, the peaks are off center, with a bulk of scores clustering at one end, and a tail trailing off at the other end. Such distributions are often described as **skewed**, and can be described in terms of the direction of the skew. When the longer tail trails off to the right, as in D and E of Figure 2.8, this is a **positively skewed distribution**. An example of an attribute that is positively skewed is *annual income*. In most countries, most people have low or moderate incomes and would cluster to the left, and the relatively small numbers in upper income brackets would be distributed in the tail. When a skewed distribution has a long tail pointing to the left (Figure 2.8, F), this is a **negatively skewed distribution**. For example, if we constructed a frequency polygon for the variable *age at death*, we would have a negatively skewed distribution: Most people would be at the far right side of the distribution, with relatively few people dying at a young age.

Skewness and modality are independent aspects of a distribution's shape. As Figure 2.8 shows, a distribution can be multimodal and skewed (D), or multimodal and symmetric (B and C)—as well as unimodal and skewed (E and F), or unimodal and symmetric (A).

Statisticians have developed methods of quantifying a distribution's degree of skewness. These skewness indexes are rarely reported in research reports, but they can be useful for evaluating whether statistical tests that are described later in this book are appropriate. A skewness index can readily be calculated by most statistical computer programs in conjunction with frequency distributions. The index has a value of 0 for a perfectly symmetric distribution, a positive value if there is a positive skew, and a negative value if there is a negative skew. For the heart rate data (Figure 2.7), the skewness index is −.20, indicating a very modest negative skew.

TIP: *In SPSS, if you request information about skewness within the Frequency procedure, you will get a value for both the skewness index and a standard error (a concept discussed more fully later in this book). As a rough guide, a skewness index that is more than twice the value of its standard error can be interpreted as a departure from symmetry. In our example, the skewness index of −.20 was smaller than the standard error (.24), indicating that the heart rate distribution is not markedly skewed.*

Kurtosis

A third aspect of a distribution's shape concerns how pointed or flat its peak is—that is, the distribution's **kurtosis**. Two distributions with different peakedness are superimposed on one another in Figure 2.9. Distribution A in this figure is more peaked,

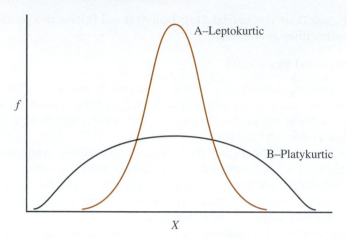

FIGURE 2.9   Example of distributions with different kurtoses.

and would be described as a **leptokurtic** (from the Greek word *lepto*, which means thin) **distribution**. Distribution B is flatter, and is a **platykurtic** (from the Greek word *platy*, which means flat) **distribution**.

As with skewness, there is a statistical index of kurtosis that can be computed when computer programs are instructed to produce a frequency distribution. For the kurtosis index, a value of 0 indicates a shape that is neither flat nor pointed (e.g., distribution A in Figure 2.8). Positive values on the kurtosis statistic indicate greater peakedness, and negative values indicate greater flatness. For the heart rate data displayed in Figure 2.8, the kurtosis index is −.55 (with a standard error of .48), indicating a distribution that is only slightly more platykurtic than leptokurtic.

The Normal Distribution

A distribution that has special importance in statistical analysis is the normal distribution (also known as the *bell-shaped curve*, *normal curve*, or *Gaussian distribution*). A **normal distribution** is one that is unimodal, symmetric, and not too peaked or flat. Figure 2.8 (A) illustrates a distribution that is normal. The normal distribution was given its name by the French mathematician Quetelet who, in the early 19th century, noted that many human attributes—such as height, weight, intelligence, and so on—appeared to be distributed according to this shape. Most people are in the middle range with respect to say, height, with the number tapering off at either extreme: Few adults are under 5 feet tall, for example, and similarly few are over 7 feet tall. Much more will be said about the normal distribution in subsequent chapters.

TIP: *Because of the importance of normal distributions in statistical analysis, some computer programs have a command that allows researchers to examine visually the extent to which their data approximate a normal distribution. For example, SPSS has an option to display the actual distribution for a variable, with a normal distribution superimposed, as illustrated in Figure 2.6. When this option is selected, it can readily be seen how "far off" the distribution is from being normal.*

RESEARCH APPLICATIONS OF FREQUENCY DISTRIBUTIONS

Readers who have some experience reading research reports in professional journals may have noticed that most journal articles do not present entire frequency distributions in either tabular or graphic form. This does not mean, however, that frequency distributions are unimportant in data analysis. This section examines some of the main reasons for constructing frequency distributions, and offers suggestions for reporting frequency distribution information in reports.

The Uses of Frequency Distributions

There are many reasons for constructing frequency distributions within a research context, several of which are described here. Many of these reasons correspond to activities from the first two rows of Figure 1.4, the data analysis flow chart described in Chapter 1.

1. *Becoming familiar with the dataset*   Most researchers routinely begin their data analysis by instructing a computer program to construct frequency distributions on all or most variables in their dataset. Researchers want to make sense of their data, and a good place to begin is to inspect the data after they have been organized in frequency distributions. The initial inspection usually involves tabled displays, as in Figure 2.1.

2. *Cleaning the data*   Data that have been entered into a computer file for subsequent analysis almost always contain some errors. One aspect of **data cleaning** involves a search for **outliers**—that is, values that lie outside the normal range of values for other cases. Outliers can be found by inspecting the values in a frequency distribution, with special scrutiny of the highest and lowest values. For some variables, outliers are legitimate. For example, a question about sample members' annual income might yield responses primarily in the $20,000 to $200,000 range, but a response of $2 million could be legitimate. In many cases, however, outliers indicate an error in data entry that needs to be corrected. There are also situations in which frequency distributions reveal a code that is impossible. For example, Figure 2.10 presents a frequency distribution for responses to the question, "Have you had a mammogram in the past 12 months?" In this example, only the codes 1 (yes) and 2 (no) are valid responses. The codes 3 and 5 are **wild codes** resulting from data entry errors. In this situation, the researcher would need to identify the four cases with the improper codes (three cases coded 3 plus one case coded 5), determine the correct codes, and then make the needed corrections. After data cleaning is completed, a new set of frequency distributions should be run to make sure that the problems have been corrected as intended.

> **TIP:** *Within SPSS, you can get help with outliers through the commands Analyze → Descriptive Statistics → Explore → Statistics for the variable in question. This will show the five highest and five lowest values, and the case numbers with these values in the data file so that corrections, if needed, can readily be made.*

3. *Inspecting the data for missing values*   Researchers strive for a *rectangular matrix* of data—data for all participants for all key variables. This ideal is seldom achieved, and so researchers must decide how to handle missing values. The first step is to determine the extent of the problem by examining frequency distributions on a variable-by-variable basis. In Figure 2.10, only one case (1% of

Frequencies

Mammogram in past year?

		Frequency	Percent	Valid Percent	Cumulative Percent
Valid	Yes	23	23.0	23.2	23.2
	No	72	72.0	72.7	96.0
	3	3	3.0	3.0	99.0
	5	1	1.0	1.0	100.0
	Total	99	99.0	100.0	
Missing	System	1	1.0		
Total		100	100.0		

FIGURE 2.10 SPSS printout of a frequency distribution with wild codes and missing data.

the sample) had a missing value (in this case, a "system missing" or blank) on the mammogram question. Methods of addressing missing data problems are discussed in Chapter 14.

4. *Testing assumptions for statistical tests*   As discussed in subsequent chapters, many widely used inferential statistics are based on a number of assumptions. In statistics, an **assumption** is a condition that is presumed to be true and, when ignored or violated, can lead to misleading or invalid results. Many inferential statistics assume, for example, that variables in the analysis (usually the dependent variables) are normally distributed. Frequency distributions and the associated indexes for skewness and kurtoses provide researchers with information on whether the key research variables conform to this assumption—although there are additional ways to examine this, as will be discussed in later chapters. When variables are not normally distributed, researchers have to choose between three options: (1) Select a statistical test that does not assume a normal distribution; (2) Ignore the violation of the assumption—an option that is attractive if the deviation from normality is modest; or (3) Transform the variable to better approximate a distribution that is normal. Various **data transformations** can be applied to alter the distributional qualities of a variable, and the transformed variable can be used in subsequent analyses. Some data transformation suggestions are shown in Table 2.4.

5. *Obtaining information about sample characteristics*   Frequency distributions are used to provide researchers with descriptive information about the background characteristics of their sample members. This information is often of importance in interpreting the results and drawing conclusions about the ability to generalize the findings. For example, if a frequency distribution revealed that 80% of study participants were college graduates, it would be imprudent to generalize the findings to less well-educated people.

6. *Directly answering research questions*   Although researchers typically use inferential statistics to address their research questions, descriptive statistics are sometimes used to summarize substantive information in a study. For example, Lauver, Worawong, and Olsen (2008) asked a sample of primary care patients what their health goals were. They presented several descriptive tables with frequency and relative frequency (percentage) information. For instance, as their primary health goal, 40% of participants ($N = 24$) said they wanted to get in better shape and 30% ($N = 18$) wanted to lose weight. Only 6.7% ($N = 4$) mentioned the desire to manage stress as their primary goal.

TABLE 2.4 Data Transformations for Distribution Problems

Problem	Type of Transformation	SPSS Function[a, b]
Positive skew, moderate	Square root	$newvar = SQRT\ (var)$
Positive skew, substantial	Base 10 logarithmic	$newvar = LG10\ (var)$
Positive skew, severe	Inverse	$newvar = 1 \div var$
Negative skew, moderate	Reversed square root	$newvar = SQRT\ (K - var)$
Negative skew, substantial	Reversed base 10 logarithmic	$newvar = LG10\ (K - var)$
Negative skew, severe	Reversed inverse	$newvar = 1 \div (K - var)$

[a]Within SPSS, a new variable would be created through the Transform → Compute Variable command. The new variable (*newvar*) would be set equal to a mathematical function of the original variable (*var*). The SQRT and LG10 functions are in the "Arithmetic" function group of the Compute Variable dialog box.

[b]K is a value from which each score is subtracted, such that the smallest score = 1; K is set equal to the highest score value in the distribution + 1.

The Presentation of Frequency Information in Research Reports

Frequency distributions are rarely presented in full in research journal articles because of space constraints and because full distributional information is rarely of interest. Tables and figures take a lot of space and are usually reserved for presenting more complex information. Take, for example, the marital status information shown in Table 2.3 and in graphic form in Figures 2.3 and 2.4. This information could be more efficiently reported as text:

> Nearly half (49.6%) of the sample was married, while 22.0% had never been married, 19.6% were divorced or separated, and 8.8% were widowed.

Note that results are always reported in the past tense, not the present tense. Results reflect measurements taken on a sample of study participants at a particular time in the past.

The publication guidelines of the American Psychological Association (2001) advise that tables should not be used for simple data presentations (e.g., one column by five or fewer rows, or two columns by two rows). Frequency information is most likely to be presented in a table or figure when *several* variables are being reported simultaneously, or when there is a time dimension.

> **TIP:** *Whenever you include tables or figures in a report, they should be numbered (e.g., Table 1, Figure 2), and cited in the text of the report.*

Tables with frequency information often are used to summarize the background characteristics of study participants. For example, Liu and co-researchers (2008) studied the effects of age and sex on health-related quality of life among patients with kidney transplantation. Table 2.5, an adaptation of a table in their report, shows frequency distributions for three background variables. Two variables, sex and race, are nominal-level variables. Age is a ratio-level variable, shown here in a grouped frequency distribution with five class intervals. This method of presentation is efficient, because it provides readers with a quick summary of important sample characteristics.

Researchers are most likely to present substantive frequency information in tables or graphs when there are several variables that have the same codes or score

TABLE 2.5 Example of Table with Frequency Distribution Information for Sample Description

Participants' Characteristics	Number	%
Sex		
Male	72	52.2
Female	66	47.8
Age		
25–34	20	14.5
35–44	31	22.5
45–54	44	31.9
55–64	30	21.7
≥65	13	9.4
Race		
White/Caucasian	106	76.8
Other	32	23.2
Total Number	138	

Adapted from the study by Liu et al. (2008) of patients with kidney transplantation, using information from their Table 1 (p. 85), titled "Samples and Demographic Data."

values, so that an entire matrix of frequency information can be presented simultaneously. For example, Kennedy-Malone, Fleming, and Penny (2008) studied prescribing patterns among gerontologic nurse practitioners. Their report included a table (an abbreviated, adapted version of which is shown in Table 2.6) that showed the frequency with which the nurse practitioners in their sample prescribed 29 medications deemed inappropriate for people aged 65 and older. Such a matrix, with multiple medications and three response categories, presents a wealth of descriptive frequency information in a compact format.

In summary, frequency information is often presented in the text of a research report—typically as percentages—rather than in graphs or tables. Yet, when multiple variables or multiple data collection points can be presented simultaneously, a

TABLE 2.6 Example of Frequency Distributions for Multiple Variables

Medications Prescribed Inappropriately by Gerontological Nurse Practitioners (N = 234)			
Medication[a]	**Never** %	**Occasionally** %	**Frequently** %
Diphenhydramine (Benadryl)	44	48	8
Cyclobenzaprine (Flexeril)	55	39	6
Amitriptyline (Elavil)	60	35	5
Ticlopidine (Ticlia)	74	23	3
Diazepam (Valium)	80	18	2
Chlorzoxazone (Parafon Forte)	90	9	1
Propantheline	98	2	0

[a]A selected, illustrative list; the original table included 29 medications

Adapted from Table 4 in Kennedy-Malone et al. (2008), titled "GNPs Patterns of Inappropriate Prescribing Based on the 1997 Modified Beers Criteria."

frequency graph or table can be quite efficient. Even though graphs require considerable space, they do have an arresting quality that captures people's attention, and so are preferred in any type of oral presentation where space constraints are not an issue. They also can be very effective if used sparingly in reports to emphasize or clarify important pieces of information.

Tips on Preparing Tables and Graphs for Frequency Distributions

Although frequency distributions are not often presented in tables or graphs in research reports, following are a few tips for preparing them. Some of these tips also apply to displays of other statistical information that we discuss in subsequent chapters.

- When percentage information is being presented, it is generally not necessary (or desirable) to report the percentages to two or more decimal places. For example, a calculated percentage of 10.092% usually would be reported as 10.1% or, sometimes, 10%.
- In reporting percentages, the level of precision should be consistent throughout a specific table or figure. Thus, if the percentages in a distribution were 10.1%, 25%, and 64.9%, they should be reported either as 10%, 25%, and 65% *or* 10.1%, 25.0%, and 64.9%.
- A reader should be able to interpret graphs and tables without being forced to refer to the text. Thus, there should be a good, clear title and well-labeled headings (in a table) or axes (in a graph). With frequency information, the table should include information on the total number of cases (N) on which the frequencies were based. Acronyms and abbreviations should be avoided or explained in a note.
- Occasionally there is a substantive reason for showing how much missing information there was. For example, if we were asking people about whether they used illegal drugs, it might be important to indicate what percentage of respondents refused to answer the question. In most cases, however, missing information is not presented, and only valid percentages are shown.

TIP: *If you are preparing figures or charts for a poster or slide presentation at a conference, charts created by programs like SPSS, Excel, or Word may suffice. However, for publication in journals, it may be necessary to hire a graphic artist to create professional images. You can also consult books such as those by Few (2004) or Wallgren, Wallgren, Persson, Jorner, and Haaland (1996) for additional guidance on how to prepare statistical graphs.*

Research Example

Almost all research reports include some information on frequencies or relative frequencies. Here we describe a published study that used frequency information extensively.

Study: "Physical injuries reported in hospital visits for assault during the pregnancy-associated period" (Nannini et al., 2008).

Study Purpose: The purpose of this research was to describe patterns of physical injuries reported on hospital visits for assault among women during their pregnancy or postpartum period.

Research Design: Using hospital records (linked to natality records) in Massachusetts during the period 2001 to 2005, the researchers obtained data for a sample of 1,468 women for 1,675 hospital visits for assault. The first physical injury was noted for each visit that had a physical injury diagnostic code (N = 1,528 visits).

Key Variables: The hospital records data were used to describe the distribution of physical injuries by body region and nature of the injury. The variable *body region*, a nominal-level variable, had five categories: head and neck, spine and back, torso, extremities, and unclassifiable. *Nature of injury*, another categorical variable, had six categories: fracture, sprain, open wound, contusion, system wide, and other. The researchers also had data regarding the women's characteristics, including race/ethnicity and marital status (nominal variables), education

(ordinal), and age (ratio level, but shown in a grouped frequency distribution with five class intervals: <20, 20–24, 25–29, 30–34, and 35+).

Key Findings: The women in this sample of assaulted pregnant or postpartum women tended to be young (64.0% were under age 25) and single (82.6% were unmarried). The distribution of injuries indicated that the women's head and neck were the most commonly injured body regions (42.2% overall). Injuries to the torso were observed for 21.5% of the pregnant women and 8.7% of the postpartum women. In terms of nature of the injury, the most prevalent type was contusions, observed for 46.5% of the women.

Summary Points

- A **frequency distribution** is a simple, effective way to impose order on data. A frequency distribution orders data values in a systematic sequence (e.g., from lowest to highest), with a count of the number of times each value was obtained. The sum of all the frequencies (Σf) must equal the sample size (N).
- In a frequency distribution, information can be presented as **absolute frequencies** (the counts), **relative frequencies** (that is, **percentages**), and **cumulative relative frequencies** (cumulative percentages for a given value plus all the values that preceded it).
- When there are numerous data values, it may be preferable to construct a **grouped frequency distribution**, which involves grouping together values into **class intervals**.
- Frequency distribution information can be presented in graphs as well as in tables. Graphs involve plotting the score values on a horizontal axis (the **X axis**) and frequencies or percentages on the vertical axis (the **Y axis**).
- Nominal (and some ordinal) data can be displayed graphically in **bar charts** or **pie charts**, while

interval and ratio data are usually presented in **histograms** or **frequency polygons**.
- Data for a variable can be described in terms of the *shape* of the frequency distribution. One aspect of shape is **modality**: A **unimodal** distribution has one peak or high value, but if there are two or more peaks it is **multimodal**.
- Another aspect of shape concerns symmetry: A **symmetric distribution** is one in which the two halves are mirror images of one another.
- A **skewed distribution** is asymmetric, with the peak pulled off center and one tail longer than the other. A **negative skew** occurs when the long tail is pointing to the left, and a **positive skew** occurs when the long tail points to the right.
- A third aspect of a distribution's shape is **kurtosis**: Distributions with sharp, thin peaks are **leptokurtic**, while those with smooth, flat peaks are **platykurtic**.
- A special distribution that is important in statistics is known as the **normal distribution** (bell-shaped curve), which is unimodal and symmetric.

Exercises

The following exercises cover concepts presented in this chapter. Appendix C provides answers to Part A exercises that are indicated with a dagger (†). Exercises in Part B involve computer analyses using the datasets provided with this textbook, and answers and comments are offered on this book's Web site.

PART A EXERCISES

† **A1.** The following data represent the number of times that a sample of nursing home residents who were aged 80 or older fell during a 12-month period.

0	3	4	1	0	2	0	1	2	0
1	0	0	1	2	5	0	1	0	1
0	2	1	0	1	1	3	2	1	0
1	3	1	1	0	4	6	1	0	1

Construct a frequency distribution for this set of data, showing the absolute frequencies, relative frequencies, and cumulative relative frequencies.

† **A2.** Using information from the frequency distribution for Exercise A1, answer the following:

(a) What percentage of the nursing home residents had at least one fall?

(b) What number of falls was the most frequent in this sample?

(c) What number of falls was the least frequent in this sample?

(d) What percentage of residents had two or fewer falls?

(e) What is the total size of the sample?

(f) Are there any outliers in this dataset?

A3. Draw a frequency histogram for the data shown in Exercise A1. Now superimpose a frequency polygon on the histogram. Using a ruler, measure the height and width of your graphs: Is the height about two thirds of the width?

† **A4.** Describe the shape of the frequency distribution drawn in Exercise A3 in terms of modality and skewness. Is the number of falls normally distributed?

A5. If you wanted to display information on patients' age using the data in Table 2.5, would you construct a histogram, bar graph, frequency polygon, or pie chart? Defend your selection, and then construct such a graph.

PART B EXERCISES

† **B1.** Using the SPSS dataset Polit2SetA, create a frequency distribution for the variable *racethn*. You can do this by clicking on Analyze (on the top toolbar menu), then select Descriptive Statistics from the pull-down menu, then Frequencies.

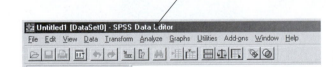

This will bring up a dialog box (this is true in almost all SPSS menu options) in which you can designate the variables of interest and specify certain statistical or output options. For this exercise, click on the variable *racethn* (the fourth variable in the list) and then click on the arrow in the middle of the dialog box to move this variable into the list for analysis. Then click OK. Based on the output you have created, answer these questions:

(a) What percentage of women in this study were "White, not Hispanic"?

(b) Does the column for "Cumulative Percent" yield meaningful information for this variable?

† **B2.** Re-run the frequency distribution for *racethn*. This time, use the toolbar with icons that is second from the top. Put the mouse pointer over the icons, from left to right. Find the icon (likely to be the fourth one) that has a "Tool Tip" that reads "Recall recently used dialogs" when you use the mouse pointer.

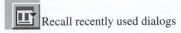 Recall recently used dialogs

Click on this icon—it will bring up a list of recently used analytic commands. The "Frequencies" command should be at the top of the list because it is the one most recently used, so using this "dialog recall" feature is a useful shortcut when running multiple analyses with different variables. For this run, when the Frequencies dialog box appears, click on the "Charts" pushbutton, and then select "Bar Chart" and "Percentages." Compare the tabled versus graphic results from Exercises B1 and B2.

† **B3.** Now execute the SPSS Frequency command once again for the variable *higrade*, highest grade of education for participants (Variable 6). (If you do this analysis right after the previous one, you will need to remove the variable *racethn* from the variable list with the arrow push button, and then move *higrade* into the list for analysis.) Examine the frequency distribution information and answer these questions:

(a) What percentage of women completed 16 years of education?

(b) What percentage of women had 10 years or less of education?

(c) How many women had exactly 12 years of education?

† **B4.** Now focus on missing data for the variable *higrade*, using the same frequency distribution output as in Exercise B3. Answer these questions:

(a) How many cases altogether had valid information, and what percentage of the overall sample did these cases represent?

(b) How many different types of missing values were there?

(c) What were the missing value codes (available by looking at the Variable View screen of the Data Editor, or in the Codebook)?

(d) What do these missing values codes mean?

† **B5.** Re-run the frequency distribution for *higrade*. This time, when the dialog box comes up, click the pushbutton for "Statistics." When a new dialog box appears that asks which statistics you would like, click the "Skewness" and "Kurtosis" options that appear in the lower right section under the heading "Distribution." Then return to the main dialog box (Click Continue) and click OK. Examine the resulting output and then answer these questions:

(a) What are the values for the skewness and kurtosis indexes?

(b) Based on the information shown on the output, would you conclude that this variable is normally distributed?

(c) How would you describe the distribution of scores?

† **B6.** Re-run the frequency distribution for *higrade* a third time. Now, when the initial dialog box opens, click the pushbutton for "Charts." When a new dialog box appears, click on "Histogram" and "With normal curve." Return to the main dialog box and click on OK. Examine the resulting output and then answer these questions:

(a) Did the SPSS program produce a histogram with original values or class intervals—and, if the latter, what class interval did the SPSS program use?

(b) Does the graph confirm your conclusions about the normality of the distribution?

† **B7.** To examine the issue of outliers, use the SPSS Explore command by clicking on Analyze in the top toolbar, then selecting Descriptive Statistics, then Explore. Move the variable *higrade* (highest grade completed) into the Dependent Variable list using the arrow; then move the variable *id* (Identification number) into the slot "Label cases by:" At the bottom left, where there are options for Display, click on Statistics. Then click on the Statistics pushbutton and click on Outliers. Then return to the main dialog box (Continue) and hit OK. Examine the table labeled Extreme Values. It will show the highest five values and the lowest five values for the designated variable—i.e., potential outliers. Answer these questions:

(a) What is the grade for the highest value? How many cases had this value? Would you consider this value an outlier?

(b) What are the grades for the lowest value? How many cases had each value? Would you consider these values outliers?

(c) What are the ID numbers for those whose highest grade completed was 1?

† **B8.** Run Frequencies for the following three demographic/background variables in the dataset: educational attainment (*educatn*, variable number 5); currently employed (*worknow*, variable 7); and current marital status (*marital*, variable 9). Create a table (in a word processing program or by hand) that would display this information, using Table 2.5 of the textbook as a model. Then write a paragraph summarizing the most salient characteristics of the sample.

3

Central Tendency, Variability, and Relative Standing

A distribution of data values for quantitative variables can be described in terms of three characteristics: its shape, central tendency, and variability. Chapter 2 discussed a distribution's shape. This chapter focuses on statistics that describe central tendency and variability, and also discusses indexes of position for scores within a distribution.

CENTRAL TENDENCY

Full frequency distributions for interval- or ratio-level variables are seldom presented in research reports because there is a more succinct, convenient way to summarize these distributions: by reporting an index of central tendency. **Central tendency** refers to the location of a "typical" data value—the data value around which other scores tend to cluster. Because a value is more likely to be typical if it is in the middle of a distribution than if it is at an extreme, the term *central tendency* has come to be used for this class of descriptive statistics.

The word *average* is the everyday term for central tendency. With regard to the heart rate data that we used to illustrate concepts in Chapter 2, we could convey more useful information by reporting the sample's average heart rate than by reporting what percentage of cases had a heart rate of 55, 56, 57, and so on. Researchers usually do not use the term *average*, because there are three alternative types of average: the mode, the median, and the mean.

The Mode

The **mode** is the numerical value in a distribution that occurs most frequently. Take, for example, the following set of values:

$$20 \quad 21 \quad 21 \quad 22 \quad 22 \quad 22 \quad 22 \quad 23 \quad 23 \quad 24$$

We can readily see that the mode is 22, because this score occurred four times—a higher frequency than for any other value. If we constructed a frequency polygon for these 10 numbers, the peak in the graph would occur at the modal value of 22. In the heart rate example, we can tell from Figure 2.7 that the mode is 66: 11 people had a heart rate of 66 bpm, and no other heart rate value occurred more frequently.

Although the mode is easy to determine, it has drawbacks as an index of central tendency. One problem is that there may be two or more modes in a single distribution— that is, the distribution might be multimodal, as in the following example:

$$20 \quad 20 \quad 20 \quad 21 \quad 22 \quad 23 \quad 24 \quad 25 \quad 25 \quad 25$$

Here, both 20 and 25 are the most frequently occurring numbers—both are considered modes. In this example, we cannot characterize the distribution with a single number if we use the mode to indicate central tendency. Another limitation is that the mode tends to be a fairly unstable index. By *unstable*, we mean that the values of modes tend to fluctuate from one sample to another drawn from the same population. Given its instability, it is difficult to attach much theoretical importance to the mode.

Because of these shortcomings, the mode is not used extensively in research, except when the researcher is interested in describing typical (modal) values for nominal-level variables. For example, using the frequency distribution information from the study by Liu and colleagues (2008) presented in Table 2.4, we could characterize the participants as follows: "The typical (modal) subject was a white, middle-aged male."

The Median

A second descriptive statistic used to indicate central tendency is the median. The **median** (sometimes abbreviated as *Mdn*) is the point in a data distribution that divides the distribution into two equal halves: 50% of the score values lie above the median, and the other 50% lie below the median. As an example, the median of the following set of values is 25:

$$21 \quad 22 \quad 22 \quad 23 \quad 24 \quad 26 \quad 26 \quad 27 \quad 28 \quad 29$$

The point that has 50% above it and 50% below it is half way between 24 and 26. Even though no one had a score of 25, the value of 25 is the median because it splits the distribution exactly into two equal halves.

To calculate the median, the data values must first be sorted, as in a frequency distribution. The median is the middle value of all cases. If there is an even number of cases, the median is the value halfway between the two middle ones, as in the preceding example where the median was 25. If there are an odd number of cases, the median is simply the value in the middle, as in the following example, where the median is also 25:

$$22 \quad 23 \quad 23 \quad 24 \quad 25 \quad 26 \quad 27 \quad 27 \quad 28$$

In this example, the median is the value in the middle, or 25. Notice that, in this example, it cannot be said that 50% of the cases are above and below 25: 4 out of 9 cases (44.4%) are above the value of 25, and 4 out of 9 cases (44.4%) are below it. However, the number 25 can be thought of as the midpoint of an interval extending between the values of 24.5 and 25.5. These are called the **real limits** of a number. Thus, to find the median in this example, we would use the midpoint between the number's real limits, or (24.5 + 25.5)/2 = 25.0.

Because the median is an index of the average *location* in a distribution of numbers, the median is insensitive to the distribution's actual numerical values. Suppose we changed the last number in the previous example:

$$22 \quad 23 \quad 23 \quad 24 \quad 25 \quad 26 \quad 27 \quad 27 \quad 128$$

Although the ninth value in the distribution has increased from 28 to 128, the median is still 25: It remains the point that divides the distribution into two equal halves. Because of this characteristic, the median is often the most useful index of central tendency when a distribution is highly skewed and one wants to find a "typical" value.

The Mean

The most commonly used index of central tendency is the **mean,** the term used in statistics for the arithmetic average. The equation for calculating the mean is as follows:

$$\overline{X} = \frac{\Sigma X}{N}$$

where $\overline{X}$ = the mean
Σ = the sum of
X = each individual data value
N = the number of cases

That is, the mean is computed by summing each individual score (ΣX), and then dividing by the total number of cases (N). The mean is symbolized either as M or $\overline{X}$—pronounced "X bar." In research reports, one is more likely to see the symbol M, whereas in statistics books $\overline{X}$ is more often used.

As an example, let us take the set of nine scores whose median was 25:

$$\overline{X} = \frac{22 + 23 + 23 + 24 + 25 + 26 + 27 + 27 + 28}{9} = 25.0$$

The value of the mean, unlike the median, is affected by every score in the distribution. Thus, although the median was unchanged at 25 when we replaced the 9th score of 28 with 128, the mean would change markedly:

$$\overline{X} = \frac{22 + 23 + 23 + 24 + 25 + 26 + 27 + 27 + 128}{9} = 36.1$$

The mean has an interesting property that underscores why it is a good index of central tendency: *The sum of the deviations of all scores from their mean always equals zero.* That is, if the mean is subtracted from every score in a distribution, the sum of these differences invariably is zero. As an example, consider the following numbers, which have a mean of 5.0: 9, 7, 5, 3, and 1. Now, if we subtract the mean from each score, we would obtain five **deviation scores.**

Score		Mean		Deviation Score
9	−	5	=	4
7	−	5	=	2
5	−	5	=	0
3	−	5	=	−2
1	−	5	=	−4

When the deviation scores are added, we obtain the sum of 0. It is this property of the mean—the fact that it balances the deviations above it and below it—that makes the mean an important index of central tendency.

Comparison of the Mode, the Median, and the Mean

In a normal distribution, the mode, the median, and the mean have the same value, as illustrated in Figure 3.1. Distributions of real data, however, are rarely perfectly normal, and thus the values of the three indexes of central tendency are typically not exactly the same. When this is the case, the researcher must decide which index to report.

The mean is usually the preferred, and most widely reported, index of central tendency for variables measured on an interval or ratio scale. The mean has many desirable features, including the fact that it takes each and every score into account. It is also the most stable index of central tendency, and thus yields the most reliable estimate of the central tendency of the population.

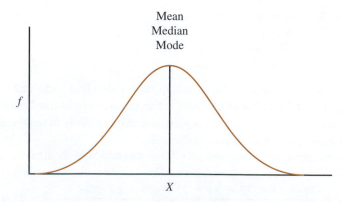

FIGURE 3.1   The mean, median, and mode in a normal distribution.

In many situations the mean's ability to capture every score value is an advantage, but sometimes this feature is a disadvantage. Suppose we collected data on the annual income of 10 study participants and obtained the following:

$17,000

$40,000

$40,000

$40,000

$52,000

$54,000

$55,000

$56,000

$60,000

$200,000

In this example, the mode is $40,000, the median is $53,000, and the mean is $61,400. Despite the fact that 90% of the sample had annual incomes of $60,000 or less, the mean is greater than this figure. Extreme scores can exert a powerful influence on the mean and result in a misleading picture of the distribution of values. Thus, when the primary aim of summarizing a distribution is to describe what a "typical" value is, the median may be preferred. In this example, the value of $53,000 (the median) does a much better job of communicating the financial circumstances of the sample than does the mean. In general, the median is a better descriptive index when the data are highly skewed or when there are extreme, but valid, outliers. The median may also be preferred for ordinal-level variables that cannot reasonably be viewed as approaching interval-level measurement (e.g., the four pressure ulcer stages in Box 1.5).

Figure 3.2 illustrates that in skewed distributions the values of the mode, the median, and the mean are different. The mean is always pulled in the direction of the long tail—that is, in the direction of the extreme scores. Thus, for variables that are positively skewed (like income), the mean is higher than the mode or the median; for negatively skewed variables (like age at death), the mean is lower.

In distributions that are close to being normal, researchers usually report only the mean. When the distribution is asymmetrical, however, researchers sometimes

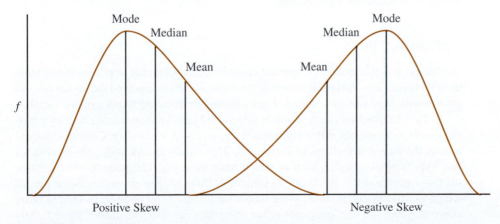

FIGURE 3.2 The mean, median, and mode in skewed distributions.

report two or more indicators of central tendency. When there are extreme values in the distribution (even if it is approximately normal), researchers sometimes report means that have been adjusted for outliers. There are several alternative methods of adjusting means, one of which is to calculate a **trimmed mean** that discards a fixed percentage (usually 5%) of the extreme values from either end of the distribution.

TIP: *The symbols for a* sample *mean (a descriptive statistic) are either* M *or* $\overline{X}$, *whereas the symbol for the* population *mean (a parameter) is the Greek letter* μ *(pronounced mew). It is conventional to use Greek letters to represent parameters, although these are rarely seen in actual research articles because researchers almost always work with samples.*

Computers and Central Tendency

Although it is not difficult to compute an index of central tendency, manual calculation can be time consuming if the sample size is large. Computers can be used to compute all major descriptive statistics.

Computing central tendency indexes in statistical software is usually simple. Because of this fact, researchers often compute all three indexes rather than making an *a priori* decision about which is preferable. For the heart rate data presented in Table 2.1, the commands to compute all three indexes using SPSS for Windows would simply involve a few more "clicks" beyond the commands to produce the frequency distribution (Figure 2.1): Analyze ➜ Descriptive Statistics ➜ Frequencies ➜ Statistics, then click mean, median, and mode under "Central Tendency." This would result in output showing that the mode is 66.00, the median is 66.00, and the mean is 65.21. With these heart rate data, we would probably report only the mean because the distribution is not skewed and the values of all three indexes are fairly close. (SPSS also computes means and other descriptive statistics in the Analyze ➜ Descriptive Statistics ➜ Descriptives procedure.)

Computer programs will compute means for all variables, regardless of their levels of measurement. If we instructed the computer to calculate the mean marital status of participants (for example, using the data in Table 2.3), it would proceed to do so, but the information would not make sense: The mean for the data in Table 2.3 is 1.876, a meaningless number. The ease with which a computer can perform calculations should not lead researchers to forego consideration of what is appropriate for the variable's level of measurement.

VARIABILITY

In addition to a distribution's shape and central tendency, another important characteristic is its variability. **Variability** refers to how spread out or dispersed the scores are—in other words, how similar or different participants are from one another on the variable.

Two distributions with identical means and similar shapes (e.g., both symmetric) could nevertheless differ considerably in terms of variability. Consider, for example, the two distributions in Figure 3.3. This figure shows body weight data for two hypothetical samples, both of which have means of 150 pounds—but, clearly, the two samples differ markedly. In sample A, there is great diversity: Some people weigh as little as 100 pounds, while others weigh up to 200 pounds. In sample B, by contrast, there are few people at either extreme: The weights cluster more tightly around the mean of 150.

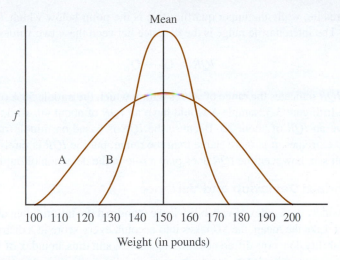

FIGURE 3.3 Two distributions with different variability.

We can verbally describe a sample's variability. We can say, for example, that sample A is **heterogeneous** (highly varied) with regard to weight, while sample B is **homogeneous**. These verbal descriptors, however, are imprecise and open to subjective interpretations. Statisticians have developed indexes that express the extent to which scores on quantitative variables deviate from one another in a distribution, several of which are described here.

The Range

The **range**, the simplest measure of variability, is the difference between the highest score and the lowest score in the distribution. In Figure 3.3, the range for sample A is about 100 (200 − 100 = 100), while the range for sample B is about 50 (175 − 125 = 50). In research reports, the range is often shown as the minimum and maximum value, without the subtracted difference score.

The range provides a quick summary of a distribution's variability, and is easy to compute. The range also provides useful information about a distribution when there are extreme values. For example, a researcher might want to know that the range of values for annual income is (to use the example presented previously) from $17,000 to $200,000 (i.e., a range of $183,000).

However, the range has drawbacks. Because the range is based on only two values, it is highly unstable. For example, in another sample of 10 people, the annual incomes might range from $40,000 to $50,000 (a range of only $10,000). Another problem is that the range tends to increase with sample size: the larger the sample, the greater the likelihood that an extreme value will be obtained. It is more likely, for example, that a sample of 1,000 people will include a millionaire than a sample of 10 people. Because of these limitations, the range is rarely used as the only descriptive index of variability.

Interquartile Range

The median is the score at the 50th *percentile*: it is the point below which 50% of the cases fall. As we describe later in this chapter, percentiles can be computed at any point in a distribution. The **interquartile range** or *IQR* is a variability index calculated on the basis of **quartiles.** The lower quartile (Q_1) is the point below which 25%

of the scores lie, while the upper quartile (Q_3) is the point below which 75% of the scores lie. The interquartile range is the distance between these two values, or:

$$IQR = Q_3 - Q_1$$

Thus, the *IQR* indicates the range of scores within which the middle 50% of the score values lie. In Figure 3.3, sample A would have an *IQR* of about 40, while sample B would have an *IQR* of about 20. Because the *IQR* is based on middle-range cases rather than extremes, it is more stable than the range, but the *IQR* is rarely reported. As we shall see, however, the *IQR* does play a role in the detection of outliers.

The Standard Deviation and Variance

The most widely used index of variability is the **standard deviation** (often abbreviated as **SD** or *s*). Like the mean, the *SD* takes into account every score in a distribution.

Variability concerns differences among scores, and thus an index of variability necessarily captures the degree to which scores are different from one another. In the range and *IQR*, this notion of differences is indicated by a minus sign, designating the difference between two values. The *SD* is also based on differences—in this case, differences between every score and the value of the mean. Thus, the first step in calculating a standard deviation is to calculate deviation scores. The formula for a deviation score (often symbolized as *x*) is:

$$x = X - \overline{X}$$

For example, if a person weighed 200 and the average weight of the sample were 150, that person's deviation score would be 50.

Indexes of central tendency are useful because they offer a single numerical value that describes the "average" score in a distribution. Researchers also want as an index of variability a single number that describes the "average" amount of dispersion. This might lead you to surmise that a good indicator of variability could be obtained by summing the deviation scores and dividing by the number of cases, to obtain an average deviation. However, as we have already seen, the sum of deviation scores is always equal to 0, i.e., $\Sigma x = 0$.

The standard deviation addresses this problem by squaring the deviation scores before summing them and dividing by the number of cases. Then, to return to the original unit of measurement, the square root is taken. The formula for the *SD* is:

$$SD = \sqrt{\frac{\Sigma x^2}{N - 1}}$$

The computation of a standard deviation is illustrated in Table 3.1. The first column shows the weights of 10 people. At the bottom of this first column, the mean is computed to be 150.0 pounds. In the second column, a deviation score for each person is calculated by subtracting the mean of 150.0 from each original weight value. In the third column, each deviation score is squared, and the sum of these squared deviation scores (x^2) is calculated to be 6,000. At the bottom of the table, the *SD* is computed: 6,000 is divided by nine (the number of cases minus one)[1], and then the square

---

[1] Some books show the *SD* formula with *N* rather than *N* – 1 in the denominator. *N* is appropriate for computing the *SD* for population values, and is sometimes used for computing the *SD* with sample data if there is no intent to estimate population values. When population parameters are of interest, statisticians have shown that it is appropriate to use *N* – 1 in the denominator. Statistical programs use *N* – 1 rather *N* in computing *SDs*.

TABLE 3.1 Example of the Computation of a Standard Deviation

X	$x = X - \bar{X}$	$x^2 = (X - \bar{X})^2$
110	−40	1600
120	−30	900
130	−20	400
140	−10	100
150	0	0
150	0	0
160	10	100
170	20	400
180	30	900
190	40	1600
$\Sigma X = 1500$	$\Sigma x = 0$	$\Sigma x^2 = 6000$

$\bar{X} = 1500/10$

$\bar{X} = 150.0$

$$SD = \sqrt{\frac{6000}{9}} = \sqrt{666.67} = 25.820$$

root is taken to bring the index back to the original units. The value of the *SD* of the weights for the 10 people is 25.820 (or, rounding to one decimal place, 25.8).

What does the number 25.8 represent? While it is easy for most people to understand that the average weight in this example is 150.0, it is less easy to understand the meaning of a standard deviation of 25.8. There are several ways to explain the concept of an *SD*.

The *SD* of 25.8 signifies the "average" deviation from the mean. The mean indicates the best single point in the distribution for summarizing a set of values, but the *SD* tells us how much, on the average, the values deviate from that mean. The smaller the *SD*, the better is the mean as the summary of a typical score. To take an extreme case, if all 10 people in our example weighed 150 pounds, the *SD* would be 0, and the mean of 150.0 would communicate perfectly accurate information about all the participants' weights. At the other extreme, suppose the first five people weighed 100 and the last five people weighed 200. In this case of extreme heterogeneity, the mean would still be 150.0, but the *SD* would be 52.7.

An *SD* is often easier to interpret in a comparative context. For example, looking back at Figure 3.3, distributions A and B both had a mean of 150, but sample A would have an *SD* of about 20, while sample B would have an *SD* of about 10. The *SD* index communicates that sample A is much more heterogeneous than sample B.

Another way in which the *SD* can be interpreted concerns the evaluation of any single score in a distribution. In our example of 10 subjects' weights, the *SD* was 25.8. This value represents a "standard" of variability against which individual weights can be compared. People with weights that are greater than 1 *SD* away from the mean (i.e., less than 124.2 pounds or more than 175.8 pounds) have weights that are farther away from the mean than the average. Conversely, weights between 124.2 and 175.8 pounds are closer to the mean than the average.

When data values are normally distributed, the standard deviation can be used in an even more precise way to evaluate individual values. In a normal distribution,

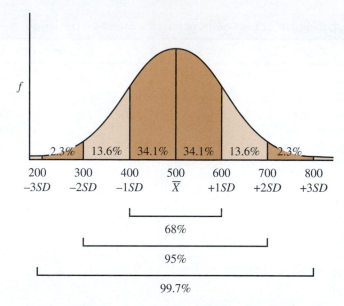

FIGURE 3.4   Standard deviations in a normal distribution.

there are approximately 3 *SD*s above the mean, and 3 *SD*s below it, as shown in Figure 3.4. This figure shows a distribution of scores with a mean of 500 and an *SD* of 100, which is similar to the distribution of scores for many standardized tests such as the SAT or the Graduate Record Examination (GRE). When data are normally distributed, a fixed percentage of cases fall between the mean and distances from the mean, as measured in *SD* units. Sixty-eight percent of the cases fall within 1 *SD* of the mean: 34% are above the mean and 34% are below it. In the example shown in Figure 3.4, nearly seven out of every 10 people obtained a score between 400 and 600. A full 95% of the cases fall within 2 *SD*s of the mean. Only a small percentage of cases (about 2.5% in each tail) are more than 2 *SD*s away from the mean. With this information, it is easy to interpret an individual score. A person with a score of 600, for example, obtained a higher score than 84% of the sample (i.e., 50% below the mean and 34% between the mean and 1 *SD* above it).

The *SD* is often cited in research reports in conjunction with the mean, and is the most widely used descriptive index of variability. However, another index of variability, called the variance, plays an important role in inferential statistics. The **variance** is simply the value of the standard deviation before the square root is taken, as in the following formula:

$$Var = \frac{\Sigma x^2}{N - 1} = SD^2$$

In the example shown in Table 3.1, the variance is 666.67 (6000 ÷ 9), which is 25.820^2. Because the variance is not in the same measurement units as the original data—in this example, it is in pounds squared)—the variance is rarely used as a descriptive statistic.

TIP: *The symbol for the population standard deviation (a parameter) is the Greek letter σ (sigma), but you will rarely, if ever, see this symbol in research reports.*

Statistics

Heart Rate in Beats per Minute

N	Valid	100.0000
	Missing	.0000
Mean		65.2100
Median		66.0000
Mode		66.0000
Std. Deviation		4.4953
Variance		20.2080
Range		19.0000
Percentiles	25	62.0000
	50	66.0000
	75	68.0000

FIGURE 3.5 SPSS printout of basic descriptive statistics.

Computers and Variability

In SPSS and other user-friendly statistical software, commands to calculate indexes of variability are simple. The SPSS commands to compute the range, the *SD*, and the variance are within the "Frequencies" (and also "Descriptives") routine; the sequence is the same as for the central tendency indexes, except that different selections would be made in the "Statistics" dialog box.

Researchers usually instruct the computer to calculate indexes of central tendency and variability simultaneously. In SPSS, we selected the following statistics within the Frequencies procedure for the heart rate data shown in Table 2.1: mode, median, mean, standard deviation, variance, range, and quartiles (i.e., the 25th, 50th, and 75th percentiles). Figure 3.5 presents the printout that resulted. The Frequencies command in SPSS does not directly compute the *IQR*, but from the information about the 25th and 75th quartile in Figure 3.5, we could calculate the *IQR* as 6.0 (68.0 − 62.0 = 6.0). Later we will see that SPSS computes the *IQR* in a procedure for detecting outliers.

RELATIVE STANDING

The central tendency and variability statistics discussed thus far allow researchers to describe an entire distribution, but there are better indexes for interpreting individual scores. In this section, we briefly discuss two indexes that provide information about the position—or relative standing—of an individual score value within a distribution of scores.

Percentile Ranks

One approach to expressing relative standing is to calculate the percentile rank of a score. The percentage of scores in the distribution that fall at or below a given value is the **percentile rank** of that value. For example, in the distribution of heart rate values, the percentile rank of the value 68 bpm is 75. That is, 75% of the scores in this distribution are at or below 68. As a rough approximation, a percentile rank is comparable to the cumulative percentage of a score value in a frequency distribution. In Figure 2.1, which shows the heart rate distribution, 76% of the scores were at or below 68. The reason the cumulative percentage is not *exactly* the same as the percentile rank of 75 is because there were multiple values of 68 in this dataset.[2]

If we start with a percentile in mind, we can also determine which *score* corresponds to that percentile. A **percentile** is equal to one 100th of the distribution. We have already seen that the median divides a distribution into two equal halves, that is, at the 50th percentile. *Quartiles* divide the distribution into quarters, with 25% of the scores falling at or below the 25th percentile, and so on. *Deciles* divide the distribution into tenths. As we shall see, percentiles are the basis for creating a graph that can nicely summarize certain features of a distribution. Within SPSS, you can determine the score value corresponding to any specified percentile within the "Frequencies" routine.

Standard Scores

Percentile ranks provide an ordinal measure of relative standing. Another index of relative standing, the standard score, provides information not only about rank but also distance between scores. **Standard scores** are scores that are expressed in terms of their relative distance from the mean. Researchers most often use standard scores to make their data values more interpretable. For example, SAT scores are actually standard scores—they do not represent the number of questions a person answered correctly on the test.

A standard score (often called a **z-score**) is easy to compute once the mean and standard deviation have been calculated. The formula is as follows:

$$z = \frac{X - \overline{X}}{SD}$$

That is, for each person, the deviation score (the raw score minus the mean) is divided by the standard deviation to yield a standard score. This converts all raw scores to *SD* units: A raw score that is 1 *SD* above the mean would be a *z* score of $+1.0$, while a raw score 2 *SD*s *below* the mean would be a *z* score of -2.0. A score directly at the mean would be a standard score of 0.0. The mean of a distribution of *z* scores is necessarily 0, and the *SD* is always 1. The shape of the distribution of *z* scores is identical to the shape of the original distribution of scores.

As an example, consider once again the heart rate data. As we saw, the mean of the distribution is 65.21 and the *SD* is 4.50 (Figure 3.5). The standard score for a person with a heart rate of 70 would be 1.06 ($z = [70.00 - 65.21] \div 4.50 = 1.06$). A heart rate of 70 is just slightly greater than 1 *SD* above the mean. A raw score of 56, by contrast, would equate to a *z* score of -2.05, about two standard deviations *below* the mean.

Sometimes it is more convenient to work with standard scores that do not have negative numbers or decimals. Standard scores can be transformed to have *any* desired mean and standard deviation. As an example, SAT and GRE scores are transformed *z* scores that have a mean of 500 and an *SD* of 100. Many widely used cognitive and personality tests (such as the Wechsler IQ test) are standardized to have a mean of 100 and an *SD* of 15. The formula for converting raw scores to this particular standard score scale is as follows:

$$\text{Standard Score}_{100,15} = \left(\left(\frac{X - \overline{X}}{SD} \right) \times 15 \right) + 100$$

---

[2] Determining the exact percentile rank of a score is complex. Those interested in the formula should consult statistics textbooks such as those by McCall (2000) or Jaccard and Becker (2001).

In other words, the z score $((X - \bar{X}) \div SD)$ is multiplied by 15 (the desired SD for the standardized scores), and the result is added to 100 (the desired mean). On this particular scale, a raw score of 70 bpm for the heart rate data would equate to a standard score of 115.9 ($1.06 \times 15 + 100 = 115.9$). If we wanted to transform z scores on a scale like the GRE or SAT, we would substitute the SD of 100 for 15 as the multiplier in the preceding formula, and the mean of 500 would replace the addend of 100. On this scale, a heart rate value of 70 bpm would be a standardized score of 606 ($1.06 \times 100 + 500 = 606$) in this sample.

TIP: *It does not make particularly good sense to convert heart rate data to standard scores because the raw data are in units that are directly interpretable. However, scores on many tests and psychological scales whose units are not inherently meaningful may be easier to understand when the raw scores have been standardized, especially for group comparisons.*

We saw earlier that, for normal distributions, there is a fixed percentage of cases within SD units of the mean, so individual standard scores can readily be interpreted for normally distributed variables (Figure 3.4). A GRE score of, say, 700, is 2 SD units above the mean of 500, and so a score of 700 is higher than 97.7% of the scores on this test (50% below the mean, plus another 47.7% between 500 and 700).

Z scores can be computed with a simple command within many computer programs. For example, to convert the variable *hartrate* to z scores, you would use the Analyze → Descriptive Statistics procedure and click on the box that says "Save standardized values as variables." This would add a new variable to the end of your data file—in this case, that variable is automatically called *zhartrat*. The value for this new variable would be computed for every case in the file, and the mean and SD of this new variable would 0.0 and 1.0, respectively. If you wanted your standard score to have a mean other than 0 and an SD other than 1.0, you would do this by creating a new variable yourself using the Compute Variable procedure.

TIP: *The most commonly used transformed standard scores are those with means of 500 with SDs of 100; means of 100 with SDs of 15; and means of 50 with SDs of 10. Standard scores with means of 50 and SDs of 10 are sometimes called* **T scores.**

RESEARCH APPLICATIONS OF CENTRAL TENDENCY AND VARIABILITY

Descriptive indexes of central tendency and variability are widely used by researchers. This section examines some of the major applications of these indexes and discusses methods of effectively displaying such information in research reports.

The Uses of Central Tendency and Variability Indexes

For variables that are measured on an interval or ratio scale (and for many ordinal-level variables as well), researchers routinely compute indexes of central tendency and variability, paying particular attention to the mean and SD. We have already seen that the mean and SD have an important application in the creation of standard scores. A few of the other major reasons for using such indexes are described in the following section.

1. *Understanding the data*   Researchers often develop a better understanding of their data by examining their main study variables descriptively. Means and *SDs* (in addition to frequencies and percentages) are almost always computed for major variables measured on interval- or ratio-level variables before undertaking more complex analyses. In research reports, researchers often present information about central tendency and variability to orient readers before reporting the results of inferential statistics. For example, Budin and colleagues (2008) undertook a randomized controlled trial that tested alternative interventions to promote emotional and physical adjustment among patients with breast cancer. Before reporting their main findings (which involved multivariate inferential statistics), they presented a descriptive table that summarized the means, *SDs*, and ranges on their dependent variables (scores on scales of psychological well-being, health, and social adjustment) for each treatment group at baseline.

2. *Evaluating outliers*   In the previous chapter, we described how researchers can use frequency distribution information to identify possible outliers, but more can now be said on this matter. Outliers are often identified in relation to the value of a distribution's *IQR*. By convention, a *mild outlier* is a data value that lies between 1.5 and 3.0 times the *IQR* below Q_1 or above Q_3. An *extreme outlier* is a data value that is more that three times the *IQR* below Q_1 or above Q_3. For example, for the heart rate data, the *IQR* is 6 and the score at Q_1 is 62. A mild lower outlier would be any value between 44 ($62 - [3 \times 6]$) and 53 ($62 - [1.5 \times 6]$), and an extreme outlier would be a value less than 44—or, at the other end of the distribution, above 86. In our data distribution (see Figure 2.1), there are no outliers. A graph called a **boxplot** (or *box and whiskers plot*) is a useful way to visualize percentiles and to identify outliers. The left panel (A) of Figure 3.6 shows the boxplot for the original heart rate data for 100 people. A boxplot shows a box that has the 75th percentile as its upper edge (here, at 68) and the 25th percentile at its lower edge (here, at 62). The horizontal line through the middle of the box is the median (here, 66). The

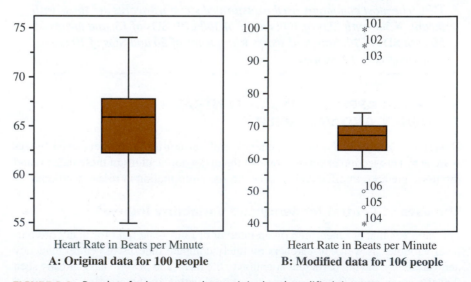

FIGURE 3.6 Boxplots for heart rate data: original and modified datasets.

"whiskers" that extend from the box show the highest and lowest values that are not outliers, in relation to the *IQR*, as defined earlier. This graph confirms that there are no outliers in the original dataset. To illustrate what a computer-generated boxplot shows when there *are* outliers, we added six extreme values to the original dataset: 40, 45, and 50 at the lower end and 90, 95, and 100 at the upper end. Panel B of Figure 3.6 shows the resulting boxplot. The six data values that we added all are shown as outliers—outside the outer limits of the whiskers. Mild outliers are shown with circles: Case number 106 with a value of 50 and case number 105 with a value of 45 are mild outliers, for example. Cases that are extreme outliers are shown with asterisks. When there are outliers, the first thing to do is to see if they are legitimate values, or reflect errors in data entry. If they are true values, researchers can decide on whether it is appropriate to make adjustments, such as trimming the mean. (In SPSS, a lot of diagnostic information, including boxplots and the value of *IQR*, is available through the Analyze ➜ Descriptive Statistics ➜ Explore procedure).

3. ***Describing the research sample***   As noted in Chapter 2, it is important to carefully describe major background characteristics of study participants so that the findings can be properly interpreted. Many sample characteristics are more succinctly described through indexes of central tendency than through frequencies. For example, Holditch-Davis, Merrill, Schwartz, and Scher (2008) studied factors that predicted wheezing in prematurely born infants. Their sample description included information about means and *SD*s for such ratio-level characteristics as the infant's gestational age, birthweight, days on mechanical ventilation, and number of neurologic insults.

4. ***Answering research questions***   When a study is descriptive, researchers are sometimes able to answer their research questions directly through the computation of descriptive statistics such as indexes of central tendency and variability. For example, one of the aims of a study by Miller, Alpert, and Cross (2008) was to describe levels of obesity in nurses from six regions of the United States. They reported the means, medians, standard deviations, and ranges for values of the body mass index (BMI) for 760 nurses who participated in the study, by their state of residence.

The Presentation of Central Tendency and Variability in Research Reports

Measures of central tendency and variability are reported in the vast majority of research reports. They are usually reported either directly in the text or in tables. Means are occasionally presented in graphic form.

Decisions about presenting information in tables or in the text should be based primarily on efficiency. If only one or two descriptive statistics are being reported (for example, the sample's mean age and mean number of days hospitalized), it is probably better to present this information in the text. However, if there are descriptive statistics for multiple variables that are conceptually related, a table is likely to be the most effective method of presentation. At a minimum, researchers typically report means and *SD*s, and often ranges as well. If the number of cases varies from one variable to the next, the *N*s should also be presented. If a data distribution is skewed, medians may be preferred in lieu of (or in addition to) means.

Graphs are most likely to be used to display central tendency information when the researcher wants to emphasize contrasts. For example, boxplots are sometimes presented for two or more groups of participants (e.g., experimentals versus controls). Graphs are also used to great advantage to plot means over time. Mean values

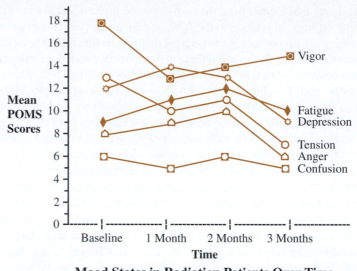

Mood States in Radiation Patients Over Time

FIGURE 3.7 Example of a graph plotting means over time.

typically are plotted on the *Y* (vertical) axis, while the time periods are plotted along the *X* (horizontal) axis. Occasionally, researchers display this information in a histogram-type format with bars drawn to a height indicating a mean value. More often, however, means are plotted using dots that are connected by a straight line, creating a **line graph**. For example, suppose we were interested in studying the mood states of cancer patients who received radiation therapy over a 3-month period. Using the Profile of Mood States (POMS), which consists of six subscales, we could collect data on patients' moods prior to radiation and then at 1, 2, and 3 months after treatment. Mean scores on the POMS subscales over time could then be displayed in a graph, such as the one shown in Figure 3.7.

Tips on Preparing Tables with Central Tendency and Variability Indexes

Here are some suggestions for enhancing the presentation of central tendency and variability indexes in tables.

- It is usually better not to combine in one table variables for which different types of descriptive statistics are appropriate. For example, if some variables are better described with percentages (nominal-level variables), while others are better described using means (interval- or ratio-level variables), two separate tables may be necessary. The exception is that a single table is often used for displaying the background characteristics of a sample, regardless of the level of measurement of the variables.
- Readers can usually compare numbers down a column more readily than across a row. For this reason, variable names are usually listed along the left in the first column, together with any needed information about the unit of measurement (e.g., grams, years, etc.). The descriptive statistics being presented are named across the top row. Table 3.2, which we describe in the next section, exemplifies this format.

TABLE 3.2 Example: Table Showing Central Tendency and Variability

	Mean	*SD*	Range of Values
Age (years)	81.0	8.4	—
Number of comorbidities	8.8	2.5	—
Mini-Mental State Examination Score	16.0	5.6	—
Cortisol, 9–9:30 A.M. (μg/dL)	0.48	0.32	0.07–1.35
Cortisol, noon–4:30 P.M. (μg/dL)	0.19	0.05	0.05–0.51
Cortisol, 6:45–7:15 P.M. (μg/dL)	0.29	0.22	0.07–0.79

Adapted from Table 1 of Woods et al. (2008). The table was titled "Resident characteristics, age, gender, MMSE, co-morbidities, and salivary cortisol for the UWM ($N = 22$) and UCLA ($N = 16$) studies." Only data for the University of Wisconsin Milwaukee site (UWM) are shown here.

- There are no rules for ordering the variables that appear in a table of descriptive statistics. If there is a meaningful conceptual ordering (for example, dependent variables might be ordered to correspond to a set of hypotheses), this is a highly effective approach. If the values of the statistics themselves can be meaningfully ordered (e.g., in ascending or descending order of the means), this is advantageous to the reader. For example, Polit and Beck (2008) studied whether there was gender bias in nursing research—i.e., whether participants in nursing studies are disproportionately female. One table showed the mean percentage female for studies in different nursing specialty areas, listed in order of declining mean values.

- Researchers have adopted several different conventions for displaying means and *SD*s in tables. One option is to list the means and *SD*s in separate columns, as in Table 3.2. Sometimes, to save space, researchers place the *SD* in parentheses directly next to the mean. For example, the first entry in Table 3.2 would then be 81.0 (8.4). A third method is to present the *SD* next to the mean, preceded by "±" (e.g., 81.0 ± 8.4).

- In tables with central tendency and variability information, it may be desirable to display other information at the same time. For example, in addition to the actual range of score values, researchers sometimes include the theoretical range (i.e., the minimum and maximum score that is possible for the measure being used). When variables have been measured by psychosocial scales (e.g., measures of depression, self-esteem, and so on), researchers sometimes present the reliability coefficients[3] of the scale in the same table as the means and *SD*s.

- Means and *SD*s are usually reported to one or two decimal places. Greater precision is almost never necessary. Within a column of information, the level of precision should be the same.

---

[3] A **reliability coefficient** is a quantitative index of how reliable or consistent a measure is. Reliability indexes are discussed in Chapters 9 and 13.

Research Example

Indexes of central tendency and variability are reported in the vast majority of research reports. Below we provide a brief summary of the descriptive statistics reported in a nursing study.

Study: "Using saliva to measure endogenous cortisol in nursing home residents with advanced dementia" (Woods et al., 2008)

Study Purpose: The researchers cited studies suggesting that elevated cortisol could amplify dementia neuropathology in certain areas of the brain. The purpose of their study was to assess the feasibility of saliva collection for measuring cortisol in nursing home residents with advanced dementia. The research questions were: (1) Can sufficient saliva be collected? and (2) Do the cortisol values exhibit enough variability for meaningful interpretation?

Research Design: Data were collected from residents aged 65 and older who were living in nursing homes for 2 months or more in Milwaukee ($N = 22$) or Los Angeles ($N = 16$). Dementia severity was evaluated using the Mini Mental State Examination (MMSE). Salivary cortisol measurements were obtained in the morning, afternoon, and evening on a single day.

Key Variables: The researchers described their study participants in terms of sex (73% were female), age, number of medical comorbidities, and scores on the MMSE. The main outcome variables were the cortisol levels measured at different times of the day.

Key Findings: The results were similar in the two sites, so we present information here for the Milwaukee site only. Table 3.2 shows means, *SDs*, and—for cortisol values—ranges for the study variables. Participants were, on average, 81.0 years old and had 8.8 comorbidities. Their average score on the MMSE was 16.0, which is considered moderate dementia. The researchers also presented boxplots that showed cortisol levels at different times of the day for patients with different salivary profiles. The researchers concluded that cortisol assay is viable in nursing home settings and noted that the values showed range and variability, often consistent with normal adult patterns.

Summary Points

- A data distribution for a quantitative variable can be described in terms of shape, central tendency, and variability.
- Indexes of **central tendency** are numerical descriptions of a "typical" or average data value, usually from the center of the distribution. The three most widely used indexes of central tendency are the mode, the median, and the mean.
- The **mode** is the score value that occurs most frequently in a distribution.
- The **median (*Mdn*)** is the point in the distribution above which and below which 50% of the cases fall (i.e., the score at the 50th *percentile*).
- The **mean (*M* or $\overline{X}$)** is the arithmetic average, computed by adding together all score values and dividing by the number of cases. Unless data are severely skewed, the mean is the preferred index of central tendency because of its stability and utility in other statistical procedures.
- Indexes of **variability** yield a quantitative measure of how dispersed or spread out are the data values in a distribution. The most widely used indexes of

variability are the range, the interquartile range, and the standard deviation.
- The **range** is the highest score minus the lowest score.
- The **interquartile range (*IQR*)** is the score at the 75th percentile or third quartile (Q_3) minus the score at the 25th percentile or first quartile (Q_1).
- IQRs are most often used to define outliers. A *mild outlier* is a data value that lies between 1.5 and 3.0 times the *IQR*, below Q_1 or above Q_3. An *extreme outlier* is a data value that is more than three times the *IQR*, below Q_1 or above Q_3.
- The **standard deviation (*SD*)** is an index that captures how much, on average, scores deviate from the mean. It is calculated by summing all the squared **deviation scores** (each person's raw score minus the mean), dividing by $N - 1$, and then taking the square root. It is the most widely used index of variability.
- In a normal distribution, 95% of all scores fall within 2 *SDs* below and above the mean.
- The **variance** is an index of variability equal to the standard deviation, squared.

- Indicators of *relative standing* or *position* provide information about individual score values in a distribution. The percentage of scores in the distribution that fall at or below a given value is the **percentile rank** of that value. **Percentiles** divide a distribution into one hundredths, *quartiles* divide it into fourths, and *deciles* divide it into tenths.
- Another index of relative standing is the **standard score**, which is a score expressed as relative distances from the mean, in standard deviation units. A standard score (often called a **z-score**) uses this formula: $z = X$ (a score value) minus $\overline{X}$, divided by SD.

- A **boxplot** (or *box-and-whiskers plot*) is a graph based on percentiles. It shows a box whose upper and lower ends indicate the values corresponding to the 25th and 75th percentile, a horizontal line indicating the median (50th percentile), and "whiskers" or lines extending above and below the box indicating the range of values not considered outliers.
- When there are outliers, researchers sometimes make adjustments to the mean, such as calculating a **trimmed mean**, which involves calculating a mean after removing a fixed percentage of cases (e.g., 5%) from either end of the distribution.

Exercises

The following exercises cover concepts presented in this chapter. Appendix C provides answers to Part A exercises that are indicated with a dagger (†). Exercises in Part B involve computer analyses using the datasets provided with this textbook, and answers and comments are offered on this book's Web site.

PART A EXERCISES

† **A1.** The following numbers represent the scores of 30 psychiatric inpatients on a widely used measure of depression (the Center for Epidemiologic Studies-Depression scale). What are the mean, the median, and the mode for these data?

41	27	32	24	21	28	22	25	35	27
31	40	23	27	29	33	42	30	26	30
27	39	26	34	28	38	29	36	24	37

If the values of these indexes are not the same, discuss what they suggest about the shape of the distribution.

† **A2.** Find the medians for the following distributions:
(a) 1   5   7   8   9
(b) 3   5   6   8   9   10
(c) 3   4   4   4   6   20
(d) 2   4   5   5   8   9

† **A3.** For which distribution in question A2 would the median be preferred to the mean as the index of central tendency? Why?

† **A4.** The following ten data values are systolic blood pressure readings. Compute the mean, the range, the SD, and the variance for these data.

130	110	160	120	170
120	150	140	160	140

† **A5.** For each blood pressure value in question A4, compute a z score. Then, transform these z scores to standard scores with a mean of 500 and an SD of 100.

PART B EXERCISES

† **B1.** Using the SPSS dataset Polit2SetA, determine the mean, range, standard deviation, and variance for the variable *age1bir* (Participants' age at first birth). To do this, click on Analyze (on the top toolbar menu), then select Descriptive Statistics from the pull-down menu, then Descriptives. When the dialog box appears, move the variable *age1bir* into the variable list, then click the pushbutton labeled Options. Click on Mean (at the top), then Std. Deviation, Variance, and Range under "Dispersion." What are the values of these descriptive statistics?

† **B2.** Now, for the same variable (*age1bir*), determine the median, mode, and quartile values, using the Frequencies procedure (Analyze → Descriptive Statistics → Frequencies). When the dialog box appears, "uncheck" the box that says "Display Frequency Tables." (Why do you think we recommended this?) Move *age1bir* into the variable list, then click the Statistics pushbutton. In the upper left corner, for Percentiles, click quartiles. For Central Tendency, click mean, median, and mode. For Dispersion, click all options *except* Std. Error (this is explained in a later chapter). Now, answer these questions: (a) What are the values of the median and mode? (b) Are the values for the mean, SD, and so on the same as in Exercise B1? (c) What are the quartile values? (d) What is the value of the *IQR*? (e) Based on the three indicators of central tendency, what can you infer about the shape of the distribution?

† **B3.** In this next exercise, perform analyses relating to outliers, again with the variable *age1bir*. Using the Explore procedure (Analyze → Descriptive Statistics → Explore) put *age1birth* into the Dependent List when the dialog box appears, and put Identification number in the box that says "Label Cases by." Then, at the bottom left, click on "Both" for type of display, i.e., both Statistics and Plots. Click the Statistics pushbutton

and click Descriptives, Outliers, and Percentiles, then Continue. Now, back in the original dialog box, click the Plots pushbutton. Under Boxplots, click on Factor levels together, unselect stem-and-leaf plot if it is checked, then hit Continue. Now run this procedure (click OK) and answer the following questions: (a) In the table of Descriptive Statistics, what is the value of the trimmed mean? What percent of outliers does SPSS trim in calculating this statistic? Is the trimmed mean different from the untrimmed mean? (b) Does this table indicate the value of the *IQR*—and, if so, is the value the same as your own calculations in Exercise B2? (c) Does the skewness index in this table suggest a skew? If so, in which direction? (d) What does the kurtosis index in this table suggest? (e) Looking at the Percentile Table (ignoring information on Tukey's Hinges), what age is at the 5th percentile? What age is at the 95th percentile? Explain the bearing of these values on the calculation of the trimmed mean. (f) Looking at the table for Extreme Values, what is the highest value, and which case corresponds to that value? What is the lowest value, and which case corresponds to that value? (g) Looking at the boxplot, are there any outliers? Are there outliers at the lower end (below Q_1)? If so, how many—and are they "mild" or "extreme"? Are there outliers at the upper end (above Q_3)? If so, how many—and are they "mild" or "extreme"? (h) Are the outliers and extreme values at either end plausibly *real* values, or do you think they represent data entry errors?

† **B4.** In this exercise, you will create a new variable (*crowded*) and then generate *z* scores for that variable. The new variable will be an index of how crowded participants were in their residences. To create *crowded*, you will instruct the computer to divide the number of rooms in the household (*rooms*) by the total number of people living in the household (*hhsize*). So, if there are two people living in four rooms, the value of *crowded* would be 2.0 (i.e., two rooms per person). In SPSS, when new variables are created they are automatically put at the end of the file, unless you take steps for a different placement, which we do not explain here. From the main toolbar, click Transform, then select Compute. In the dialog box, type the name of the new variable

(*crowded*) in the box labeled New Variable. Click the pushbutton directly below this (Type & Label) and give the variable a longer label that will appear on output (e.g., Number of rooms per person in HH). Now, on the right side of the dialog box, you need to instruct the computer how to calculate this new variable. Find *rooms* in the list, and click on the right arrow to move this variable into the box that says "Numeric expression." Next, type in a slash (/), which is the symbol for division. Then, from the variable list, find *hhsize* and use the arrow to insert it into the expression. The expression should read "rooms / hhsize." Now click OK to create the variable, setting crowded equal to number of rooms divided by household size. Now run Analyze → Descriptives Statistics → Descriptives for *crowded*. In the opening dialog box, click the option that says "Save standardized values as variables." When you have done this, run Descriptives again for the new standard score, which will appear as the last variable in the file. Then answer the following questions: (a) What is the mean and *SD* for the variable *crowded*? What is the range? What does this information mean? (b) What is the name that SPSS assigned to the standard score it created for *crowded*? (c) What is the mean and *SD* for the standard score variable? (d) Now look in the Data Editor and find the two new variables in Data View. What is the value of *crowded* and the standard score for crowded for the first person in the file? Explain the sign (positive or negative) on her standard score.

† **B5.** Run descriptive statistics on the following variables in the Polit2SetA dataset: *age, age1bir, higrade, hhsize*, and *income*. Create a table summarizing the results, using Table 3.2 as a model—or elaborate on it by adding other descriptive statistics. Then write a paragraph summarizing the information in the table.

B6. Select a variable from the Polit2SetB dataset that is an interval-level or ratio-level variable. Do some basic descriptive statistics (means, *SD*s, etc.) for the selected variable, and run the Explore procedure to examine outliers. Write a paragraph summarizing what you learned about the variable.

Bivariate Description: Crosstabulation, Risk Indexes, and Correlation

Most research questions are about relationships between two or more variables. For example, when scientists study whether smokers are more likely than nonsmokers to develop lung cancer, they are asking if there is a relationship between smoking and lung cancer. When nurse researchers ask whether primiparas are more likely than multiparas to request epidural analgesia, they are studying the relationship between parity and requests for pain relief.

The univariate descriptive statistics we have discussed thus far do not concern relationships: They are used to describe one variable at a time. Most of the remainder of this book describes inferential statistical tests that allow us to make inferences about relationships within the population. This chapter discusses methods of *describing* relationships in a research sample by means of **bivariate descriptive statistics**.

CROSSTABULATION

Suppose we were interested in comparing men and women patients with regard to their rate of re-admission into a psychiatric hospital within 1 year of discharge. In this example, there are two research variables—gender and readmission status—and both are dichotomous, nominal-level variables. Two frequency distributions would tell us, first, how many men and women were in the sample, and second, how many sample members were or were not readmitted within 1 year of discharge. To describe the relationship between the two variables, we would

TABLE 4.1 Contingency Table for Gender/Readmission Status Example

Readmission Status	Gender		Total
	Male	**Female**	**Total**
Readmitted	15 (30.0%)	10 (20.0%)	25 (25.0%)
Not Readmitted	35 (70.0%)	40 (80.0%)	75 (75.0%)
Total	50	50	100

crosstabulate the two variables in a **contingency table** (or **crosstabs table**), which is essentially a two-dimensional frequency distribution. Table 4.1 presents a hypothetical contingency table for our example.

To construct a contingency table, we array the categories of one variable horizontally across the top (in this example, gender), and the categories of the second variable vertically along the left (here, readmission status). This creates the **cells** for the contingency table, that is, the unique combination of the two variables. The number of cells is the number of categories of the first variable multiplied by the number of categories of the second. There are four cells (2 × 2) in the present example.

Next, cases are allocated to the appropriate cell. That is, men who were readmitted are tallied in the upper left cell, women who were readmitted are tallied in the upper right cell, and so on. Once all sample members have been properly allocated, frequencies and percentages can be computed for each cell. In this example, we see in Table 4.1 that men were somewhat more likely than women to be readmitted to a psychiatric hospital within 1 year of discharge (30% versus 20%, respectively).

Contingency tables are easy to construct and they communicate useful information. The commands for instructing the computer to prepare a contingency table are straightforward as well—although thought needs to be given to which variable to put in the rows and which in the columns. Note that in Table 4.1, the percentages were based on gender: 30.0% of the men (15 ÷ 50) and 20.0% of the women (10 ÷ 50) were readmitted. We could also have calculated percentages based on readmission status. For example, we could say that 60.0% of all patients readmitted were men (15 ÷ 25), or that 53.3% of those *not* readmitted were women (40 ÷ 75). Computers can be instructed to compute all possible percentages.

As an example, suppose we were interested in comparing women who were either married or not married at childbirth with regard to a subsequent diagnosis of postpartum depression (PPD). A fictitious contingency table for 100 women (Figure 4.1) has been created to demonstrate how to read a printout from a crosstabulation. We created this figure in SPSS through the Analyze ➜ Descriptive Statistics ➜ Crosstabs commands, but we added shading to facilitate our discussion. Let us begin with the overall percentages. In the bottom (shaded) row we see that 19 women (19.0%) were not married and 81 (81.0%) were married. In the far-right (shaded) column we see that 20 women (20.0%) were diagnosed with PPD, and 80 women (80.0%) were not. These are sometimes referred to as the **marginal frequencies**. Both the row totals and the column totals add up to the grand total of 100 cases (100%), shown in the bottom right corner.

As in the previous example, there are four cells (2 × 2) where the two variables intersect because both variables in Figure 4.1 are dichotomous. In the printout, each cell contains four pieces of information, which we describe for the first (upper left) cell, shaded in darker blue. According to the output, eight of the 100 women in this sample were unmarried *and* experienced postpartum depression. The next number is

Crosstabs

PPD Diagnosis * Marital Status Crosstabulation

			Marital Status		
			Not Married	Married	Total
PPD Diagnosis	Yes	Count	8	12	20
		% within PPD Diagnosis	40.0%	60.0%	100.0%
		% within Marital Status	42.1%	14.8%	20.0%
		% of Total	8.0%	12.0%	20.0%
	No	Count	11	69	80
		% within PPD Diagnosis	13.8%	86.2%	100.0%
		% within Marital Status	57.9%	85.2%	80.0%
		% of Total	11.0%	69.0%	80.0%
	Total	Count	19	81	100
		% within PPD Diagnosis	19.0%	81.0%	100.0%
		% within Marital Status	100.0%	100.0%	100.0%
		% of Total	19.0%	81.0%	100.0%

FIGURE 4.1 SPSS printout of a crosstabulation (shading added).

the percent within PPD diagnosis, which is the row percentage: 40.0% (8 ÷ 20) of the women who were depressed were not married. The third number in the cell is the percent within marital status, which is the column percentage: 42.1% (8 ÷ 19) of the unmarried women had a PPD diagnosis. Finally, the fourth number is the total percentage: of the 100 sample members, 8.0% were unmarried and depressed. The output shows how to read these numbers by indicating the order of the information, just to the left of the first cell: Count; % within PPD Diagnosis; % within Marital Status; and % of Total.

The most important pieces of information in this particular table are the column percentages for the cells: They tell us that substantially more of the unmarried women (42.1%) than those who were married (14.8%) experienced postpartum depression. When the computer is instructed to display the independent variable in the columns, as in this example, it is usually the column percentages that are of greatest interest. For creating a table for a report, the independent variable is typically used as column headings.

Contingency tables such as these are used with nominal-level variables, but they are also appropriate if the variables are ordinal-level with a small number of categories. For example, if the PPD diagnosis was classified as *severe PPD, mild PPD,* or *no PPD,* the variable would be ordinal level. When crossed with marital status, the resulting six-cell contingency table (3 × 2) would describe the relationship between marital status and severity of PPD.

RISK INDEXES

Clinical decision making based on research evidence has become an important issue in the current EBP environment, and several descriptive statistical indexes can aid such decision making. These **risk indexes** are important because they facilitate the interpretation of risks (and risk reduction) within a context. If an intervention reduces the risk of an adverse outcome ten times over, but the initial risk is minuscule, the intervention may be impractical if it is costly. Both absolute change (the actual amount of difference) and relative change (comparisons between groups or conditions) are important in clinical decision making.

The indexes described in this section involve two dichotomous nominal-level variables. Data of this type might be generated in several research situations, but here we consider three. Some research is designed to identify the factors that put people at special risk of a negative outcome. The goal of such research might be to educate people about the risk or to identify at-risk people who might benefit from a special intervention. One example is prospective research on smoking as a risk factor (smokers versus nonsmokers) and subsequent lung cancer as an outcome (lung cancer versus no lung cancer). In retrospective case-control studies, the goal is similarly to identify risk, but in this design, researchers start with the adverse outcome (lung cancer versus no lung cancer) and then examine prior smoking practices in both groups. A third situation involves interventions designed to reduce risk—such as a nurse-led smoking cessation intervention. In this situation, receipt of the intervention is one dichotomous variable (received versus did not receive it) and smoking status after the intervention is the other (smoking versus not smoking).

TIP: *Researchers sometimes dichotomize interval- or ratio-level variables so they can calculate these risk indexes. This strategy is especially useful if there are clinically important thresholds or cutoff points for a risk variable. For example, values for the body mass index (BMI) could be used to designate whether a person is or is not obese, based on a standard BMI cutpoint of 30.*

Risk indexes such as those we discuss in this section are not always presented in statistics textbooks—and, in fact, they are infrequently reported in nursing journal articles. Readers can sometimes use information in articles to calculate these indexes if full crosstabulation information has been presented. Indeed, there are many Web sites that will calculate the indexes for you if you do not have raw data but rather are working with cell percentages such as those described in the previous section. We suspect that, because of the high visibility of EBP, increasing numbers of researchers will report these indexes in the years ahead, and so we discuss ways to calculate them from raw data.

TIP: *Various Web sites on the Internet provide assistance in calculating indexes described in this section, including the University of British Columbia's Clinical Significance Calculator (http://www.spph.ubc.ca/calc/clinsig.html), or the Evidence-Based Emergency Medicine Web site (http://www.ebem.org/nntcalculator.html).*

One of the terms often associated with the risk indexes is *exposure*—i.e., exposure to risk. People with the risk factor are in the *exposed* group, and those without the risk are in the *not exposed* group. For example, in a study of fall risk in relation to cognitive impairment among nursing home residents, those *with* a cognitive impairment would be in the exposed group, and those *without* cognitive impairment would be in the not exposed group. In studies of interventions designed to reduce risk or negative outcomes, we can conceptualize the control group as being "exposed" to ongoing risk, under the hypothesis that the intervention is beneficial and reduces risk. In

TABLE 4.2 Indexes of Risk in a 2 × 2 Table

Risk Factor	Outcome		Total
	Yes (Undesirable Outcome)	No (Desirable Outcome)	
Yes, exposed to risk (Or, *not* given an intervention—Controls)	a	b	a + b
No, not exposed to risk (Or, given an intervention—Experimentals)	c	d	c + d
TOTAL	a + c	b + d	a + b + c + d

Absolute Risk, risk-exposed or control group (AR_E)	$= a \div (a + b)$
Absolute Risk, nonexposed or experimental group (AR_{NE})	$= c \div (c + d)$
Absolute Risk Reduction (ARR)	$= AR_{NE} - AR_E$
Relative Risk (RR)	$= AR_E \div AR_{NE}$
Relative Risk Reduction (RRR)	$= ARR \div AR_{NE}$
Odds, risk-exposed or control group ($Odds_E$)	$= a \div b$
Odds, nonexposed or experimental group ($Odds_{NE}$)	$= c \div d$
Odds Ratio (OR)	$= \dfrac{Odds_E}{Odds_{NE}}$
Number Needed to Treat	$= 1 \div ARR$

this situation, being in the treatment group corresponds to nonexposure (i.e., protection from risk factors that would typically be present without the intervention).

In the situation we have described, we could construct a 2 × 2 contingency table with four cells, as depicted in Table 4.2. This table labels the four cells in the contingency table so that computations for the risk indexes can be explained. *Cell a* is the number of people with an undesirable outcome (e.g., death) in a risk-exposed (or control) group; *cell b* is the number with a desirable outcome (e.g., survival) in the risk-exposed group; and *cells c* and *d* are the two outcome possibilities for a non–risk exposed (or intervention) group. We can now explain the meaning and calculation of several indexes that are of particular interest to clinicians.

Note that the computations shown in Table 4.2 require the independent variable (risk exposure) to be in the rows, and the outcome to be in the columns—*This is exactly the opposite of how we recommended arranging variables in our previous discussion on crosstabs.* This reverse ordering of variables is recommended within SPSS (Norušis, 2008) for the computation of several key risk indexes. Moreover, the variables should be coded such that the smaller code for the independent variable is associated with greater hypothesized risk, and that the smaller code for the dependent variable is associated with less favorable outcomes. In other words, *cell a in Table 4.2 should be where you would expect the least favorable outcomes* if you are using the formulas shown in Table 4.2 (or if you are using SPSS to calculate risk statistics). So, for example, in a smoking cessation intervention study, the control group not receiving the intervention should be coded 0 and the experimental group members receiving the intervention should be coded 1, and not vice versa (or codes 1 and 2, respectively). And if smoking status 1 month later were the outcome variable, smokers should be designated by a code 0, and nonsmokers with a code of 1—or, again, codes 1 and 2, respectively. (We discuss this a bit further later in this chapter.)

TIP: *Within major software packages, you would be able to recode your values if you did not originally follow the coding suggestions just outlined. For example, if experimentals were coded 1 and controls were coded 2, you would just need to instruct the computer to recode all 2s as 0s. In SPSS, you could do this through the Transform ➜ Recode into Same Variable command.*

Absolute Risk and Absolute Risk Reduction

Absolute risk can be computed for both those exposed to a risk factor, and for those not exposed. **Absolute risk** is simply the proportion of people who experienced an undesirable outcome in each group. We illustrate this and other indexes with our earlier data on marital status and a PPD diagnosis. In this situation, we are asking about how much risk an unmarried woman has of PPD, relative to her risk if married. Thus, in this example we have hypothesized that being unmarried is a risk factor for postpartum depression. Table 4.3 shows the crosstabulation of these two variables, with the same data as earlier—except here the PPD outcome is shown in the columns, and the risk factor (marital status) is shown in the rows. This table shows only counts and row percentages.

In this fictitious example, the absolute risk of a PPD diagnosis is 42.1% among unmarried (exposed) women ($AR_E = .421$), and 14.8% in the married (not exposed) group ($AR_{NE} = .148$). Thus, absolute risk corresponds to the row percentage for each group: $a \div (a + b)$ and $c \div (c + d)$. Women in both groups were at risk of PPD, but not being married was associated with a heightened risk of a poor psychological outcome in this sample.

The **absolute risk reduction (ARR)**, which is sometimes called the *risk difference,* is a comparison of the two risks. It is computed by subtracting the absolute risk for the nonexposed group from the absolute risk for the exposed group. This index indicates the estimated proportion of extra people who would be harmed from risk exposure—or, in an intervention study, the proportion spared from the undesirable outcome through receipt of the treatment. In our example, the value of ARR is .273 ($.421 - .148 = .273$). In other words, 27.3% of the mothers had a PPD diagnosis associated with not being married, over and above the estimated 14.8% who would have been depressed even if married.

Relative Risk and Relative Risk Reduction

The index called **relative risk (RR)**, or the **risk ratio**, is the ratio of absolute risks in the two groups. RR represents the proportion of the original risk of an adverse outcome (in our example, a PPD diagnosis) that is associated with the risk exposure. Said another way, relative risk is the probability of a bad outcome for someone with risk exposure, relative to the probability of a bad outcome without such exposure.

TABLE 4.3 Data for Risk Index Computations: Marital Staus and PPD Outcome

| | | | PPD Diagnosis | | Total |
			Yes	No	
Marital Status	Not married	Count % within PPD diagnosis	8 42.1% (a)	11 57.9% (b)	19 100.0% (a + b)
	Married	Count % within PPD diagnosis	12 14.8% (c)	69 85.2% (d)	81 100.0% (c + d)
TOTAL		Count % within PPD Diagnosis	20 20.0%	80 80.0%	100 100.0%

Absolute Risk, risk-exposed group (AR_E) $= 8 \div 19$ $= .421$
Absolute Risk, nonexposed group (AR_{NE}) $= 12 \div 81$ $= .148$
Absolute Risk Reduction (ARR) $= .421 - .148 = .273$
Relative Risk (RR) $= .421 \div .148 = 2.842$
Relative Risk Reduction (RRR) $= .273 \div .148 = 1.845$
Odds, risk-exposed group ($Odds_E$) $= 8 \div 11$ $= .727$
Odds, nonexposed group ($Odds_{NE}$) $= 12 \div 69$ $= .174$
Odds Ratio (OR) $= \dfrac{.727}{.174}$ $= 4.182$
Number Needed to Treat $= 1 \div .273$ $= 3.663$

When the value of RR is close to 1, it means that risk exposure and outcomes are not related—the two groups are expected to have similar outcomes.

To compute an RR, the absolute risk for risk-exposed people (AR_E) is divided by the absolute risk for nonexposed people (AR_{NE}). In our fictitious example, the RR is $.421 \div .148 = 2.842$. This means that the risk of postpartum depression was nearly three times as high for unmarried as for married women. RR, which can be computed within SPSS as part of the Crosstabs procedure, is one of the most frequently used risk indexes.

Another index that is sometimes used when evaluating the effectiveness of an intervention is the **relative risk reduction (RRR)**. RRR is the estimated proportion of risk associated with risk exposure that is reduced when there is no exposure—or, in the context of an intervention, it is the estimated proportion of baseline risk that is reduced as a result of the treatment. This index is computed by dividing the ARR by the absolute risk for the risk-exposed group. In our example, RRR $= .273 \div .148 = 1.845$. This means that being married decreased the relative risk of a PPD diagnosis by 185%, compared to being unmarried.

Odds and the Odds Ratio

The odds ratio is among the most widely reported index among those described in this section, but it is less intuitively meaningful than the RR as an index of risk. The term "odds" is most frequently used in the context of gambling, like a horse's odds of winning a major stakes race, or the odds of rolling "snake eyes" (two ones) with a pair of dice. The **odds**, in the context of healthcare outcomes, is the proportion of people in each group *with* the adverse outcome relative to those *without* it. In our example, the odds of PPD for the unmarried group is 8 (the number who had a PPD diagnosis) divided by 11 (the number who did not), or .727. The odds for the married group is 12 divided by 69, or .174. The **odds ratio (OR)** is the ratio of these two odds, or 4.182 in our example (i.e., .727 ÷ .174). The estimated odds of being depressed postpartum are about four times higher among unmarried than among married women in this sample. Like RR, when the value of an OR is close to 1, the risk factor and the outcome are not related.

The odds ratio can be computed in SPSS within the Crosstabs procedure. The printout for our example is shown in Figure 4.2. (For the moment, ignore the confidence interval information in the right columns—confidence intervals are explained in the next chapter). This output shows that the OR is 4.182—the same value we computed manually. The RR for having a PPD diagnosis is shown next, with the label "For cohort PPD Diagnosis = Yes." This index indicates the relative risk of having a PPD diagnosis, given the status of being unmarried. The RR of 2.842 is the same value we obtained with manual calculations. The next entry in the output ("For cohort PPD Diagnosis = No") can be ignored in the present example—it represents the relative risk of *not* having a PPD diagnosis (.680), given a nonmarried status.

Number Needed to Treat

One other index of interest in the current evidence-based practice environment is the **number needed to treat (NNT)**. This index is especially useful in the context of an intervention—it represents an estimate of how many people would need to receive a treatment to prevent one undesirable outcome. The NNT is computed by dividing 1 by the value of the absolute risk reduction. In our example, ARR = .273, and so NNT is 3.663—although it is not a particularly meaningful index in this context. It suggests that between three and four unmarried women would need to marry to avoid one PPD diagnosis. Although not useful in this example, the NNT is obviously important when the independent variable is a treatment, and there is an interest in understanding how many treated people would yield an improved outcome. The NNT is valuable for decision makers because it can be integrated with monetary information to assess whether an intervention is likely to be cost effective.

Risk Estimate

	Value	95% Confidence Interval	
		Lower	Upper
Odds Ratio for Marital Status (Not Married/ Married)	4.182	1.395	12.535
For cohort PPD Diagnosis = Yes	2.842	1.353	5.969
For cohort PPD Diagnosis = No	.680	.458	1.008
N of Valid Cases	100		

FIGURE 4.2 SPSS printout of risk indexes (shading added).

Example of ARR, RR, and NNT:

Nakagami and colleagues (2007) evaluated the effectiveness of a new dressing containing ceramide 2 for preventing persistent erythema and pressure ulcers in bedridden older patients. The study involved 37 patients in Japan, who were administered the dressing, at random, to either the right or left greater trochanter for 3 weeks. No dressing was applied to the opposite side, which served as the control condition. The results indicated that the incidence of persistent erythema was lower on the intervention side than on the control side. The absolute risk reduction was about 24%. The RR index was .18 and NNT was 4.11. That is, for four people receiving the special dressing, the incidence of persistent erythema would be reduced by one.

Risk Index Issues

Some additional guidance and discussion may be helpful in interpreting the various risk indexes and selecting which one to use. One issue concerns Table 4.2, which is set up with the expectation that the worst outcome would be in cell a, as recommended within SPSS (Norušis, 2008). In fact, this is different than presentations in other textbooks, including that by one of us (Polit & Beck, 2008, Table 21.8). In that book and other books on EBP (e.g., DiCenso, Guyatt, & Ciliska, 2005), the table is set up to have the worst expected outcome in cell c, which results when an intervention group is in the top row and a control group is in the bottom row. In such presentations, "exposure" is conceptualized as exposure to a beneficial treatment, not to a risk factor. As we will see, both arrangements are perfectly fine—as long as you pay attention to what the resulting risk index values mean.

In our example, we coded not married as "1" and married as "2" so that the unmarried women would be in the top row. If we reversed the coding of these two groups, then in a computer analysis the values for married women would be in the top row rather than in the bottom one. If married women were in the top row, the row percentages would not, of course, change—and hence, the values of absolute risk of PPD would remain the same: .421 for unmarried women and .148 for married women. But now, to compute the RR, instead of dividing .421 by .148, we would do the reverse (.148 ÷ .421), and this would yield an RR of .352 instead of 2.842. The result is actually identical: Instead of saying unmarried women were about three times as likely to have PPD as married women, the RR value of .352 means that married women are about one third as likely to have PPD as unmarried women. When interpreting indexes like RR or OR, it is important to look at absolute values, like the row percentages (AR).

There has been a lot of discussion about whether to report RR or OR values in reports. Certainly, relative risk is much easier to grasp than the odds ratio. As DiCenso and colleagues (2005) noted, "As clinicians, we would like to be able to substitute the relative risk, which we intuitively understand, for the odds ratio, which we do not understand" (p. 412). This statement reflects the fact that *odds* is a gambling concept not widely grasped in the healthcare community, let alone the concept of a ratio of odds. Interestingly, however, the value of the OR and RR are frequently quite similar, and this is especially true when the consequences of risk exposure is low, or the beneficial effect of an intervention is modest. In other words, when the absolute risk reduction is smaller, the two indexes are closer in value.

To illustrate, suppose that in our earlier example only four rather than eight of the 19 unmarried women was diagnosed with PPD—i.e., 21.1% rather than 42.1%

had the diagnosis. In this situation, ARR would decrease from .27 to .06. The value of RR (1.42) is now quite close to the value of the OR (1.53).

TIP: *The odds ratio, and not the RR, should be used when the study design is a retrospective case-control design. For RCTs and prospective studies, either the OR or the RR can be used, although the RR may be preferred for interpretive reasons.*

One final point is that relative risk should not be interpreted without taking absolute risk into consideration, because similar RR values can be associated with quite different ARR values. For example, suppose that both unmarried and married women had half the risk of a PPD diagnosis as was observed in Table 4.3. In other words, only four out of 19 unmarried women (21.1%) and six out of 81 married women (7.4%) had a PPD diagnosis. ARR, in this case, is .137—half of what it was initially, and NNT also changes, doubling to 7.30. Yet, RR remains unchanged (2.84). Thus, in making clinical decisions—for example, about the cost effectiveness of implementing an intervention—both relative and absolute risk need to be considered.

CORRELATION

A **correlation** refers to a bond or connection between variables—variation in one variable is systematically related to variation in the other. Correlation analysis is a useful way to describe the direction and magnitude of a relationship between two variables. For example, correlation analysis can be used to address the question, To what extent is respiratory function related to anxiety levels in patients with chronic obstructive pulmonary disease? Or, What is the magnitude of the relationship between measurements of resting energy expenditure using indirect calorimetry and the Fick method?

Variables are correlated with one another when there is a relationship between them. Correlations between two variables can be plotted graphically, but are more often reported through an index that summarizes the extent and direction of a relationship. We describe graphic procedures first because they help us to visualize why correlation coefficients are useful in describing **linear** (straight line) **relationships** that have a constant rate of change between the variables.

Scatterplots

The relationship between two variables that have been measured on an interval or ratio scale can be displayed graphically on a **scatterplot** (or *scatter diagram*). Such a graph plots the values of one variable (X) on the X axis, and simultaneously plots the values of a second variable (Y) on the Y axis. As an example, suppose that for every hour that students volunteered to work at a school-based clinic, a sponsor donated $1 toward the school's athletic fund. Figure 4.3 presents data for hours worked (X) and dollar amounts donated (Y) for 10 students. The first student volunteered 1 hour, and so the amount of the donation was $1. The tenth student volunteered 10 hours, resulting in a $10 donation. Figure 4.3 also shows a scatterplot of these data. Each dot on the plot is a data point for the two variables (e.g., the dot at the intersection of 1 hour on the X axis and $1 on the Y axis is the data point for student number 1). This graph shows that there is a straight line relationship between X and Y. Algebraically,

Student	Data Hours (X)	Donation (Y)
1	1	$1
2	2	$2
3	3	$3
4	4	$4
5	5	$5
6	6	$6
7	7	$7
8	8	$8
9	9	$9
10	10	$10

FIGURE 4.3 Scatterplot for volunteer/donation example.

we can say that $X = Y$: The value of X always equals the value of Y. If a student worked 20 hours, the donation would be $20. The relationship between X and Y is called a **perfect relationship**, because we need only know the value of X to know or predict the value of Y, and vice versa.

Researchers rarely study variables that are perfectly related, and so scatterplots of actual research data are seldom so orderly as the one in Figure 4.3. Figure 4.4 presents a scatterplot with some fictitious data for two variables for which the relationship is strong, but not perfect. Let us say that X is nursing students' test scores on a 10-question midterm statistics test and Y is their scores on a 10-question final exam. (The letters on the graph correspond to students a–j, and are shown here to help identify each data point.) We cannot perfectly predict values of Y based on values of X, but nevertheless students who performed well on the midterm also tended to do well on the final.

Student	Data Midterm (X)	Final (Y)
a	2	3
b	6	7
c	5	6
d	9	8
e	7	9
f	9	10
g	3	4
h	4	6
i	1	2
j	4	5

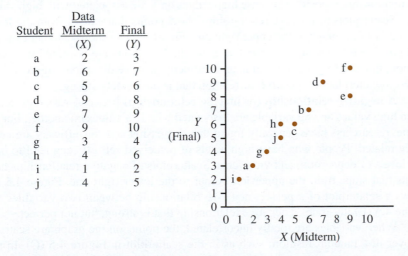

FIGURE 4.4 Scatterplot of students' test scores.

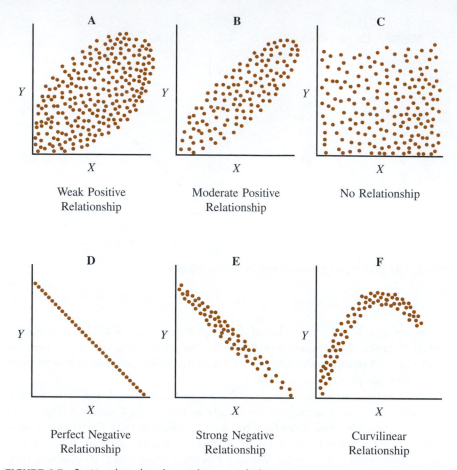

FIGURE 4.5   Scatterplots showing various correlations.

Scatterplots show both the magnitude and direction of relationships. The scatterplot in Figure 4.4 illustrates a strong **positive relationship**. The relationship is strong because the data points fall closely together along a straight diagonal line; The relationship is positive because high values on *X* are associated with high values on *Y*. Scatterplots of positive relationships show points that extend from the lower left corner of the graph to the upper right one. Figure 4.5 (A) shows another example of a positive relationship, but one that is weak: The points are scattered in a loose fashion, though the general trend is in a distinctly positive direction. Figure 4.5 (B) shows a scatterplot of a positive correlation that is moderately strong.

A **negative relationship** (or **inverse relationship**) between variables occurs when high values on one variable are associated with low values on another. For example, researchers have generally found that depression and self-efficacy are negatively related: People who have high levels of perceived self-efficacy tend to have low levels of depression, and vice versa. Scatterplots of negative relationships have points that slope from the upper left corner to the lower right one. Figure 4.5 (D) shows a scatterplot of a perfect negative relationship between two variables and Figure 4.5 (E) illustrates a negative relationship that is strong, but not perfect.

When variables are totally uncorrelated, the points on the graph are scattered all over in a random fashion, such as in the scatterplot in Figure 4.5 (C). In this situation, a person with a high score on *X* is equally likely to have a low or a high score on Y. For example, if we were to construct a scatterplot showing the relationship between nurses' height and their degree of burnout, we might expect a graph such as this one: There is no reason to expect tall nurses to be more (or less) burned out than short nurses.

Another type of relationship is shown in Figure 4.5 (F). This scatterplot illustrates a **curvilinear relationship.** In this situation, a straight line does not adequately characterize the relationship between the variables. Scores on Y increase as the scores on X increase, but only to a certain point, and after that point the scores on Y decline. As an example, there may be a curvilinear relationship between the number of hours slept and self-reported energy levels: Perceived energy would likely increase with increasing amounts of sleep, but at some point a large number of hours of sleep might reflect a physiological condition associated with low energy.

Correlation Coefficients

Although correlations between two variables can readily be graphed, researchers are more likely to describe correlations by a statistic called a **correlation coefficient**. Correlation coefficients, like scatterplots, indicate both the magnitude and direction of a linear relationship between two variables. Because they are expressed numerically, correlation coefficients are more precise about magnitude than scatterplots, to which we usually attach broad verbal labels such as "weak" or "moderately strong."

Correlation coefficients are indexes whose values range from -1.00 through .00 to $+1.00$. Negative values (from -1.00 to $-.01$) indicate negative relationships, while positive values (from $+.01$ to $+1.00$) indicate positive relationships. A correlation coefficient of .00 indicates no relationship between the variables.

The **absolute value** (the numerical value without any sign) of the correlation coefficient indicates relationship strength. The smaller the absolute value, the weaker the relationship. For example, $-.90$ indicates a very strong relationship, while $+.45$ indicates a moderate relationship. When two variables are perfectly and positively correlated (as in Figure 4.3), the correlation coefficient is $+1.00$. Perfect negative correlations are expressed as -1.00.

PEARSON'S r   The most widely used correlation index is the **Pearson product-moment correlation coefficient** (also called **Pearson's r**), a statistic that is appropriate when two variables are measured on an interval or ratio scale, or on a level that approximates interval characteristics. Other correlation indexes are described later in this book.

Correlation coefficients are usually calculated by computer rather than manually. However, manual computation, though laborious, is not difficult. There are several alternative formulas for computing Pearson's r. We offer the following equation:

$$r_{xy} = \frac{\Sigma(X - \overline{X})(Y - \overline{Y})}{\sqrt{\Sigma[(X - \overline{X})^2][(Y - \overline{Y})^2]}}$$

where r_{xy} = the correlation coefficient for variables X and Y
Σ = the sum of
X = an individual value for variable X
$\overline{X}$ = the mean for variable X
Y = an individual value for variable Y
$\overline{Y}$ = the mean for variable Y

TABLE 4.4 Calculation of Pearson's *r*

Student	1 X	2 $(X-\bar{X})$	3 $(X-\bar{X})^2$	4 Y	5 $(Y-\bar{Y})$	6 $(Y-\bar{Y})^2$	7 $(X-\bar{X})(Y-\bar{Y})$
a	2	−3	9	3	−3	9	9
b	6	1	1	7	1	1	1
c	5	0	0	6	0	0	0
d	9	4	16	8	2	4	8
e	7	2	4	9	3	9	6
f	9	4	16	10	4	16	16
g	3	−2	4	4	−2	4	4
h	4	−1	1	6	0	0	0
i	1	−4	16	2	−4	16	16
j	4	−1	1	5	−1	1	1
	$\Sigma X = 50$ $\bar{X} = 5.0$		$\Sigma = 68$	$\Sigma Y = 60$ $\bar{Y} = 6.0$		$\Sigma = 60$	$\Sigma = 61$

$$r_{xy} = \frac{\Sigma(X-\bar{X})(Y-\bar{Y})}{\sqrt{[\Sigma(X-\bar{X})^2][\Sigma(Y-\bar{Y})^2]}}$$

$$\Sigma(X-\bar{X})(Y-\bar{Y}) = 61$$
$$\Sigma(X-\bar{X})^2 = 68$$
$$\Sigma(Y-\bar{Y})^2 = 60$$

$$r_{xy} = \frac{61}{\sqrt{68 \times 60}} = \frac{61}{\sqrt{4080}} = \frac{61}{63.8745} = .955$$

Although this formula looks complex, it basically involves manipulating deviation scores for the two variables.[1] An example is completely worked out in Table 4.4, using the data for students' scores on the statistics midterm and final exam (see Figure 4.4).

The first step in computing *r* with this formula is to compute the means for *X* and *Y*, which are shown as 5.0 and 6.0, respectively (columns 1 and 4 in Table 4.4). Deviation scores are then obtained for each student (columns 2 and 5), and then each deviation score is squared (columns 3 and 6). The **cross products** of the two deviation scores are calculated in column 7. That is, the deviation score for variable *X* is multiplied by the deviation score for variable *Y* for each student. The individual values in columns 3, 6, and 7 are then summed, and these sums are the elements required in the correlation formula. As shown at the bottom of Table 4.4, the value of *r* in this example is .955, which is a very strong, positive correlation.

When a computer is used to calculate the Pearson *r* statistic, the command is usually simple. For example, in SPSS, the commands for correlating two variables would be Analyze ➡ Correlate ➡ Bivariate, followed by instructions on which variables should be correlated.

INTERPRETATION OF CORRELATION COEFFICIENTS Correlation coefficients directly communicate magnitude, but there are no straightforward guidelines for interpreting the strength of a correlation coefficient. For example, if nurses measured patients' body temperatures with two thermometers, they might find a correlation coefficient between the two values in the vicinity of .99. In this context, if the correlation

---

[1] In fact, we can simplify the appearance of the formula by using the symbols for deviation scores:

$$r_{xy} = \frac{\Sigma xy}{\sqrt{(\Sigma x^2)(\Sigma y^2)}}$$

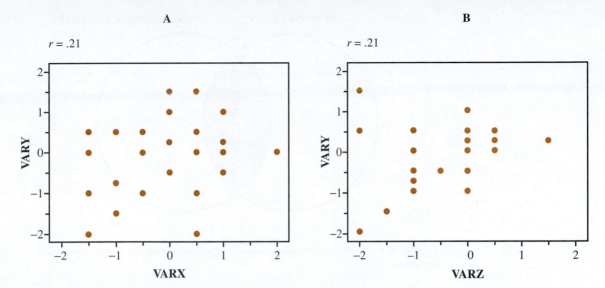

FIGURE 4.6   SPSS printout of two scatterplots.

between the two instruments was found to be .80, the correlation would be considered unacceptably low. On the other hand, the correlation between self-efficacy and depression is probably in the vicinity of $-.40$, and in this situation, a correlation of $-.80$ would be considered extremely high. Correlations between variables of a psychosocial nature rarely exceed .50.

Scatterplots are sometimes useful in interpreting correlation coefficients when the magnitude is modest. A low correlation coefficient could reflect a weak relationship between two variables, or a relationship that is not linear. For example, two computer-generated scatterplots are presented in Figure 4.6. These scatterplots (created in SPSS through the Graphs ➜ Legacy Dialogs ➜ Scatterplot commands) use standard scores as the data values rather than actual raw scores, so the means of all variables are 0. Graph A and B, which plots VARX against VARY, suggests a weak relationship. There is only the barest suggestion that the variables are positively correlated and, in fact, the correlation coefficient is only $+.21$. The correlation coefficient for the two variables in graph B of Figure 4.6 (VARY and VARZ) is the same ($r = +.21$), but the nature of the relationship is different. VARY and VARZ have a fairly strong positive relationship at all points below the means of the two variables. Above the mean of 0, however, the two variables seem related in a loosely negative direction. Because the relationship is not linear, r does not adequately summarize the pattern.

An interesting feature of a correlation coefficient is that its square (r^2) is a direct indication of the proportion of the variability in one variable that can be accounted for or explained by variability in a second variable. For example, if the correlation coefficient describing the relationship between SAT scores (X) and nursing students' grades (Y) is .50, we can say that 25% ($.50^2$) of the variability in students' grades is explained by variability in SAT scores. This relationship is depicted graphically in Figure 4.7. In this figure, the two circles represent the total amount of variation in the two variables, and the hatched area indicates how much of the variation in grades is "explained" by variation in SAT scores (i.e., 25%). The remaining 75% of the variability in grades is influenced by other factors (e.g., motivation, prior experience, idiosyncrasies of faculty grading, and so on). If the correlation between the two variables were perfect (if the student

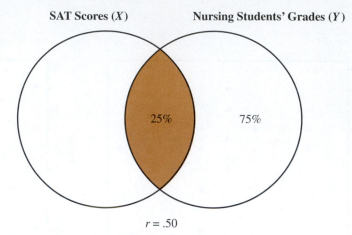

SAT Scores (X)   **Nursing Students' Grades (Y)**

25%   75%

$r = .50$

FIGURE 4.7 Illustration of percentage of explained variability in two correlated variables.

with the highest SAT scores obtained the highest grades, the second highest scorer got the second highest grades, and so on), the two circles would overlap completely.

It must be emphasized that when a researcher finds that two variables are correlated, this does not imply that one variable *caused* the other. For example, if we found a negative correlation between physical functioning and depression, we could not conclude that having low physical functioning causes people to become depressed. Nor can we conclude that being depressed reduces people's physical functioning. Either of these might be true, but it might also be that both are caused by some other factor (e.g., older age or an illness). Researchers must always be cautious when drawing inferences of a **causal relationship** from correlations. Even a very strong correlation between two variables provides no evidence that one variable caused the other.

Example of correlations:

Fredland, Campbell, and Han (2008) studied relationships between violence exposure and health outcomes in urban adolescents. They used sophisticated statistical methods for their main theory-testing analyses, but also presented a table with intercorrelations among 14 variables. The correlations ranged in direction and magnitude. For example, scores on a measure of personal violence correlated moderately with a measure of community violence ($r = .37$) but not with scores on a coping scale ($r = -.01$). The strongest correlation was between scores on two subscales of the Pediatric Symptom Checklist, the "Internalizing Symptoms" and "Attention-Getting Symptoms" subscales ($r = .58$).

RESEARCH APPLICATIONS OF BIVARIATE DESCRIPTIVE STATISTICS

Bivariate descriptive statistics are a useful means of summarizing the relationship between two variables. This section examines some of the major applications of bivariate descriptive statistics and discusses methods of effectively displaying such information.

The Uses of Bivariate Descriptive Statistics

Most studies concern the relationship between two or more variables. Researchers rely primarily on inferential statistics that are discussed in subsequent chapters, but bivariate descriptive statistics are also used widely. A few of the major uses for these statistics are discussed here.

1. *Understanding the data*   As with other descriptive statistics, bivariate descriptive statistics are often used in preliminary analyses to help researchers better understand their data when more complex analyses are planned. For example, many sophisticated multivariate techniques build on correlational techniques, and it is useful to first look at correlations descriptively. In research reports, correlations among major study variables are sometimes displayed prior to presenting the results of inferential statistics. For example, Tullai-McGuinness (2008) studied factors that predict nurses' job satisfaction in home healthcare environments, using multivariate statistical procedures in her main analysis. However, she first presented a table that showed correlation coefficients between job satisfaction and nurses' characteristics, such as their age, education, and years of experience.

2. *Cleaning the data*   When checking to make sure that data are accurate, researchers often undertake **consistency checks**, which primarily involve crosstabulations to make sure that patterns of data are reasonable. For example, a researcher might crosstabulate the variable *sex* with the variable for *number of times pregnant*. If the data reflected that a male had a pregnancy, then the researcher would need to determine which variable (*sex* or pregnancies) had incorrect values for the case with the error.

3. *Describing the research sample*   As indicated in the previous two chapters, researchers report the major background characteristics of their study participants. Researchers often describe background traits for subgroups within the sample, not just for the sample as a whole. In other words, researchers crosstabulate background characteristics with a variable that is relevant to the study, such as *sex* or diagnosis. For example, Gies, Buchman, Robinson, and Smolen (2008) evaluated the effects of a nurse-directed smoking cessation program for hospitalized adults. Before discussing their results on program effectiveness, they presented a descriptive table that crosstabulated participants' treatment group status (experimental versus control) with demographic characteristics (e.g., *sex*, marital status, type of health problem).

4. *Developing and refining an instrument*   Correlation coefficients are often used to help researchers make decisions when they are developing a new instrument to measure a construct. For example, suppose we were interested in measuring loneliness among nursing home residents, and found existing scales unsuitable. We might begin by developing an **item pool** of 30 to 40 items (e.g., agree/disagree type items) and then administering them to a sample of 100 nursing home residents on a trial basis. A score on the scale would be computed for each resident by adding together responses to the items. To evaluate whether each item was contributing properly to the scale, we would compute correlation coefficients between responses to individual items and the total scale score, and between responses to all pairs of items. Items are often discarded (or revised) if the item-total correlation coefficient is less than .50 or if an interitem correlation is less than .30. As a research example, Bu and Wu (2008) developed a scale to measure nurses' attitudes toward patient advocacy. They pilot tested their preliminary 74-item scale with

a sample of 60 nurses, and made revisions (including the deletion of two items) based on low interitem and item-total correlations.

5. *Answering research questions*   Researchers sometimes use methods described in this chapter to answer their research questions—but, more frequently, they rely on inferential statistics when the focus is on relationships between variables. Risk indexes are sometimes calculated in a descriptive fashion by clinicians who want to answer questions about the relative benefit of an intervention or the relative risk of different exposures. In most cases, however, they compute descriptive indexes of risk, like the OR or NNT, based on data generated in a study that relied on inferential statistics.

The Presentation of Bivariate Descriptive Statistics in Research Reports

Bivariate descriptive statistics are sometimes reported directly in the text of a research report. For example, a researcher might report that the correlation between subjects' preoperative heart rate and scores on an anxiety scale was .43. Whenever bivariate statistics are used to describe multiple variables simultaneously, however, the information is usually presented in tables with highlights mentioned in the text.

When a contingency table results in only four cells, as in Table 4.1, the information can be efficiently summarized in a sentence (e.g., "Twenty percent of the women, compared with 30% of the men, were readmitted to the psychiatric hospital within 1 year of discharge"). When there are six or more cells, tables may be less confusing and more informative than a textual presentation. Tables are especially effective for summarizing crosstabulations for multiple variables simultaneously. For example, in the previously mentioned smoking-cessation study by Gies and colleagues (2008), their first table presented crosstabulations for treatment group status crossed by six different demographic variables. The amount of information shown in this table would have been hard to digest if it had been reported narratively in the text of the report.

Occasionally, researchers present three-dimensional contingency tables. A three-dimensional crosstabulation involves crossing two nominal (or ordinal) variables, separately for different categories of a third variable. For example, Welch, Miller, and James (2008) examined factors influencing breast and cervical cancer screening in a sample of over 27,000 American women. One of their tables crossed screening behaviors (six categories, based on length of time since last screening) with age groups (three age groups) for three types of screening (clinical breast exam, mammography, and PAP test)—a $6 \times 3 \times 3$ table. We condensed their table by collapsing screening behaviors into three categories, and omitting clinical breast exam data (Table 4.5). Note that the percentage information shown is column percentages (using age group frequencies as the basis of the calculations), and not row percentages (which would use screening behavior frequencies as the basis).

Correlation coefficients are often displayed in a two-dimensional **correlation matrix**, with a list of variables along both the top row and in the left-hand column of the table. The correlation coefficients between each pair of variables are then placed at the intersections of the relevant column and row. Usually, the same variables are listed in both the columns and rows of the correlation matrix, which efficiently shows the correlations between all combinations of variables.

Table 4.6 presents a fictitious example of a correlation matrix, showing intercorrelations among three dimensions of pain, and a total pain score, for a sample of hospitalized adolescents. This table lists the four variables in the first column, and the top row designates the numbers corresponding to the variables. The first (upper-left)

TABLE 4.5 Example of a 3 × 3 × 2 Contingency Table

Type of Cancer Screening	18–39 Year Olds n (%)	40–64 Year Olds n (%)	Older than 64 Years n (%)
Mammography			
Never screened	6,942 (75.1)	1,775 (10.0)	781 (8.2)
Screened within prior 24 months	1,533 (16.6)	13,335 (74.7)	7,147 (75.3)
Screened 25+ months ago	772 (8.3)	2,727 (15.3)	1,567 (16.5)
PAP Test			
Never screened	508 (5.5)	306 (1.7)	672 (7.3)
Screened within prior 24 months	7,769 (84.3)	13,638 (76.9)	4,839 (52.3)
Screened 25+ months ago	936 (10.2)	3,802 (21.4)	3,740 (40.4)
Total Number of Women	9,247	17,836	9,495

Adapted and abridged from Table 1 in Welch et al.'s (2008) report. The table was titled "Breast and Cervical Cancer Screening among Behavioral Risk Factor Surveillance System Survey, 2005."

entry of 1.00 simply shows that sensory pain scores are perfectly correlated with themselves. In our example, all the diagonal values are 1.00, indicating perfect self-correlations. The next entry in the first column indicates the correlation between the sensory (variable 1) and affective (variable 2) dimensions of pain ($r_{12} = .73$), and so on. This table shows that all pain measures were positively correlated. Total pain was substantially correlated with sensory pain ($r_{14} = .92$); however, the correlation between the sensory and evaluative dimensions of pain was rather modest ($r_{13} = .33$).

In terms of graphic presentations, we have seen that correlations between two variables can be displayed graphically in a scatterplot. However, scatterplots are rarely included in research reports because correlation coefficients summarize linear relationships more succinctly and also more precisely.

Descriptive crosstabulations of two variables can be presented in graphic form, and are particularly useful for conference presentations. Figure 4.8A shows our earlier crosstabulated data on marital status and PPD diagnosis in a **clustered bar chart**. In the right panel (Figure 4.8B) the same information is presented in a **stacked bar chart**. Both figures were created by SPSS within the Graphs ➜ Legacy Dialogs ➜ Bar Chart procedure.

TABLE 4.6 Example of a Correlation Matrix for Measures of Dimensions of Pain in a Sample of Hosptialized Adolescents ($N = 200$)

Dimension of Pain	1	2	3	4
1 Sensory Pain	1.00			
2 Affective Pain	.73	1.00		
3 Evaluative Pain	.33	.35	1.00	
4 Total Pain	.92	.83	.50	1.00

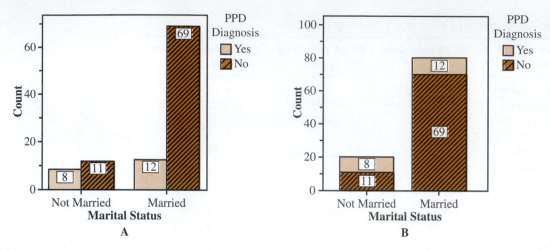

FIGURE 4.8   SPSS printouts of clustered (A) and stacked (B) bar charts for marital status and PPD data.

Tips on Preparing Tables with Bivariate Descriptive Statistics

As with any statistical tables, it is important to construct tables of bivariate descriptive statistics so that they are clear, informative, and concise. We offer some suggestions to guide table construction for displaying bivariate statistics.

- When bivariate descriptive statistics are being displayed, it is usually useful to set up the table to facilitate cross-row comparisons. For example, when two or more groups are being compared (e.g., experimental versus control, men versus women) the groups are usually displayed along the top row. Group status is often the study's independent variable. This format is especially convenient—in terms of fitting the rectangular format of journal pages—when the number of groups is fewer than the number of categories of the second variable. Moreover, in a contingency table, it is psychologically easier to read a table with percentages that add to 100% down a column rather than across a row, as in Table 4.1.
- Researchers vary in the level of precision shown in tables with bivariate descriptive statistics. It is usually adequate to present percentages to one decimal place (e.g., 45.8%).
- Correlation coefficients usually are reported to two decimal places (e.g., $r = .61$, $r = -.06$) Greater precision is rarely necessary. There should *not* be a leading zero, that it, coefficients should be reported as .40, not 0.40. When the correlation coefficient is positive, the plus sign can be omitted.
- When correlations are presented in a correlation matrix, the diagonal (i.e., the intersection of variable 1 with variable 1, variable 2 with variable 2, etc.) can have the values 1.00, indicating that all variables are perfectly correlated with themselves, as in Table 4.6. Researchers sometimes omit this information because it is not informative—they either leave the diagonal blank or insert dashes. Occasionally researchers insert information about the scales' reliability coefficients (see Chapters 9 and 13) in the diagonal. The meaningful correlation coefficients can appear either below the diagonal, as in Table 4.6, or above it.

Research Example

Here we briefly summarize some bivariate descriptive results from a study about nurses in Missouri.

Study: "Gender differences in discipline of nurses in Missouri" (Evangelista and Sims-Giddens, 2008)

Study Purpose: The purpose of this study was to examine patterns of formal license disciplinary actions against male and female nurses in the state of Missouri, where 7.5% of nurses are male. Disciplinary actions in that state take the form of censure (public reprimand); probation (restrictions for a specified time period); suspension (license is placed on hold for up to three years); and revocation.

Methods: The researchers extracted their study data from the discipline lists of the Missouri Board of Nursing for a 48-month period. Their data included information on the nurse's gender, type of license (LPN or RN), type of infraction, and type of disciplinary action taken, for 627 cases.

Analysis: Although the researchers used various inferential statistics, their report was rich in bivariate descriptive statistics. Crosstabs were a key approach, in which nurses' gender was crosstabulated with type of infractions and disciplinary actions taken.

Key Findings: The researchers found that males received 18.9% of the disciplinary actions over the 4-year period—a 2.5 greater share than their representation in nursing. Drug use accounted for a high percentage of disciplinary actions for both males and females, as shown in Table 4.7. Gender differences were most pronounced for relatively infrequent types of infraction. For example, the rates for males were more than twice as high as those for women for such infractions as abuse of a patient (7.6% of male infractions, 1.8% of female infractions) and sexual contact with a patient (males, 3.4%, females, 1.2%). By contrast, female rates were more than double that of males for forgery (3.1% versus 0.8%, respectively). There were also several infractions that were committed exclusively by female nurses, such as alcohol use on the job (2.4%) and leaving post without notification (1.6%). The researchers presented a clustered bar chart in their report, which showed the relationship between nurse's gender and type of disciplinary action taken. Female nurses (30%) were more likely than male nurses (20%) to be censured. Conversely, a higher percentage of infractions by males (19%) than by females (10%) resulted in license revocation. Disparities in disciplinary actions led the researchers to suggest further explorations of the roles of nursing culture and societal view on gender in the disciplinary process.

TABLE 4.7 Top Eight Disciplined Infractions in Missouri, by Nurse's Gender

Type of Infraction	Males n (%)	Females n (%)	Total N (%)
Drug abuse at work	36 (30.3)	117 (23.0)	153 (24.2)
Drug abuse off work	15 (12.6)	63 (12.4)	78 (12.4)
Violating a prior Board agreement	9 (7.6)	46 (9.1)	55 (8.8)
Working with lapsed license	2 (1.7)	36 (7.1)	38 (6.1)
Care errors	4 (3.4)	32 (6.3)	36 (5.7)
Medication errors	8 (6.7)	26 (5.1)	34 (5.4)
Providing care without physician order	2 (1.7)	26 (5.1)	28 (4.5)
Documentation errors	8 (6.7)	19 (3.7)	27 (4.3)
All other infractions[a]	35 (29.4)	143 (28.1)	178 (28.4)
Total	119 (100.0)	508 (100.0)	627 (100.0)

[a]There were 20 other types of infractions, each of which represented under 4% of all infractions (e.g., murdering a patient, falsifying documents, theft, sexual contact with a patient).

Abridged and adapted from Table 1 of Evangelista & Sims-Giddens (2008). The table was titled "Disciplined infractions by gender, within gender, and percentage of total infractions."

Summary Points

- **Bivariate descriptive statistics** are used to describe relationships between two variables.
- A **contingency** (or **crosstabs**) **table** is a two-dimensional frequency distribution that **crosstabulates** the frequencies of two nominal-level (or ordinal-level) variables.
- The number of **cells** in a contingency table is the number of categories of the first variable multiplied by the number of categories of the second (e.g., $2 \times 3 = 6$ cells).
- Each cell in a contingency table contains information about the counts and percentages for the specified crosstabulated categories. Percentages can be computed as *row percentages, column percentages,* or overall percentages.
- Statistical **risk indexes** have been developed to describe risk exposure and intervention effects, and are useful for facilitating clinical decisions. Most risk indexes are appropriate for 2×2 situations, such as when two groups (e.g., experimental versus control) are compared on a dichotomous outcome (e.g., alive/dead).
- **Absolute risk** is an index that expresses what percentage of those in a risk-exposed (or control) group (AR_E) experience an adverse outcome, and what percent in a nonexposed (or experimental) group (AR_{NE}) experience the bad outcome.
- **Absolute risk reduction (ARR)** expresses the estimated proportion of people who would be spared from an adverse outcome by nonexposure to the risk (or receipt of an intervention).
- **Relative risk (RR)** is the estimated proportion of the original risk of an adverse outcome that occurs in association with the risk exposure (or, failure to get an intervention).
- **Relative risk reduction (RRR)** is the estimated proportion of risk associated with exposure that is reduced when there is no exposure to the risk factor—or, in the context of an intervention, the estimated proportion of risk that is reduced as a result of the intervention.
- The **odds** is the proportion of people *with* an adverse outcome relative to those *without* it, and the

odds ratio (OR) is the ratio of the odds for the at-risk versus not at-risk (or treated versus untreated) groups.
- The **number needed to treat (NNT)** is an estimate of how many people would need to receive an intervention (or avoid risk exposure) to prevent one adverse outcome.
- A **correlation** is a bond or connection between variables. Correlation analysis is most often used to describe the magnitude and direction of **linear relationships** between two variables measured on an interval or ratio scale.
- Relationships between two variables can be graphed on a **scatterplot**, which plots values of one variable along the X axis and simultaneously plots values of the second on the Y axis.
- In a scatterplot, the points on the graph cluster closely along a straight diagonal line when the correlation is strong. Lines sloping from the lower left corner to the upper right corner reflect **positive relationships**—high values on the first variable are associated with high values on the second. Lines sloping from the upper left to the lower right reflect **negative relationships**—high values on one variable are associated with low values on the other.
- Researchers usually compute a **correlation coefficient** to efficiently summarize the magnitude and direction of linear relationships.
- Correlation coefficients range from -1.00 for a perfect negative relationship through $.00$ for no relationship to $+1.00$ for a perfect positive relationship.
- A **perfect relationship** occurs when the values of one variable can be used to perfectly predict the values of the second. The greater the absolute value of the coefficient, the stronger the relationship.
- The most widely used correlation coefficient is the **Pearson product moment correlation**, also referred to as **Pearson's *r***.
- A **correlation matrix** is a two-dimensional display that shows correlation coefficients between all pairs of variables.

Exercises

The following exercises cover concepts presented in this chapter. Appendix C provides answers to Part A exercises that are indicated with a dagger (†). Exercises in Part B involve computer analyses using the datasets provided with this textbook, and answers and comments are offered on this book's Web site.

PART A EXERCISES

† **A1.** The following data designate whether or not patients complied with a medication regimen (1 = yes, 2 = no), for an experimental group that participated in a special intervention designed to promote perceived mastery over health events, and a "usual care" control group:

Experimental 1 2 2 1 1 1 2 1 2 1 2 1 1 1 2
Control   2 2 1 2 2 2 1 2 1 2 2 1 1 2 2

Construct a contingency table for these data, computing both row and column percentages for each of the four cells.

† **A2.** Examine the results in Table 4.7. (a) Are the percentages shown in this table row percentages or column percentages? (b) Compute the percentages the opposite way, and then answer this question: Given that males represent 7.5% of all licensed nurses in Missouri, which (if any) infractions in the table were committed by males at a rate lower than their representation among nurses in that state? (c) Based on the recomputed percentages in Exercise A2b, for which infraction were male nurses most notably overrepresented?

† **A3.** The contingency table below presents fictitious data regarding an intervention to reduce pressure ulcers in nursing home residents. Using these data, compute AR_E, AR_{NE}, ARR, RR, RRR, OR, and NNT.

	Pressure Ulcer	No Pressure Ulcer	Total
Control Group	15	35	50
Experimental Group	5	45	50
Total	20	80	100

A4. Below are values for diastolic and systolic blood pressure for 10 people:

Diastolic 90 80 90 78 76 78 80 70 76 74
Systolic   130 126 140 118 114 112 120 110 114 116

Construct a scatterplot that shows the relationship between the variables. Verbally describe the direction and magnitude of the relationship.

† **A5.** Compute the correlation coefficient (Pearson's r) to summarize the relationship for the blood pressure data presented in question A4. How accurate was your verbal description of the scatterplot, as compared to the value of the coefficient?

PART B EXERCISES

† **B1.** The SPSS dataset Polit2SetB has a number of health-related variables. Use this dataset to create a contingency table that crosstabulates the women's poverty status (*poverty,* coded 1 for those below the poverty line and 2 for those above it) with a four-category ordinal variable indicating how frequently the women felt highly stressed in the prior month (*stressed*). To do this, select Analyze → Descriptive Statistics → Crosstabs. When the dialog box appears, move the variable *stressed* (Variable #20) into the slot for Rows, and move the variable *poverty* (Variable # 9) into the slot for Column. Click the pushbutton labeled Cells, and click Observed under Counts, and Row and Column under Percentages. Click Continue and then OK to execute the procedure. Then answer the following questions: (a) What percentage of women was below the poverty level? (b) What percentage of women was stressed almost all the time? (c) What percentage of women above the poverty level was stressed none of the time? (d) What percentage of women who were stressed none of the time was below the poverty level? (e) How would you characterize the women in the cell with the greatest frequency?

† **B2.** Using the same SPSS dataset (Polit2SetB), run a crosstab between poverty status (*poverty*) and current smoking status (*smoker,* Variable #15, which is coded 0 for nonsmokers and 1 for smokers). This time, check the box on the opening dialog box that says "Display clustered bar charts." Run this procedure twice, putting poverty status as the row variable for one run, and as the column variable for the second run. Which chart do you think does a better job of characterizing the relationship between poverty and smoking?

† **B3.** This exercise involves producing risk index statistics, again using the dataset Polit2SetB. Run the SPSS Crosstabs procedure, using poverty status (*poverty*) as the risk exposure variable—i.e., inserting it as the row variable. Then find Variable #43 toward the end of the variable list (*health*), which is a health status variable that dichotomized answers to a question that asked women to self-rate their health. Those who said they were in good, very good, or excellent health are coded 1, while those who said they were in fair or poor health were coded 0. Use *health* as the column variable in the Crosstabs. Click on the Cells pushbutton, and click on Row under Percentages. Then hit Continue and click the pushbutton for Statistics. On the right-hand side, click on the option for Risk, then click Continue and OK. Then answer these questions: (a) What is the absolute risk of being in fair-to-poor health for women below the poverty level and above the poverty level? (b) What is the odds ratio for the effect of exposure to poverty (versus nonexposure) on the outcome of fair-poor health? (c) What is the relative risk of exposure to poverty (versus nonexposure) on the outcome

of fair-poor health? (d) State what the relative risk index means.

† **B4.** Create a correlation matrix with four variables in the Polit2SetB dataset. The four variables are Variables #11, 18, 44, and 45: Number of visits to the doctor in the past 12 months (*docvisit*); body mass index (*bmi*); standardized score on the Short-Form Health Survey or SF12, Physical health component subscale (*sf12phys*); and standardized score on the Short-Form Health Survey, Mental health component subscale (*sf12ment*). The SF-12 is a brief, widely used measure of health status. In this dataset, standardized T scores were created using national norms based on a national mean of 50.0 and an SD of 10.0. For both subscales, higher scores represent more favorable health. To produce a correlation matrix, use Analyze ➜ Correlate ➜ Bivariate. Move the four variables into the variable list. The type of correlation should be set to Pearson. Click on the Options pushbutton, and select means and standard deviations under Statistics and Exclusion of cases pairwise under Missing Values. Then run the analysis and answer the following questions based on the output, ignoring information labeled "Sig. 2-tailed": (a) On the SF-12 subscales, were women in this sample, on average, about as healthy—both physically and mentally—as people nationally?

(b) Are the correlations in the matrix presented above or below the diagonal? (c) What is shown in the diagonal in the SPSS output? (d) What is the strongest correlation in the matrix? (e) What is the weakest correlation in the matrix? (f) Which variable included in this analysis is most strongly correlated with the women's body mass index (*bmi*)?

† **B5.** Run crosstabs to describe the relationship between women's current employment status and health-related characteristics in this sample of low income women, using the following variables in the Polit2SetB dataset: currently employed (*worknow*), does not have health insurance (*noinsur*), smokes cigarettes (*smoker*), health limits ability to work (*hlthlimt*), and in fair-poor health (*health*). Create a table summarizing the results, comparing women who were or were not working with regard to unfavorable health outcomes. Then write a paragraph summarizing the information in the table.

B6. Select several interval-level or ratio-level variables from the Polit2SetB dataset (or one of the other two datasets included with this book) and do some basic descriptive statistics (means, *SD*s, etc.) for the selected variable. Then do a correlation matrix to explore relationships among the variables. Write a paragraph summarizing what you learned about the variables.

Statistical Inference

Descriptive statistics allow researchers to depict the characteristics, circumstances, and behaviors of their samples. Most research question, however, are not about the attributes of the particular people who comprise a sample, but rather about a larger population.

Suppose, for example, a researcher hypothesized that transcutaneous nerve stimulation is an effective means of reducing pain from a surgical incision during wound dressing. Fifty patients in an experimental group are given electrical stimulation before and during wound dressing, while 50 patients in a control group get usual care. Participants in both groups rate their pain on a visual analog scale, where the values can range from 0 (no pain) to 100 (maximum pain). Using descriptive statistics, the researcher determines that the mean pain rating is 72.0 and 77.0 in the experimental and control group, respectively. At this point, the researcher can *only* conclude that the particular 50 people in the experimental group perceived less pain, on average, than the particular 50 people in the control group. The researcher does not know whether the five-point average difference in pain ratings would be observed in a new sample, and therefore cannot conclude that the transcutaneous nerve stimulation is an effective treatment for alleviating pain. Because researchers almost always want to be able to generalize beyond their sample to some broader population, they apply inferential statistics. **Inferential statistics** allow researchers to draw conclusions about population parameters, based on statistics from a sample.

We all make inferences regularly, and every inference contains some uncertainty. For example, when we eat at a new restaurant and are served a meal that we do not enjoy, we may infer that the restaurant is mediocre.

Our conclusion may be erroneous—perhaps we ordered the one dish on the menu that is below the restaurant's normal standards. We could only be certain about the restaurant's overall quality by tasting every menu item.

Similarly, when a researcher makes inferences using inferential statistics, there is always a risk of error. Only by obtaining information from populations can researchers have complete confidence that their conclusions are accurate. Because researchers seldom collect data from an entire population, they use a statistical framework that allows them to assess how likely it is that the conclusions based on sample data are valid. This framework uses the **laws of probability**.

FUNDAMENTALS OF PROBABILITY

In the hypothetical study to test the effectiveness of the transcutaneous nerve treatment for alleviating pain, there are two mutually exclusive possibilities:

H_0: The intervention is *not* effective in reducing pain.

H_1: The intervention *is* effective in reducing pain.

The first possibility is the **null hypothesis**. The null hypothesis (symbolized in statistics books as H_0) states that there is no relationship between the independent variable (the transcutaneous nerve treatment) and the dependent variable (pain). The **alternative hypothesis** (H_1) is the actual research hypothesis, which states the expectation that there *is* a relationship between the independent and dependent variables. In the population of all surgical patients, only one of these possibilities is correct.

The researcher in this example observed a five-point average difference in pain ratings between the experimental and control groups. By using inferential statistics, the researcher would be able to determine *how probable it is that the null hypothesis is false*. Probability is a complex topic, with different rules for different situations. In this section we present only an overview of probability theory, to establish a basis for understanding the fundamental principles of statistical inference.[1]

Probability of an Event

When we flip a normal, two-sided coin, one of two possible outcomes can occur: We can obtain a head, or we can obtain a tail. The probability (p) of some event, such as obtaining a head on a coin toss, can be defined as the following ratio:

$$p(\text{event}) = \frac{\text{number of ways the specified event can occur}}{\text{total number of possible events}}$$

In the coin toss example, we can use this ratio to determine the probability that heads will come up:

$$p(\text{heads}) = \frac{1 \text{ head}}{2 \text{ possible events (heads or tails)}} = \frac{1}{2}$$

Probabilities are expressed as proportions, so we can say that the probability of heads (or tails) is .50. (In everyday parlance, we might say that there is a 50-50 chance of having the coin come up heads.) On a six-sided die, the probability of rolling, say, a 3 is 1/6, or .17. In a normal, shuffled deck of 52 cards, the probability of randomly

---

[1] A fuller explication of probability is presented in several statistical textbooks, such as those by Gravetter & Wallnau (2008), and Jaccard & Becker (2001).

drawing the queen of spades is 1/52, or .02. A probability always ranges from .00 (completely impossible) to 1.00 (completely certain).

The probability of an event can also be interpreted with a "long run" perspective. For example, in 100,000 coin tosses, we would expect 50,000 heads. Over the long run, with a large enough number of trials, the proportion of heads should be .50.

Some readers may have noticed that probability is similar in form to relative frequencies, as discussed in Chapter 2. For example, in the frequency distribution of patients' marital status shown in Table 2.3, the relative frequency of "single" patients was:

$$\frac{\text{number of times the event "single" occurred}}{\text{number of possible occurrences of marital status}} = \frac{55}{250}$$

The relative frequency of single patients is .22. The probability of randomly selecting a given value from a known distribution equals the relative frequency of that value, and so the probability of randomly selecting a single person from the sample of 250 patients is .22.

Probability of Consecutive Events

Another situation involves predicting the probability of *consecutive* events. For example, we might want to determine the probability of obtaining heads twice in a row on two independent coin tosses. The *multiplicative law* in probability provides a formula for this situation:

$$p(\text{A and then B}) = p(\text{A}) \times p(\text{B})$$

where A is the first independent event
       B is the second independent event

In the coin toss example, the probability of two consecutive heads is:

$$p(\text{heads and then heads}) = p(\text{heads}) \times p(\text{heads})$$
$$p(\text{heads and then heads}) = .50 \times .50 = .25$$

In the same fashion, the probability of three consecutive heads is:

$$p(3 \text{ consecutive heads}) = p(\text{heads}) \times p(\text{heads}) \times p(\text{heads})$$
$$p(3 \text{ consecutive heads}) = .50 \times .50 \times .50 = .125$$

Knowing this formula, we could calculate the probability for all possible outcomes in consecutive coin tosses. Table 5.1 presents a partial listing of outcomes, focusing primarily on the probability of obtaining consecutive heads. In the first toss, the probability of heads (H) and tails (T) is, in each case, .50. The far-right column shows that the probability of obtaining *either* heads or tails is 1.00—that is, it is 100% certain that one of these outcomes will occur. In the second toss, the probability of two consecutive heads (HH) is .25, as is the probability of heads then tails (HT), tails then heads (TH), or two tails (TT). From the third toss on, the table shows only probabilities for consecutive heads. The probability of five consecutive heads, for example, is .031. Fewer than five times out of 100 would we expect to obtain five heads in a row.

TABLE 5.1 Probabilities in Coin Toss Example

No. of Coins Tossed	Possible Outcomes and Probabilities				Total Probability
1	H = .50	T = .50			1.00
2	HH = .25	HT = .25	TH = .25	TT = .25	1.00
3	HHH = .125	All others combined = .875			1.00
4	HHHH = .063	All others combined = .937			1.00
5	HHHHH = .031	All others combined = .969			1.00
6	HHHHHH = .016	All others combined = .984			1.00
7	HHHHHHH = .008	All others combined = .992			1.00
8	HHHHHHHH = .004	All others combined = .996			1.00
9	HHHHHHHHH = .002	All others combined = .998			1.00
10	HHHHHHHHHH = .001	All others combined = .999			1.00

H = Heads
T = Tails

We can use this table to test the hypothesis that a coin is biased (for example, that it has two heads, or is weighted to turn up heads more often than tails). Our hypotheses may be stated formally as follows:

H_0: The coin is fair.

H_1: The coin is biased.

To test the hypothesis that the coin is biased, we obtain some data by tossing the coin ten times. Let us assume that we obtained 10 heads. We can consult Table 5.1 to learn how probable this outcome is. The table indicates that the probability of getting 10 consecutive heads is .001. That is, by chance alone we would obtain 10 heads on 10 consecutive tosses only once in 1,000 times. We might then decide to reject the null hypothesis, concluding that there is a high probability that the coin is biased.

This example is similar to procedures used in statistical inference. Researchers use probability tables to assess whether an observed outcome (e.g., a five-point difference in average pain ratings) is likely to have occurred by chance, or whether the outcome had a high probability of reflecting a true outcome that would be observed with other samples from the same population. Based on information in probability tables, researchers make decisions to accept or reject the null hypothesis.

Probability as an Area

As noted earlier, probability is similar to relative frequencies. Just as relative frequencies can be graphed in histograms or frequency polygons, so too can probabilities be graphed in **probability distributions**. For example, suppose we graphed the probability of obtaining 1, 2, 3, 4, 5, and 6 dots on the roll of a single die. For each number, the probability would be 1/6, or .167. Figure 5.1 presents a histogram of the probability of obtaining one to six dots on a single roll of one die.

The area within the histogram is exactly 1.0 (i.e., 6 × .167), the total of all the probabilities that a die will yield a number between one and six. From this distribution, we can determine various probabilities from the area within the histogram.

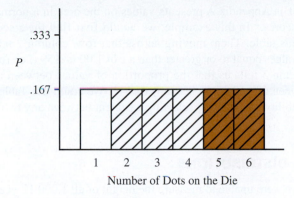

FIGURE 5.1 Probability distribution of dots in the roll of one die.

For example, the probability of rolling a five *or* a six (the shaded area on Figure 5.1) is .333 (2 ÷ 6). The probability of obtaining a number greater than one on a single roll (the hatched area) is .833 (5 ÷ 6).

Probability distributions can also be constructed for continuous variables, and are sometimes called *probability density functions*. Suppose, for example, we collected data on the heights of a population of 1,000 12-year-old children and constructed a frequency polygon (Figure 5.2). The mean (μ) of this population distribution is 60.0 inches, and the standard deviation (σ) is 5.0 inches. What is the probability that a randomly selected child from this population would be, say, 65 inches tall or taller? The shaded area in the right tail of this figure, corresponding to heights 65 inches or greater, is approximately 16% of the total area under this curve. The proportion of 12-year-old children who are 65 inches or taller can be regarded as the probability that one child selected at random from this population of 1,000 children will be at least 65 inches tall. In other words, $p = .16$ in this example.

How did we determine that heights of 65 inches or greater account for 16% of the distribution? When data values are normally distributed (or approximately so), the area under a curve can be determined by converting raw scores to standard scores and consulting an appropriate table. Using the formulas presented in Chapter 3, we can calculate the standard score (*z* score) as:

$$z = \frac{X - \overline{X}}{SD} = \frac{65.0 - 60.0}{5.0} = \frac{5.0}{5.0} = 1.0$$

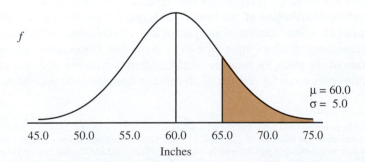

FIGURE 5.2 Hypothetical distribution of heights for a population of 1,000 12-year-old children.

Table A.1 in Appendix A presents values on the area in a normal distribution for various z scores.[2] In this example, we would first find the z score of 1.00 in column 1 of this table. Then, moving across that row, column 2 tells us that the proportion of values equal to or greater than a z of 1.00 is .159 (i.e., roughly 16% of the area). Column 3 tells us that the proportion of values between a z of 0.0 and 1.0 (here, between 60 and 65 inches tall) is .341. We could use Table A.1 to determine the probability of randomly selecting a student between any two heights in the distribution.

SAMPLING DISTRIBUTIONS

Suppose that we were unable to measure the height of all 1,000 12-year-old children in our hypothetical population, but that instead we had to rely on data from a sample. If we randomly selected 25 children and measured their height, would the obtained sample mean be exactly 60.0 inches? We *might* by chance obtain a mean of 60.0, but it would also be possible to obtain such means as 60.6, or 58.8, or 62.2. A sample statistic is often unequal to the value of the corresponding population parameter because of **sampling error**.

Sampling error reflects the tendency for statistics to fluctuate from one sample to another. The amount of sampling error is the difference between the obtained sample value and the population parameter. A researcher does not, of course, know the amount of sampling error: If the population parameter were known, there would be no need to estimate it with data from a sample. Inferential statistics allow researchers to estimate how close to the population value the calculated statistic is likely to be. The concept of **sampling distributions**, which are actually probability distributions, is central to estimates of sampling error.

Characteristics of Sampling Distributions

To understand sampling distributions, you need to imagine an activity that would never actually occur. Suppose that we randomly selected 25 12-year-old children from the population of 1,000 children, and calculated their mean height. Now consider replacing the 25 children, drawing another sample of 25 children, and calculating another mean. Table 5.2 shows the means and the sampling error—the sample mean minus the population mean of 60.0—for 20 such samples. We can see that the sampling error ranges from very small amounts (0.1 inch) to much larger amounts (2.1 inches). Now suppose we repeated the process of selecting new samples of 25 children and calculating their mean height over and over again, an infinite number of times. If we then treated each sample mean as a new "data point," we could plot these means in a frequency polygon. The hypothetical distribution, shown in Figure 5.3, is a **sampling distribution of the mean**—a theoretical probability distribution of the means of an infinite number of samples of a given size from a population. There is a different sampling distribution for every sample size. For example, the sampling distribution of the mean for samples of 25 children is different from the sampling distribution of the mean for samples of 50 children from the same population.

---

[2] Table A.1 is an abbreviated table that shows a selected number of z score values. For z scores falling between values shown in this table (e.g., a z of .13), interpolation can be used as a rough estimate, or a fuller table can be consulted (e.g., Gravetter & Walnau, 2008; Jaccard and Becker, 2001). There are also interactive Internet sites that allow you to immediately determine the area of interest—use the search term "z table" or "normal distribution table." Here is one such Web site: http://davidmlane.com/hyperstat/z_table.html.

TABLE 5.2 Sample Means of Heights in Inches in 20 Random Samples of 25 Children Drawn from a Population of 1,000 12-year-old Children

Sample Mean	Sampling Error	Sample Mean	Sampling Error
$\overline{X}$	$\overline{X} - \mu$	$\overline{X}$	$\overline{X} - \mu$
61.0	1.0	59.9	−0.1
59.4	−0.6	60.4	0.4
58.9	−1.1	61.1	1.1
62.1	2.1	59.7	−0.3
60.3	0.3	60.2	0.2
59.8	−0.2	58.0	−2.0
60.1	0.1	61.7	1.7
59.6	−0.4	59.6	−0.4
58.8	−1.2	59.1	−0.9
60.9	0.9	59.4	−0.6

Sampling distributions are theoretical because, in practice, no one draws an infinite number of samples from a population. Their characteristics can be modeled mathematically, however, and have been determined by a formulation known as the **central limit theorem**. This theorem stipulates that the mean of the sampling distribution is identical to the population mean. In other words, if we calculated the mean heights for an infinite number of samples of 25 children drawn from the population of 1,000 12-year-old children, the average of all the sample means would be exactly 60.0, as shown in Figure 5.3. Moreover, the average sampling error—the mean of the $(\overline{X} - \mu)$s—would always equal 0. As we see in Table 5.2, some sample means overestimated the population mean, and others underestimated it. With an infinite number of samples, the overestimates and underestimates would cancel each other out.

Another feature of sampling distributions is that if the score values in the population are normally distributed, the sampling distribution of the mean will also be normal. Moreover, even if the distribution of scores in the population is *not* normal, the sampling distribution will increasingly approach being normal as the size of the sample on which the distribution is based gets larger. Because sampling distributions usually approximate a normal distribution, we can make probability statements about the likelihood of obtaining various sample means based on information about the area under the curve. Before we can do so, however, we need to determine the standard deviation of the sampling distribution.

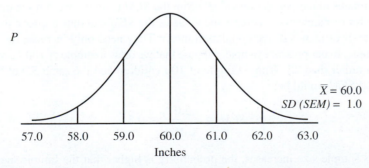

FIGURE 5.3 Sampling distribution of heights for samples of 25 12-year-old children.

Standard Error of the Mean

The standard deviation of a sampling distribution of the mean has a special name: the **standard error of the mean** (*SEM*). The term "error" indicates that the sample means in the distribution contain some error as estimates of the population mean—sampling error. The term "standard" signifies that the *SEM* is an index of the average amount of error for all possible sample means. The smaller the *SEM*, the more accurate are the sample means as estimates of the population value. The larger the *SEM*, the greater the probability that a sample mean will be a poor estimate of the population mean.

Most sampling distributions are approximately normal, and so we can use the *SEM* to estimate the probability of obtaining a sample mean in a specified range. Figure 5.3 shows that with samples of 25, the distribution of sample means for heights of 12-year-old children has a standard deviation (i.e., an *SEM*) = 1.0. As noted in Chapter 3, 95% of the values in a normal distribution lie within about ± 2 *SD*s of the mean. Thus, we can estimate that the probability is .95 that the mean height of a sample of 25 children will lie between 58.0 and 62.0. In other words, about 95% of all sample means randomly selected from the population would be within 2 inches of the true parameter, given a sample of 25 children. Only 2.5% of the sample means would be less than 58.0 and only 2.5% would be greater than 62.0—a total of 5% of the area of the sampling distribution, located in the two tails.

With information about the *SEM*, researchers can interpret a sample mean relative to the population mean. But, since researchers do not actually construct sampling distributions, how can the *SEM* be calculated? How, for example, did we know that the *SEM* for the distribution in Figure 5.3 is 1.0? Fortunately, statisticians have developed a formula for estimating the actual *SEM* based on data from a single sample:

$$SEM = \frac{SD}{\sqrt{N}}$$

where *SEM* = estimated standard error of the mean
  SD = standard deviation of the sample
  N = number of cases in the sample

In our current example, suppose that the *SD* for our sample of 25 students is 5.0. We can use this formula to calculate the following estimate of the *SEM*:

$$SEM = \frac{5.0}{\sqrt{25}} = 1.0$$

Thus, the estimated standard deviation of the sampling distribution is 1.0.

The smaller the *SEM*, the greater is the confidence that researchers have in their estimates of the population value. From the *SEM* formula, we can see that there is a way for researchers to decrease the value of the *SEM* and thus improve the accuracy of their estimates of the population mean: They need only increase the size of their sample. In our present example, suppose that we drew a sample of 100 12-year-old children rather than 25. With a sample of 100 children and the same *SD* of 5.0, the estimated *SEM* would be:

$$SEM = \frac{5.0}{\sqrt{100}} = 0.5$$

As sample size increases, the probability is higher that the sample mean will be close to the value of the population mean. This is because having a large *N* promotes the likelihood that extreme cases (very short children and very tall children) will cancel each other out.

The formula for the *SEM* also indicates that the greater the homogeneity of the population (i.e., the smaller the *SD*), the smaller is the standard error of the mean. If the *SD* of the sample had been 2.5 inches rather than 5.0 inches, the estimated *SEM* would be:

$$s_{\bar{x}} = \frac{2.5}{\sqrt{100}} = 0.25$$

Thus, small samples and a heterogeneous population lead to large *SEM*s; conversely, large samples and a homogeneous population increase the likelihood that the sampling error will be small. Researchers cannot control population heterogeneity, but they can increase the precision of their estimates by using large samples.

> **TIP:** *The standard error of the mean is sometimes abbreviated as SE in journals or as* $s_{\bar{x}}$ *in some statistics books. In SPSS, values of* **SEM** *are labeled Std err or Std error.*

ESTIMATION OF PARAMETERS

Statistical inference consists of two types of approach: estimation of population parameters and testing of hypotheses. In both cases, the overall goal is the same: to use data from a sample to draw inferences about populations, and in both cases the concepts of sampling distributions and standard errors are central features. Yet, there are important differences in these approaches.

In nursing journals, the hypothesis-testing approach has predominated, but that situation is changing. The emphasis on EBP has heightened interest among clinicians in learning not only whether a hypothesis was supported (via traditional hypothesis tests) but also the estimated parameter value and the accuracy of the estimate (via parameter estimation). Many medical journals *require* estimation information because it is seen as more useful, reflecting the view that this approach offers information about both clinical and statistical significance (e.g., Braitman, 1991; Sackett, Straus, Richardson, Rosenberg, and Haynes, 2000).

In this section we present an overview of parameter estimation and offer examples based on one-variable descriptive statistics. We expand this discussion later in the book within the context of specific statistical tests.

Confidence Intervals

Parameter estimation is used to estimate a population value, such as a mean, relative risk index, or a mean difference between two groups (e.g., experimental vs. control). Estimation can take two forms: point estimation or interval estimation. **Point estimation** involves calculating a single statistic to estimate the parameter. For example, if we drew a sample of 25 students and calculated the mean height to be 61.0 inches (the first sample mean in Table 5.2), this would be our point estimate of the population mean.

The problem with point estimates, which are simply descriptive statistics, is that they offer no context for interpreting their accuracy. How much confidence can we place in the value of 61.0 as an estimate of the parameter? A point estimate gives no information regarding the probability that it is correct or close to the population value.

An alternative to point estimation is to estimate a range of values that has a high probability of containing the population value. For example, it is more likely that the population mean lies between 59.0 and 63.0 than that it is *exactly* the calculated sample mean of 61.0. This is called **interval estimation** because the estimate is an interval of values.

Interval estimation involves constructing a **confidence interval (*CI*)** around the point estimate. (The upper and lower limits of the *CI* are called *confidence limits*.) A *CI* around a sample mean communicates a range of values for the population value, and the probability of being right. That is, the estimate is made with a certain degree of confidence of capturing the parameter.

TIP: *Confidence intervals address one of the key EBP questions for appraising evidence that we noted in Box 1.1: How precise is the estimate of effects?*

Confidence Intervals Around a Mean

Probability distributions such as those discussed earlier are used to construct *CIs* around a sample mean, using the *SEM* as the basis for establishing the confidence limits. Let us assume that we know that the true value of the SEM in our example is 1.0, and that we also know that the heights in the population of 1,000 children are normally distributed. (The true value of the *SEM* is denoted with a Greek symbol, i.e., $\sigma_{\bar{x}}$.) We can then use the normal distribution to construct a *CI*. By convention, researchers most often calculate a 95% *CI*. As noted earlier, 95% of the scores in a normal distribution lie within about ± 2 *SD*s from the mean. More precisely, 95% of the scores lie within 1.96 *SD*s above and below the mean. We can now build a 95% *CI* by using the following formula:

$$95\% \ CI = (\overline{X} \pm (1.96 \times \sigma_{\bar{x}})$$

where $\overline{X}$ = the sample mean

$\sigma_{\bar{x}}$ = the actual *SEM* of the sampling distribution

This statement indicates that we can be 95% confident that the population mean lies between the confidence limits, and that these limits are equal to 1.96 times the true standard error, above and below the sample mean. In the present example, the confidence limits would be:

$$95\% \ CI = (61.0 \pm (1.96 \times 1.0))$$
$$95\% \ CI = (61.0 \pm 1.96)$$
$$95\% \ CI = (59.04 \leq \mu \leq 62.96)$$

The last statement indicates that the confidence is 95% (i.e., the probability is .95) that the population mean (μ) lies between 59.04 and 62.96. (Strictly speaking, it is more accurate to interpret a *CI* in terms of long-range performance: Out of 100 sample means with samples of 25 children, 95% of such *CIs* would contain the population mean.)

Researchers can control the risk of being wrong by establishing different **confidence levels**. The 95% confidence level is most often used, but researchers sometimes want less risk of making an error. With a 95% confidence level there is a 5% risk, but with a 99% confidence level, there is only one chance in 100 of making an error. There is, however, a tradeoff: The price for lower risk is less precision—that is, the *CI* is wider. In a normal distribution, 99% of the scores lie within 2.58 *SD*s of the mean. Thus, the formula for a 99% *CI* is:

$$99\% \ CI = (\overline{X} \pm (2.58 \times \sigma_{\overline{x}}))$$

In the present example, the 99% *CI* would be:

$$99\% \ CI = (61.0 \pm (2.58 \times 1.0))$$
$$99\% \ CI = (61.0 \pm 2.58)$$
$$99\% \ CI = (58.42 \le \mu \le 63.58)$$

With a 99% *CI*, researchers reduce the risk that the interval will not contain the population mean, but the interval is larger. With the 95% interval, the range between the confidence limits is just under 4 inches. With a 99% *CI*, the range of possible values for the population mean is more than 5 inches—about a 30% decrease in precision. In most research situations, a 95% *CI* is adequate, but when important decisions about individuals are being made, a 99% *CI* may be required.

Confidence Intervals and the *t* Distribution

In the preceding example, we stipulated an assumption that generally is untenable: We assumed we knew that the true *SEM* (σ_x) for the sampling distribution was 1.0. Knowing the true *SEM* made it possible for us to use values from the normal distribution (1.96 for the 95% *CI*) to calculate the confidence limits. This is because when σ_x is known and we calculate a *z* score for the sample mean, we are calculating the *exact* number of *SEM*s that the sample mean is from the mean of the sampling distribution. When we use an estimated *SEM*, we need a different distribution.

In most cases, especially if the sample size is large, the normal curve provides a good approximation. In the present example, however, the sample size of 25 is not particularly large. When the true *SEM* is not known but is estimated from sample data—as will almost always be the case—a different theoretical distribution, known as the *t* **distribution**,[3] should be used to compute *CI*s.

In standard form, the *t* distribution is similar to a normal distribution: It is bell shaped, symmetrical, and has a mean of 0.0. However, the exact shape of the *t* distribution is influenced by the number of cases in the sample. There is a different *t* distribution for every sample size. Figure 5.4 shows that when $N = 5$, the shapes of the *t* and the normal distributions differ: The tails of the *t* distribution are fatter, for example, which means that you have to go out farther into the tails to capture 95% of the area. This, in turn, means that the *CI* based on the *t* distribution will be wider. Figure 5.4 also shows that when the sample size is 30 (or larger), the normal and *t* distributions are similar.

Statisticians have developed tables for the area under the *t* distribution for different sample sizes and probability levels. Such a table is presented in Table A.2 of Appendix A. To use this table, you must first select a confidence level, which are shown in the third row. Values for the 95% confidence level are shown in the third column, which is shaded. Values for other confidence levels, such as the 99% confidence level, are also shown in this table. To use this table, we must enter at the

---

[3] The *t* distribution is a theoretical distribution that was developed by W. S. Gossett, who wrote under the name of Student. For this reason, the distribution is sometimes referred to as *Student's t distribution*.

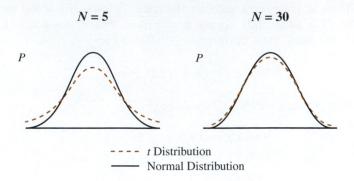

- - - - - *t* Distribution
———— Normal Distribution

FIGURE 5.4   Comparison of the normal and *t* distributions with *N* = 5 and *N* = 30.

appropriate row based on the number of degrees of freedom, labeled with the abbre-viation *df* in the first column. We will explain this concept later in this chapter. For now, it is important only to know that degree of freedom is equal to the sample size, minus 1 (*N* − 1).

Now we can construct the appropriate *CI* for the example of 25 12-year-old children whose mean height is 61.0 inches. The formula for the *CI*s when the true *SEM* is estimated from sample data is:

$$95\% \ CI = (\overline{X} \pm (t \times SEM))$$

where $\overline{X}$ = the sample mean
   t = tabled *t* value at 95% *CI* for *df* = *N* − 1
   SEM = the calculated *SEM* for the sample data

In our example, the calculated value of *SEM* is 1.0, and Table A.2 tells us that the value of *t* for the 95% *CI* with 24 degrees of freedom (25 − 1) is 2.06. Thus, we would obtain the following calculation:

$$95\% \ CI = (61.0 \pm (2.06 \times 1.0))$$
$$95\% \ CI = (61.0 \pm 2.06)$$
$$95\% \ CI = (58.94 \leq \mu \leq 63.06)$$

We can be 95% confident that the mean height of our population of 12-year-old children is between about 58.9 and 63.1. If we return to the sample means in Table 5.2, we find that, in fact, only one of the 20 sample means (62.1) would *not* have a 95% *CI* that captures the population mean of 60.0. The confidence limits for the sample mean of 62.1 (the fourth mean in the first column) would be 60.04 and 64.16. Researchers generally accept the risk that their *CI*s do not include the popula-tion mean 5% of the time.

TIP: *There are several ways to compute* CIs *around a mean within SPSS. The simplest way is to use Analyze → Descriptive Statistics → Explore. If you click on the Statistics pushbutton on the opening dialog box, you will have an option to designate the* CI *value. A 95%* CI *is the default, i.e., the option automatically used unless it is overriden by the analyst.*

Confidence Intervals Around Percentages and Risk Indexes

Confidence intervals can be constructed around all of the descriptive statistics we discussed in preceding chapters, including percentages (or proportions) and risk indexes. Consider, for example, this question: "What percentage of nursing home residents with an indwelling urinary catheter develops urinary tract infection?" This question calls for an estimated percentage, which is the same as the absolute risk index, as described in Chapter 4. The estimate will be more useful if it is reported within a 95% CI.

For percentages based on nominal-level dichotomous variables, as implied in the above question (exposed/not exposed to catheterization and positive/negative for infection), the applicable theoretical distribution is not a normal distribution, but rather a **binomial distribution**. A binomial distribution is the probability distribution of the number of "successes" (e.g., heads) in a sequence of independent yes/no trials (e.g., a coin toss), each of which yields "success" with a specified probability.

Using binomial distributions to build CIs around a proportion is computationally complex and is almost always done by computer, and so we do not provide any formulas here, nor are there tables for binomial distributions in the Appendix. Interactive Web sites that calculate risk indexes typically calculate 95% CIs automatically, and statistical software like SPSS also includes CI information with risk index values. For example, it may be recalled from Chapter 4 that the relative risk of a diagnosis of postpartum depression (PPD) for unmarried compared to married women was 2.842—a nearly threefold risk of PPD. Figure 4.2 shows that the confidence limits for the 95% CI around this RR statistic were 1.353 and 5.969. This means that we can be 95% confident that relative risk of PPD for unmarried women in the population from which this sample was drawn lies somewhere between 1.35 (a 35% increase in risk over married women) and 5.97 (a six-fold increased risk).

Although we do not present formulas or tables for the binomial distribution, certain features of CIs around proportions are worth noting. First, the CI is rarely symmetric around the sample proportion. For example, if two out of 20 sample members were "positive" for an outcome, such as urinary tract infection, the estimated population proportion would be .10 and the 95% CI for the proportion would be from .012 to .317, which is wider above than below .10. As the population proportion shifts from .50 to higher or lower values, the binomial distribution changes shape, becoming positively skewed for probabilities less than .50, and negatively skewed for probabilities greater than .50.

Second, the width of the CI depends on both sample size and the value of the proportion. The smaller the sample, and the closer the sample proportion is to .50, the wider the CI. For example, with a sample size of 30, a 95% CI for a proportion of .50 has a range of .374 (from .313 to .687), while that for a proportion of .10 has a range of only .188 (from .021 to .265).

Finally, the CI for a proportion never extends below .00 or above 1.0, but a CI can be constructed around an *obtained* proportion of .00 or 1.0. For example, if zero out of our 30 patients had a urinary tract infection, the estimated proportion would be .00 and the 95% CI would be from .000 to .116.

All of the indexes of risk described in the previous chapter, such as the ARR, RR, OR, and NNT, should be presented with CI information. The computed value of these statistics from study data represents a "best estimate" of the population values, but CIs convey information about the plausibility that the estimate is accurate. Formulas for constructing CIs around the major risk indexes are presented in an appendix of DiCenso et al. (2005) and Sackett et al. (2000), but interactive Web sites are the easiest way to construct CIs when risk indexes are computed for a study in which you do not have direct access to the actual data, such as in a published report.

Example of confidence intervals around percentages and odds ratios:

Carruth, Browning, Reed, Skarke, and Sealey (2006) examined the percentage of farm women who failed to obtain cervical cancer screening (Pap smear) in three southern states, using data from a sample of over 2,300 women. The researchers reported failure rates (percentages of women who failed to obtain a Pap smear in a 3-year period) for women from the three states, along with 95% *CI* values. For all women in Louisiana, the failure rate was 27.9% (95% *CI* = 24.5, 31.3), whereas in Texas the rate was 19.6% (95% *CI* = 15.6, 22.6). Odds ratios were calculated for failure rates in relation to various potential risk factors, such as age, ethnicity, and education. For example, the OR for white (versus nonwhite) women was 0.79 (95% *CI* = 0.47, 1.33). The *CI* included 1.0, which indicates that ethnicity was likely unrelated to failure rates.

HYPOTHESIS TESTING

Hypothesis testing is a second approach to inferential statistics. Hypothesis testing involves using sampling distributions and the laws of probability to make an objective decision about whether to accept or reject the null hypothesis. Although we have seen a few examples of null hypotheses in this chapter, we elaborate on this concept because of its importance in hypothesis testing.

The Null Hypothesis

Researchers usually have research hypotheses about expected relationships between variables. The predicted relationship can be expressed verbally in a number of ways. The following are examples of **research hypotheses** that predict a relationship between an independent and a dependent variable:

1. Length of time in labor will be *different* for women in an upright position *from* that for women in a recumbent position.
2. Oncology patients who have high levels of fatigue will be *more* depressed *than* patients with less fatigue.
3. Catecholamine production (measured by vanillymandelic acid excretion) is *related to* a patient's level of stress.

The italicized phrases in these hypotheses (different from, more than, related to) embody the nature of the predicted relationship. These are the types of hypotheses that researchers typically seek to support with their data. Research hypotheses cannot, however, be tested directly. It is the null hypothesis, which states the *absence* of a relationship, that is tested statistically. For instance, in the third example the researcher would test the null hypothesis that catecholamine production is *un*related to patients' stress levels.

Hypothesis testing, which is based on rules of negative inference, *begins with the assumption that the null hypothesis is true*. For example, in the coin toss example discussed earlier, we assumed that the coin was fair. We then collected data through coin tosses and used the results to inform our decision about the probability that this assumption was valid. We concluded, after obtaining 10 heads in a row, that the coin was probably biased and so we rejected the null hypothesis.

The null hypothesis is analogous to the basic assumption of innocence in English-based systems of criminal justice: Just as an accused criminal is assumed to be innocent until proven guilty, in research situations variables are also assumed to be "innocent" of any relationship until there is sufficient evidence to

The real situation is that the Null (H_0) is:

	True	**False**
True **(Null Accepted)**	**Correct Decision** Probability = $1.0 - \alpha$	**Type II Error** (False Negative) Probability = β
False **(Null Rejected)**	**Type I Error** (False Positive) Probability = α	**Correct Decision** Probability = $1.0 - \beta$

Researcher decides that the Null (H_0) is:

FIGURE 5.5 The four outcomes of statistical decision making.

the contrary. In the justice system, the null and alternative hypotheses may be formally stated as follows:

H_0: The accused is innocent of committing the crime.

H_1: The accused is guilty of committing the crime.

In criminal proceedings, the concept of *reasonable doubt* is important, and again there is a parallel in statistical inference. When a judge instructs a jury to find a defendant innocent if there is reasonable doubt that he or she committed the crime, the judge is, in effect, asking the jurors to decide if $p = 1.0$ that the accused is guilty. In the justice system, however, there is no objective cutoff point for determining how much doubt is reasonable. In hypothesis testing, researchers establish a fixed probability as their criterion for "guilt" and "innocence."

Another important difference between hypothesis testing and the justice system concerns the language associated with decisions. Lawyers and judges often talk about requiring *proof* that the accused is guilty. Researchers, however, do not use the term *proof*, unless they obtain data from a population—in which case, inferential statistics would not be needed. The rejection of a null hypothesis through statistical testing does not prove that the research hypothesis is valid; it constitutes *evidence* that the null hypothesis is probably incorrect. There remains a possibility that the null is true even though it is rejected.

Type I and Type II Errors

Because statistical inference is based on sample data that are incomplete, there is always a risk of error. Figure 5.5 summarizes the four possible outcomes of statistical decision making. When the null hypothesis is true (i.e., there really is no relationship between the independent and dependent variables in the population), and researchers conclude that the null is true, the correct decision has been made, as shown in the upper left cell of the figure. Similarly, when the null hypothesis is really false and researchers decide to reject the null (lower right cell), the correct decision is made again.

Researchers can commit two types of errors, as shown in the shaded cells of the figure. The first is incorrectly rejecting a true null hypothesis. For example, the null may state that there is no relationship between women's body position and their length of time in labor. If the researcher incorrectly rejects this null hypothesis, erroneously concluding on the basis of sample data that length of time is higher in, say, the recumbent position, then a **Type I error** has been committed. A Type I error is, in effect, a false positive.

Researchers can also commit an error by incorrectly accepting a false null hypothesis. For example, if the researcher concludes that women's length of time in labor is the same in both positions, when in fact labor time is really higher in the recumbent position, then a **Type II error** (false negative) has been committed.

The consequences of making statistical errors can be most readily conveyed with a drug-testing analogy. A Type I error might result in a totally ineffective drug being used to treat a disease. But a Type II error might prevent a truly effective drug from coming onto the market.

Controlling the Risk of Errors

Researchers do not, of course, realize when a Type I or Type II error is committed. Only by knowing population values would researchers be able to definitively conclude that the null hypothesis is true or false.

Researchers can, however, control the probability of committing an error. Type I errors can be controlled through the **level of significance**, which is the probability level established as the accepted risk of a false positive. Inferential statistics involve comparing a computed statistic against the probability in theoretical distributions. The level of significance, symbolized as α (**alpha**), indicates the area in the theoretical probability distribution that corresponds to the rejection of the null hypothesis.

The most widely accepted standard for the level of significance is the .05 level. This corresponds to the 95% confidence level we discussed in the previous section. With a .05 significance level, we are accepting the risk that out of 100 samples, we would reject a true null five times. Conversely, with $\alpha = .05$, the probability is .95 $(1 - \alpha)$ that a true null hypothesis will be accepted. These probabilities, shown in the two left-hand boxes in Figure 5.5, always total 1.0.

Researchers sometimes use a stricter level of significance. With an α of .01, the risk is that in only one out of 100 samples would we erroneously reject a true null hypothesis. With the stringent significance level of .001, the risk is even lower: In only one out of 1,000 samples would we erroneously reject the null hypothesis. In our example of tossing the coin to test for bias, we could have used this very conservative .001 criterion and still rejected the null hypothesis that the coin was fair.

Researchers can also exert some control over Type II errors, but the situation is much more complex than with Type I errors. The probability of committing a Type II error is symbolized as β (**beta**). The probability of correctly rejecting the null hypothesis when it is false $(1 - \beta)$ is the **power** of the statistical test. The risk of a Type II error is affected by many factors, such as sample size, measurement quality, the strength of underlying relationships between variables, and so on. Also, the probability of committing a Type II error increases as the risk of making a Type I error decreases. In other words, when researchers establish a strict criterion for α, they increase the probability of committing a Type II error.

We will say more about power and Type II errors in subsequent chapters, but we note here that many researchers accept a very high risk of erroneously accepting a false null hypothesis. Polit and Sherman (1990) found that many published nursing studies have insufficient power, placing them at risk for Type II errors. Although many years have elapsed since this analysis was done, a glance through nursing research articles suggests that many studies continue to be underpowered. The most straightforward method of reducing the risk of a Type II error is to increase the size of the sample: The larger the sample, the more powerful is the statistical test.

Establishing Probable and Improbable Results

By stipulating the significance level, researchers establish a decision rule. The decision is to reject the null hypothesis if the statistic being tested falls at or beyond a **critical region** (*acceptance region*) on the theoretical distribution, and to accept the null hypothesis otherwise. Decision rules should be established before the data are analyzed, to avoid bias.

The critical region corresponding to the significance level indicates what is *improbable* for a null hypothesis. An example should help to clarify this process. Suppose that we wanted to assess whether people with a fertility problem had positive or negative attitudes toward in vitro fertilization (IVF). We might ask a sample of 100 infertility patients to express their attitude toward IVF on a rating scale that ranged from 0 (extremely negative) to 10 (extremely positive). Our goal in this example is to determine whether the mean attitude for the population of infertility patients is different from 5.0, the score on the rating scale that represents neutrality. The null and alternative hypotheses are:

$$H_0: \mu = 5.0$$
$$H_1: \mu \neq 5.0$$

Suppose data from the sample of 100 patients result in a mean rating of 5.5 with an *SD* of 2.0. This mean is consistent with the alternative hypothesis (H_1), but can we reject the null hypothesis? Because of sampling error, we need to test for the possibility that the mean of 5.5 occurred simply by chance, and not because the population has, on average, a positive attitude toward IVF.

Since hypothesis testing involves an assumption that the null hypothesis is true, we can construct a sampling distribution that assumes that the population mean is 5.0. Next, we need to estimate the standard deviation of the sampling distribution—the *SEM*—using the sample *SD*:

$$SEM = \frac{2.0}{\sqrt{100}} = \frac{2.0}{10} = 0.2$$

The relevant sampling distribution is presented in Figure 5.6. Because we are using the estimated *SEM* rather than the actual *SEM*, the *t* distribution rather than the normal distribution is appropriate for establishing critical regions. In Table A.2, we

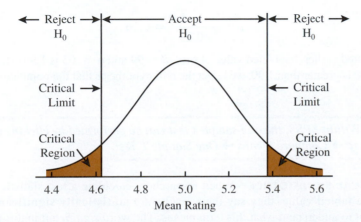

FIGURE 5.6 Critical regions in the sampling distribution: attitudes toward IVF example.

find that for a significance level of .05 and $df = 99$ ($100 - 1$), the t value is about 1.99. The limit of what is "probable" if the null hypothesis is correct is just under two standard deviations (1.99 SDs) on the sampling distribution.

The boundaries of the critical region for rejecting the null hypothesis are established by multiplying the estimated SEM by the t value—i.e., $1.99 \times .2 = .398$. As shown in Figure 5.6, the limits of what is probable if the null hypothesis is true are the points corresponding to .398 above and below the hypothesized population mean of 5.0. If our sample mean falls inside the critical limits (i.e., between 4.602 and 5.398), we would conclude that the null hypothesis has a 95% probability of being true. Our sample mean of 5.5 is beyond the critical limit—it lies in the shaded region on the distribution that indicates what is "improbable" if the null hypothesis were true. We can now accept the alternative hypothesis that patients are not, on average, neutral in their attitudes toward IVF.

Test Statistics

In practice, researchers do not construct sampling distributions and draw critical regions on them. Rather, they compute a **test statistic**, using an appropriate formula, and then compare the value of the test statistic to a value in a table. The selection of a test statistic is made on the basis of such factors as the nature of the hypothesis and the level of measurement of the variables.

In subsequent chapters, we describe numerous test statistics that can be used to test various types of hypothesis. Here, we illustrate the process of hypothesis testing using the example of patients' attitudes toward IVF, for which we would use the **one-sample t test**. For this test statistic, the formula is as follows:

$$t = \frac{\overline{X} - \mu}{SEM}$$

where $\overline{X}$ = the sample mean
μ = value of population mean for null hypothesis
SEM = the estimated standard error of the mean

We would then compare the obtained value of t resulting from this formula to the values in Table A.2 for the designated significance level and degrees of freedom. If the absolute value of the computed t statistic is greater than the tabled value, then the null hypothesis is rejected. In the example at hand, the computed value of t is as follows:

$$t = \frac{5.5 - 5.0}{0.2} = 2.50$$

As indicated earlier, the tabled value of t for $df = 99$ and $\alpha = .05$ is 1.99. Therefore, since 2.50 is greater than 1.99, we reject the null hypothesis that the population mean is 5.0.

TIP: *Within SPSS, the one-sample* t *test can be performed by clicking on Analyze → Compare Means → One Sample T Test.*

STATISTICAL SIGNIFICANCE When researchers calculate a test statistic that is beyond a tabled value, they say their results are **statistically significant**. It is important to understand what this term means. The word *significant* in this context should not be interpreted to mean *important* or *useful* or *clinically relevant*.

In statistics, *significant* means that the results are probably not attributable to chance (i.e., attributable to random fluctuations and sampling error), at a specified probability level.

By convention, any probability value (**p value**) greater than .05 (e.g., .09) is **statistically nonsignificant**. A nonsignificant result is one that could have been obtained simply by chance, i.e., with $p > .05$. In other words, a nonsignificant result is one that, on the relevant theoretical distribution, does not lie in the critical region for rejecting the null hypothesis.

There is a definite prejudice in research circles for results that are statistically significant. Researchers are often disappointed if their substantive predictions—their research hypotheses—are not supported by the data. Moreover, journal reviewers and editors are less likely to accept manuscripts when there are no statistically significant results. This prejudice is not arbitrary: It reflects the fact that nonsignificant results are ambiguous. Inferential statistics are designed to disconfirm the null hypothesis, and so there is never justification for interpreting an accepted null hypothesis as evidence of a *lack* of relationship among variables. Because of the basic framework for hypothesis testing, researchers whose substantive hypotheses are the null case (i.e., they hypothesize no relationship among variables) will have difficulty making the required inferences with traditional inferential statistics.

While there is a strong preference for statistical significance, we caution that significance does not necessarily mean that the results are important. Researchers can reduce standard errors by increasing the size of their sample, and so with a large enough sample, almost all findings are statistically significant. This does not always mean that the findings have clinical value.

ONE-TAILED VERSUS TWO-TAILED TESTS   In most situations, researchers use what are called two-tailed tests. A **two-tailed test** is one that uses both tails of a sampling distribution to determine the critical region for rejecting the null hypothesis. For example, the critical region in Figure 5.6 is found in both tails of the sampling distribution—values above 5.398 and below 4.602. The area corresponding to 5% of the probability distribution (for an α of .05) is comprised of 2.5% at the lower end and 2.5% at the upper end.

Sometimes, however, two-tailed tests are unnecessarily conservative. When researchers have a strong basis for predicting a specific *direction* for the alternative hypothesis, a one-tailed test may be appropriate. A **one-tailed test** is one in which the critical region is in only one end of the distribution.

To illustrate, suppose that we had a firm basis for hypothesizing not only that infertility patients' attitudes toward IVF are not neutral, but also that they are positive. This is referred to as a **directional hypothesis**. Our hypotheses in this example might be formally stated as follows:

$$H_0: \mu = 5.0$$
$$H_1: \mu > 5.0$$

Originally, we predicted simply that the population mean would not be neutral (not equal to 5.0). This **nondirectional hypothesis** implies that we were prepared to find mean ratings that reflected either negative attitudes or positive ones, and so we needed to look at both tails of the sampling distribution. In a one-tailed test, the critical region defining improbable values is entirely in one tail of the distribution—the tail corresponding to the alternative hypothesis. Because the entire 5% of "improbable" values is at one end with a one-tailed test, it is easier to reject the null hypothesis.

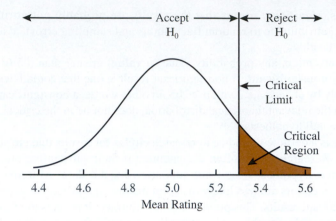

FIGURE 5.7   Critical region for a one-tailed test: attitudes toward IVF example.

Figure 5.7 illustrates this point with our example. With a two-tailed test, the mean sample score had to exceed 5.398 to be statistically significant at the .05 level. With a one-tailed test, the mean sample rating has to exceed only 5.332 to reject the null hypothesis. This value represents the hypothesized mean (5.0), plus the standard error (0.2) times the tabled value for a one-tailed test with $\alpha = .05$ and $df = 99$. Column two of Table A.2 (i.e., the column headed by .10 for a two-tailed test and .05 for a one-tailed test) indicates that the tabled t value is about 1.66. The critical limit is thus $(5.0 + (0.2 \times 1.66)) = 5.332$.

Most researchers use two-tailed tests even when their research hypotheses are directional. In research reports, if researchers do not state that statistical tests were one-tailed, then two-tailed tests can be assumed. This is a conservative approach that reduces the risk of committing a Type I error. Yet, the result is also that the risk of a Type II error increases, because one-tailed tests have more statistical power than two-tailed tests. Thus, when theory or prior research evidence strongly suggests that findings opposite to those in the directional hypothesis are virtually impossible, a one-tailed test may be justified. For example, suppose we were to test the following null hypothesis:

H_0: Hand washing has no effect on bacteria counts.

In this situation, the alternative hypothesis is directional—i.e., that hand washing reduces bacteria. It would make little sense to test the null hypothesis against the tail of the distribution implying the possibility that hand washing *increases* bacteria.

The decision to use a one-tailed test should always be based on a solid foundation of theory or prior evidence, and should be made *before* analyses are performed. It is inappropriate to compute a test statistic and then decide, based on the result, that a one-tailed test should be used.

ASSUMPTIONS   The use of statistical tests always requires certain statistical assumptions to be made. An **assumption** concerns characteristics of the population that are accepted as true without proof.

Assumptions vary according to the test statistic being used. We will note the assumptions associated with specific tests in subsequent chapters. One assumption that is common to virtually all statistical tests, however, is the assumption that study participants were independently and randomly sampled from the population. In a

random sample, every element in the population has an equal chance of being selected. Random samples have a greater likelihood than nonrandom samples of being representative of the population. Sampling errors can occur in random samples, but such sampling errors are simply the result of chance factors. Samples that are not selected by random procedures are likely to harbor **systematic bias**. When samples are biased, findings from the sample cannot be generalized to the population.

In most nursing research—or, for that matter, in most research with humans, regardless of discipline—samples are *not* randomly selected. In our hypothetical example of 100 infertility patients, it is unlikely that we could have obtained our sample by selecting 100 patients at random from *all* infertility patients. More likely, we would have obtained our sample from clients at a local infertility clinic. Even if we defined our population very narrowly as all the patients at that one clinic, the chances are pretty high that the sample would not be random. Some people, for example, would refuse to participate in the study, and nonparticipation is rarely random.

Since the assumption of independent and random observations should be met for the statistical test to be valid, what should researchers do? First, random sampling should be used whenever feasible. Second, if random sampling is not possible, researchers should consider what is reasonable to assume as the population. In essence, researchers need to ask, "From what population can this group be assumed to be a reasonably random (representative) sample?" Third, the interpretation of the findings from nonrandom samples should be conservative and cautious. In deciding whether the results of the statistical inference can be generalized to the population, researchers should look for evidence of similarities between sample characteristics and population characteristic. A final piece of advice is to **replicate** studies—that is, to repeat the study with a new sample.

For the one-sample t test, it is assumed that the values on the focal variable are independent of each other and normally distributed in the population. Fortunately, statisticians have been able to demonstrate that in most situations the t test is **robust** to violations of the normality assumption. By robust, we mean that the accuracy of decisions (the frequency of making Type I and Type II errors) is not strongly diminished when the variable's underlying distribution is not normal. Generally, small deviations from normality can be tolerated regardless of the size of the sample. Larger deviations can be tolerated as the sample size increases. Thus, if a sample is small (under 30 cases) and there is evidence that the distribution is bimodal or severely skewed, a one-sample t test should not be used.

PARAMETRIC AND NONPARAMETRIC TESTS   Statistical tests can be classified in two broad groups. Most tests described in this book are **parametric tests**, which involve estimating a parameter. The one-sample t test, a parametric test, involves estimating the population mean. Parametric tests, in general, assume that dependent variables are normally distributed in the population, and most parametric tests have other assumptions as well. Parametric statistics are applied when the dependent variable is measured on a level approximating an interval level or higher.

Nonparametric tests do not test hypotheses about population parameters. These tests are sometimes called **distribution-free tests** because they require no assumption about the shape of the distribution of variables in the population. There are nonparametric tests that are appropriate for all four levels of measurement, although nonparametric tests are most often used when the variables are measured on a nominal or ordinal scale. Nonparametric tests are generally easier computationally than parametric tests.

The use of parametric and nonparametric tests in controversial. Some people argue that if the assumptions for a parametric test are not met, then a nonparametric test should be selected. Parametric tests are generally robust to minor violations of the underlying assumptions, however, and so others argue that parametric tests are usually appropriate when the violations are modest.

Since nonparametric tests are easier to compute and have less restrictive assumptions, why would researchers ever choose a parametric test? First, the ease of computation is not much of an issue now that most statistical analyses are done by computer. Second, parametric tests are much more powerful. By powerful, we refer to the concept of power discussed earlier: the likelihood of correctly rejecting a false null hypothesis. With a given set of data, a parametric test has a higher probability of correctly rejecting the null hypothesis than when a nonparametric test is applied to the same set of data.

It seems sensible to adopt a moderate position in this controversy. When deviations from normality appear to be modest, and when the measures of the variables are approximately interval level, it is probably safe to use a parametric test. When the distribution of a variable is markedly skewed or multimodal, however—especially if the sample is small—or if the variables cannot possibly be construed as interval level, a nonparametric test may be preferable.

BETWEEN-SUBJECTS TESTS AND WITHIN-SUBJECTS TESTS Another distinction in statistical tests concerns the type of comparisons being made. Hypothesis testing involves making some type of comparison. In a one-sample *t* test, for example, we compare a sample mean against a hypothesized population value. If the hypothesis concerns the relationship between smoking and lung cancer, smokers would be compared to nonsmokers with regard to lung cancer incidence.[4]

When the comparison involves different people, the statistical test must be a **between-subjects test** (sometimes called a **test for independent groups**). For example, when men are compared to women, a test for independent groups is required because the people in the male group are not the same people as those in the female group. As another example, if a researcher compared the effects of two therapies (relaxation therapy versus music therapy) on pain levels, and randomly assigned people to either the relaxation group or the music group, a test for independent groups would again be required because people in the relaxation group did not receive the music therapy and vice versa.

Some research designs, however, involve a single group of people. For example, the researcher in the example of the two pain therapies might expose half the participants to the relaxation therapy first, followed by music therapy, while the other half would get the therapies in the reverse order. In this *crossover design*, the comparison of the two therapies is not independent, because the same people are in both groups. Another example involves a design in which people are compared before and then after some intervention to determine if there were changes. With such designs, the appropriate statistical tests are **within-subjects tests** (sometimes called **tests for dependent groups**). Both between-subjects and within-subjects tests are described in subsequent chapters.

Steps in Hypothesis Testing

The remainder of this book describes various statistical tests that are appropriate for particular research situations. Each test has a computational formula and a table corresponding to a relevant theoretical distribution. The overall process of

---

[4] The term *comparison* suggests an examination of group differences. But, in fact, whenever a researcher tests a hypothesis about a relationship between variables, the analysis involves comparisons. For example, when a researcher asks if there is a relationship between cholesterol levels and heart rate, this can be conceptualized as asking whether people with high cholesterol levels have different heart rates than people with low cholesterol levels. Correlational questions essentially involve comparisons of relative value on a continuum.

testing hypotheses, however, is basically the same, regardless of which test is used.

When the test statistic is being calculated manually, the steps in hypothesis testing are as follows:

1. *Decide which test statistic to use*   The selection of an appropriate test depends on several factors, including the type of comparison being made, the number of groups being compared, the measurement level of the variables, and the extent to which assumptions have been met. The tables on the inside covers of this book provide some guidance for selecting an appropriate statistical test. These tables will be more understandable as you progress through the book and become familiar with alternative statistical analyses.

2. *Establish the level of significance*   The criterion for the decision rule regarding rejection of the null hypothesis should be set before the analyses are undertaken. The level of significance will usually be .05.

3. *Determine whether to use a one-tailed or two-tailed test*   In most cases, a two-tailed test will be appropriate. If there is a firm basis for hypothesizing the direction of a relationship, a one-tailed test may be warranted.

4. *Calculate the test statistic*   Using data collected for the research, the test statistic is computed, using the formula associated with the selected statistical test.

5. *Determine the degrees of freedom*   **Degrees of freedom (df)** is a concept used in statistical testing to indicate the number of components that are free to vary about a parameter. This concept is difficult to grasp, but fortunately formulas for determining degrees of freedom are easy. A simple illustration may clarify what we mean by "free to vary about a parameter." Suppose we knew that the mean value of five numbers was 10.0. How many individual data values (Xs) would we need to know to have complete information about the data? The answer is four ($N - 1$): Once we know the first four values, the fifth value is fixed, given that the mean is 10.0. For example, if the first four Xs were 8, 9, 10, and 11, the fifth number would not be free to vary: It would have to be 12.

6. *Compare the computed test statistic to a tabled value*   Each statistical test has an associated theoretical distribution. Tables have been developed to indicate probability levels for different test values in the distribution for different degrees of freedom. Most tables are set up to show the critical limit of the test statistic for the most commonly used significance levels—often .05, .01, and .001. To use the tables, you must locate the appropriate α and df, and then find the value of the critical limit. Then this tabled value is compared to the computed statistic.

7. *Decide to accept or reject the null hypothesis*   If the absolute value of the computed statistic is greater than the tabled value, the null hypothesis can be rejected and the result is said to be statistically significant, at the specified probability level. If the computed statistic is smaller, then the null hypothesis is retained and the results are nonsignificant.

TIP: *The tables on the inside covers are designed to help you select the right test, but there are many online resources with decision trees and interactive guides to help as well. Examples include http://www .microsiris.com/Statistical%20Decision%20Tree/ and http://www.users .muohio.edu/houslemk/decision%20tree.htm.*

When a computer is used to perform the analyses, researchers still need to make up-front decisions (steps 1 through 3). First, researchers must select the appropriate statistical test so that the correct instructions can be given to the computer. Next, researchers should decide on a significance criterion and whether a one-tailed or two-tailed test is appropriate. The next three steps are then carried out by the computer: The computer will calculate the test statistic, determine degrees of freedom, and specify the actual probability that the null hypothesis is true. For example, the computer might indicate that the probability is .018 that the mean pain ratings for a music therapy group and a relaxation therapy group are the same. This means that fewer than two times out of 100 (18 times out of 1000) would a group difference as large as that observed be found simply as a result of chance; group differences in average pain levels have a high probability of being real. The computed probability must then be compared to the significance criterion. If α was set at .05, the result would be statistically significant because .018 reflects an outcome that is even less probable than the criterion. If α was set at .01, however, the result would be nonsignificant. Note, though, that computer-generated probability levels are usually for two-tailed tests. If a one-tailed test is desired, the probability value needs to be divided in half. In the present example, the p value would be .009 for a one-tailed test (.018 ÷ 2). Thus, the one-tailed test would pass the significance criterion of .01, whereas a two-tailed test would not.

RESEARCH APPLICATIONS

This section discusses some of the research applications of statistics discussed in this chapter, and how they are presented when they are reported in journal articles.

The Uses of Statistics Described in Chapter 5

With *CI*s added to your statistical repertoire, you can now do more than clean your data and describe your sample: You are on the road to answering research questions and developing evidence for nursing practice. Here are a few specific uses of statistics discussed in this chapter.

1. *The SEM*   Sometimes the standard error of the mean is used descriptively—in lieu of the standard deviation—to communicate information about variability. That is, some researchers present information about means for key variables, and then state the *SEM* rather than the *SD*. This does not happen very often in nursing articles, but is not uncommon in medical journals. For example, Leung and colleagues (2007) studied surgical waiting times for patients with intraocular tumors, and reported that the mean was 86.75 days, with an *SEM* of 9.44. Thus, when you are interpreting research evidence from reports in other disciplines, you should pay attention to whether means are reported with SD or SEM information.

2. *Confidence intervals around descriptive statistics*   When researchers calculate means, they do not routinely calculate *CI*s around those values. For example, if researchers described the mean age of study participants as 38.4 years, they likely would not state the *CI* around that mean, because age is not the central focus of the study. Moreover, researchers seldom ask research questions that can be answered with a mean value of an outcome for their entire sample. They are more likely to be interested in *differences* in the mean values between two or more groups, and they might report the *CI* around mean differences—a topic we discuss in the next chapter. Yet, there are circumstances in which a key study objective is to ascertain a mean value, in which case reporting the *CI* around that mean is an important tool for drawing conclusions about the precision of the

estimate of the population mean. For example, Missildine (2008) completed an interesting study of sleep and the sleep environment of older adults in acute care settings. Her purpose was to document and describe such factors as light and noise levels, sleep duration and efficiency, and so on. For all of these variables, she computed mean values (e.g., mean light levels were 6.14 lux). Given the small sample size in this pilot study, she did not compute *CI*s around her means, but it would be valuable to do so in a larger study. Risk indexes, by contrast, directly address many research questions, and are almost always reported with *CI* information. Risk indexes are different than means because they inherently encompass a comparison—they are indexes of bivariate relationships and involve the comparison of two risk groups with regard to an outcome.

3. ***One-sample t test***   Our illustration of the one-sample *t* test, which involved comparing mean ratings of IVF attitudes against a hypothetically neutral score of 5.0, was clearly contrived. In reality, one-sample *t* tests are infrequently used in nursing research, because researchers rarely have a specific value against which to test the sample mean. One exception is when there are **norms**, which are standards based on data from either a population or a large, representative sample. We present an example of a study that used one-sample *t* tests by one of this book's authors at the end of the chapter. Polit and Beck (2008) tested the hypothesis that females are overrepresented in studies conducted by nurses—i.e., that the mean proportion female in nursing studies is greater than a specific value, .50.

Presentations in Research Reports

Point estimates and *CI*s often can be reported in the text of a report. The following is an example of a statement that could be made to report a *CI*: "The mean birthweight for the infants whose mothers were addicted to heroin was 2,025 grams (95% *CI* = 2,010, 2,040)." This indicates that there is a 95% probability that the mean population birthweight for infants of heroin-addicted mothers lies between 2,010 and 2,040 grams.

Tables are convenient for displaying *CI*s for multiple means, percentages, or risk indexes simultaneously. When a series of one-sample *t* tests have been performed, they can also be presented in a table. The table that illustrates findings from Polit and Beck's (2008) study (Table 5.3) includes both *CI* and one-sample *t*-test information.

Confidence intervals—or, alternatively, *SEM*s around a mean—can also be presented graphically. To illustrate, four group means and *CI* information are shown in Figure 5.8, again using data from Polit and Beck's study. The *X* axis designates a group or subgroup variable (here, four different age groups for people participating in nursing studies), and the *Y* axis designates values of the means—i.e., the mean percentage female in nursing studies. This graph, created within SPSS (Graphs ➜ Legacy Dialogs ➜ Error Bars) uses squares to indicate the mean values, and **error bars** or brackets around the means to designate the 95% *CI*s. In this instance, a graph works well to highlight differences among the four age groups.

Tips on Preparing Tables with Information on Statistical Significance

In this section, we offer general guidance on presenting information about statistical tests in tables.

- Tables that report results from tests of statistical significance vary in content and organization, and we will present many examples for specific tests in

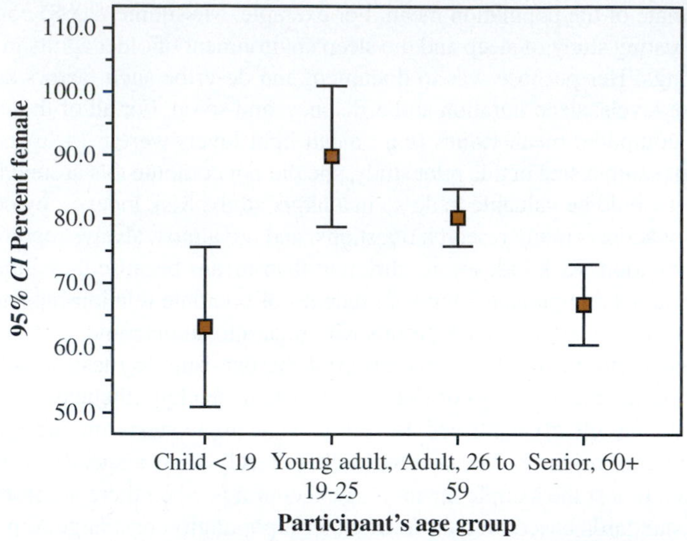

FIGURE 5.8 SPSS graph with means and 95% *CI* error bars: percentage female in study samples, by participants' age group.

chapters that follow. We can make a few general points here, however. In many cases, tables have a column headed by the name of the test statistic. The entries in the column are the values of the computed statistic. Table 5.3 illustrates this arrangement with some information from Polit and Beck's (2008) study on gender bias in nursing research. This study is described more fully in the next section. The fourth column, headed "*t*," has values of the *t* statistic for eight separate one-sample *t* tests.

- When the number of cases on which the test statistic is based varies from one variable to another, there is usually a column designating sample size or

TABLE 5.3 Example of Table with One-Sample *t* Tests and 95% *CI* Information: Mean Percentage Female in Nursing Studies by Selected Characteristics of the Study

Study Characteristic	*N* of Studies	Mean Percentage Female (*SD*)	*t*	*p*	95% *CI*, Mean Percentage Female	
					Lower Limit	*Upper Limit*
Type of Study						
Quantitative	175	73.2 (27.7)	11.06	<.001	69.0	77.3
Qualitative	74	79.1 (26.5)	9.46	<.001	73.0	85.2
Research Design, Quantitative						
Experimental/quasi-experimental	39	75.6 (35.3)	6.33	<.001	67.4	83.8
Nonexperimental	142	73.2 (27.5)	10.07	<.001	68.7	77.8
Research Tradition, Qualitative						
Grounded theory	12	80.8 (28.3)	3.78	.003	62.9	98.8
Phenomenologic	19	72.5 (33.2)	2.95	.009	56.5	88.5
Descriptive/no specific tradition	40	77.3 (24.6)	7.02	<.001	69.4	85.2
All studies	259	75.3 (27.2)	14.95	<.001	72.0	78.6

Based on data from Polit and Beck (2008).

arrangement with some information from Polit and Beck's (2008) study on gender bias in nursing research. This study is described more fully in the next section. The fourth column, headed "*t*," has values of the *t* statistic for eight separate one-sample *t* tests.

- When the number of cases on which the test statistic is based varies from one variable to another, there is usually a column designating sample size or degrees of freedom. In Table 5.3, *N* is shown in column 2. If *N* is the same throughout a table, sample size or *df* can be shown in a footnote or in the table title.

- When statistical tests have been performed, tables almost invariably present probability information. Often, as in Table 5.3, there is a separate column for the *p* values. Significant *p* values are sometimes displayed as being below the commonly used cut-off values of .05, .01, and .001, as appropriate, or as *NS* (nonsignificant). Now that most analyses are done by computer, however, it is preferable to show actual probability values (American Psychological Association, 2001), as in Table 5.3, column 5.

- An alternative to having a separate column for *p* values is to place asterisks next to the value of the test statistic to designate probability levels. In most cases, one asterisk is used to represent $p < .05$, two asterisk designates $p < .01$, and three asterisks designate $p < .001$. (There should always be a key at the bottom of the table explaining what the asterisks represent.) In Table 5.3, for example, the entries under the *t* column could have been 11.06*** for the first row (quantitative studies), and 3.78** for the fifth (grounded theory studies). When this system is used, statistics with no associated asterisks are under-

Research Example

The following example describes a study by this book's author that involved one-sample *t* tests. We describe the study and also show SPSS computer printouts (Figures 5.8 and 5.9).

Study: "Is there gender bias in nursing research?" (Polit & Beck, 2008)

Study Purpose: The purpose of this study was to test the hypothesis that females are disproportionately represented as participants in nursing studies. We also examined whether bias toward female participants, if any, was associated with characteristics of the researchers, participants, or study methods.

Methods: Data were extracted from a consecutive sample of journal articles published in four leading nonspecialty nursing research journals in 2005 and 2006. Each article was coded with regard to characteristics of the participants (e.g., predominant age group), the researchers (e.g., *sex* of the lead author), nursing specialty focus (e.g., oncology, pediatrics), and study methods (e.g., quantitative versus qualitative). The primary outcome variable for this study was the percentage of participants in each study that was female.

Analysis: The primary analyses involved a series of one-sample *t* tests that tested the hypothesis that the mean percentage female across studies was not equal to 50.0. (The null hypothesis was that the mean percentage *is* 50.0; i.e., that males and females are equally likely to participate in nursing studies.) Figure 5.9 shows SPSS output from the *t* test for the entire sample of studies. The top panel shows the number of studies in the analysis ($N = 259$), the mean percentage female across all studies (75.28), the *SD* (27.21), and the *SEM* (1.69). The bottom panel shows inferential statistics. At the top, we see that the test value = 50. That is, the null hypothesis being tested is that the mean percentage is 50, which would presumably reflect a total absence of gender bias. Then, reading from the left, we see that the value of *t* (with 258 *df*) is 14.953. For a two-tailed test, the probability of obtaining this result if the null hypothesis of a 50-50 male-female split were true is .000 (Sig. [2-tailed]). This means that the mean percentage of 75.3 would be obtained by chance alone in fewer than one in 1,000 samples of nursing studies. SPSS truncates the probability when the actual value is less than .0005, so we do not know for sure what the probability is—it could, for example, be .0004 or .000009. We do know,

T-Test

One-Sample Statistics

	N	Mean	Std. Deviation	Std. Error Mean
Percent female	259	75.27961	27.206805	1.690549

One-Sample Test

	Test Value = 50					
					95% Confidence Interval of the Difference	
	t	df	Sig. (2-tailed)	Mean Difference	Lower	Upper
Percent female	14.953	258	.000	25.279615	21.95058	28.60865

FIGURE 5.9   SPSS printout of a one-sample *t* test.

however, that a mean percentage of 75.3 is highly un-likely to merely reflect sampling fluctuations. The next entry shows that the mean difference between the obtained mean of 75.3 and the hypothesized mean of 50.0 is 25.3. The far-right entry shows that the 95% *CI* around this mean difference is 21.95 and 28.61.

Results: On average, 75.3% of study participants were female, and 38% of studies had all-female samples. The bias favoring female participants was statistically significant and persistent. A significant bias was observed regardless of methodological features, and regardless of other participant characteristics, such as their age. Table 5.3 presents some of the findings relating to study methods. As this table shows, the mean percentage female far exceeded 50.0% regardless of whether the study was quantitative or qualitative, experimental or nonexperimental, or conducted within various qualitative research traditions such as grounded theory or phenomenology. All the *t* tests in the table were statistically significant. Note that we reported the *p* levels in Table 5.3 as <.001, even though the SPSS output said that Sig. = .000. The actual probability is not zero, but it is very low, less than one in 1,000. Another thing to note is that this table shows 95% *CIs* around the mean percentage, not around the mean difference as shown on the computer printout in Figure 5.9. Thus, the table tells us that for the sample of studies as a whole, we can be 95% confident that the true mean lies somewhere between 72.0 and 78.6. The lower limit is well above 50.0, which is consistent with the results of the one-sample *t* test. Figure 5.8 shows graphic results for the mean percentage female for four age groups of participants. This figure shows that, regardless of age group, the lower limit of the 95% *CI* was greater than 50.0—although it was close to 50.0 for children under age 19 (51.0). The figure also suggests that nurse researchers were especially likely to use predominantly female samples when their study population was young adults. For studies involving participants in the 19- to 25-year-old age group—there were 11 such studies—the mean percentage female was 89.7.

TIP: *You have perhaps noticed the overlap between parameter estimation and hypothesis testing in this example. The one-sample* t *test and the 95%* CIs *provide consistent information because both were based on the t distribution and on means and* SEMs *calculated from the study data. We can see in Table 5.3 that* CIs *provide hypothesis-testing information as well as parameter estimates. The lower limits of the various 95%* CIs *were always higher than 50.0%, which corresponds to the null hypothesis, and thus indicates that the null hypothesis can be rejected. We think the two approaches complement each other nicely. The* CIs *provide useful information about the precision of our estimates, but (because the probability level was fixed at 95%), they do not convey information about how improbable the null hypothesis is. The* p *values associated with the* t *tests tell us how totally improbable it is that the true population parameter was 50.0%.*

Summary Points

- Researchers use **inferential statistics** to generalize from sample data to a broader population. Researchers are not able to make inferences about population values directly from sample data due to **sampling error**, which reflects the tendency of sample statistics to fluctuate from one sample to another, simply by chance.

- Inferential statistics use theoretical **sampling distributions** and the **laws of probability** as a basis for establishing "probable" and "improbable" research outcomes.

- The **sampling distribution of the mean** is a hypothetical distribution of the means of an infinite number of samples of a given size from a population.

- The standard deviation of a sampling distribution of means is called the **standard error of the mean** (*SEM*); it is an index of the average amount of error in a sample mean as an estimate of the population mean. The smaller the *SEM*, the more accurate are the estimates.

- An estimated *SEM* can be calculated by dividing the sample standard deviation by the square root of *N*, i.e., sample size.

- Statistical inference encompasses two broad approaches: estimation procedures and hypothesis testing. **Estimation procedures** are used to estimate population parameters.

- **Point estimation** provides a single descriptive value of a parameter (e.g., a mean, proportion, or odds ratio).

- **Interval estimation** provides a range of values—a **confidence interval** (*CI*)—between which the population value is expected to fall, at a specified probability level. Researchers establish the degree of confidence that the population value lies within this range. Most often the 95% *CI* is reported, which indicates that there is a 95% probability that the true population value lies between the upper and lower **confidence limits**.

- Confidence intervals around a mean are calculated by multiplying the sample *SEM* times a value obtained from a theoretical distribution called the *t* **distribution,** and then adding and subtracting that value from the mean. A *t* distribution is similar to a normal distribution, but has fatter tails when sample size is small. When there is information about the *actual* (not estimated) *SEM*, *z* scores and the normal distribution can be used to calculate *CI*s around a mean.

- *CI*s around a proportion or risk index involve using a theoretical distribution called the **binomial distribution.**

- **Hypothesis testing**, the alternative approach to parameter estimation, begins with an assumption that the null hypothesis is true. The **null hypothesis** (H_0) is typically a statement about the absence of a relationship between variables, while the **research hypothesis** (or **alternative hypothesis, H_1**) is the hypothesis researchers seek to support. Based on a calculated **test statistic** that is compared to values in a theoretical distribution, researchers make decisions to accept or reject the null hypothesis based on how "improbable" the calculated statistic is.

- Because decision making is based on sample data, there is always a possibility of error. When researchers incorrectly reject a null hypothesis that is true, a **Type I error** (false positive) is committed; when researchers incorrectly accept a false null hypothesis, a **Type II error** (false negative) is committed.

- Researchers establish a **level of significance**, which is the probability of making a Type I error. The two most commonly used levels of significance (often symbolized as α) are .05 and .01. With α equal to .05, the researcher accepts the risk that in five samples out of 100 the null hypothesis will be rejected when it is, in fact, true.

- The probability of committing a Type II error (symbolized as β) is more difficult to control, but large samples reduce the risk—that is, a large *N* increases the **power** of the statistical test.

- Hypothesis testing involves several steps. Researchers begin by selecting an appropriate **statistical test**, based on such factors as the level of measurement of the variables and the degree to which the data are likely to support the **assumptions** for a parametric test.

- A **parametric test** involves the estimation of a parameter, the use of data measured on an interval scale or higher, and assumptions about the distribution of the variables. A **nonparametric test** has less restrictive assumptions, and is more likely to be used when the key variables are nominal or ordinal level.

- Researchers also decide whether a **one-tailed test** (suitable for a **directional hypothesis**) is defensible, or whether a **two-tailed test**, which uses both ends of the theoretical distribution to define the **critical region** of "improbable" values, is more appropriate.
- Once researchers make preliminary decisions, a test statistic is calculated using sample data. After calculating **degrees of freedom** (*df*), researchers then consult the appropriate table. If the absolute value

of the test statistic is greater than the tabled value, the result is **statistically significant**, at the specified level of probability. This means that the obtained result is probably "real" and not likely to be the result of chance factors. A **nonsignificant** result is one in which deviations from the null hypothesis are likely to have occurred simply by chance.

- One statistical test, the **one-sample *t* test,** is used when the researcher tests the null hypothesis that the sample mean is equal to a specified value.

Exercises

The following exercises cover concepts presented in this chapter. Appendix C provides answers to Part A exercises that are indicated with a dagger (†). Exercises in Part B involve computer analyses using the datasets provided with this textbook, and answers and comments are offered on this book's Web site.

PART A EXERCISES

† **A1.** What is the probability of drawing a spade from a normal, shuffled deck of 52 cards? What is the probability of drawing five spades in a row (i.e., the probability of getting a flush in five-card poker)?

A2. Draw a histogram that graphs the probability of drawing a spade, a club, a heart, or a diamond from a normal deck of 52 cards. Shade in the area showing the probability of drawing a red card.

† **A3.** Given a normal distribution of scores with a mean of 100 and an *SD* of 10, compute *z* scores for the following score values: 95, 115, 80, and 130.

† **A4.** Based on Figure 5.2, which shows a normal distribution of children's heights with a mean of 60.0 and an *SD* of 5.0, approximately what is the probability of randomly selecting a child whose height is less than 50 inches? (Use tabled values for the normal distribution in Table A.1.)

† **A5.** If a sampling distribution of the mean had an *SEM* equal to 0.0, what would this suggest about the sample means drawn from the population—and about the scores in the population?

† **A6.** Compute the mean, the standard deviation, and the estimated standard error of the mean for the following sample data: 3, 3, 4, 4, 4, 5, 5, 5, 5, 5, 5, 6, 6, 6, 7, and 7.

† **A7.** Population A and Population B both have a mean height of 70.0 inches with an *SD* of 6.0. A random sample of 30 people is selected from Population A, and a random sample of 50 people is selected from Population B. Which sample mean will probably yield a more accurate estimate of its population mean? Why?

† **A8.** Suppose we obtained data on vein size after application of a nitroglycerin ointment in a sample of 60 patients. The mean vein size is found to be 7.8 mm with an *SD* of

2.5. Using the *t* distribution in Table A.2 (because information on the true *SEM* is not available), what are the confidence limits for a 95% *CI* around the mean? What are the confidence limits for a 99% *CI*?

† **A9.** Suppose you wanted to test the hypothesis that the average speed on a highway—where the maximum legal speed is 55 mph—is not equal to 55 mph (i.e., H_0: $\mu = 55$; H_1: $\mu \neq 55$). Speed guns are used to measure the speed of 50 drivers, and the mean is found to be 57.0, $SD = 8.0$. What is the calculated value of *t* for a one-sample *t* test? With $\alpha = .05$ for a two-tailed test, is the sample mean of 57.0 significantly different from the hypothesized mean of 55.0 (i.e., can the null hypothesis be rejected)?

† **A10.** For the problem in Question A9, would the obtained result be statistically significant with = .05 for a one-tailed test (i.e., for H_1: $\mu > 55$)?

PART B EXERCISES

† **B1.** For the exercises in this chapter, you will again be using the SPSS dataset Polit2SetB. First, run a descriptive analysis for the variable *bmi,* the body mass index for study participants. Do this within Analyze ➔ Descriptive Statistics ➔ Descriptives. Move the variable *bmi* (variable #19) into the variable list, then click the pushbutton for Options. Select the following statistics: mean, standard deviation, minimum, maximum, and standard error (S. E. mean). Then click Continue and OK to run the analysis and answer the following questions: (a) What is the mean body mass index in this sample of low-income women? (b) What is the *SD?* (c) What is the standard error of the mean? (d) Using the *SEM* and values from the *t* distribution in Table A.2, compute the value of the 95% *CI* around the mean. Now, what is the value of the 99% *CI* around the mean for BMI?

† **B2.** Now, have SPSS compute the same *CI*s around the mean of *bmi* by using the Analyze ➔ Descriptive Statistics ➔ Explore procedure. In the opening dialog box, Insert the *bmi* variable into the Dependent Variable list. Next, click

"Statistics" at the bottom left, then click on the Statistics pushbutton, where you can designate the desired confidence level. The default is 95%. Run the analysis twice, once with a 95% *CI* and another time for the 99% *CI*. How close were your manual calculations to the computer-generated statistics for the *CI*s?

† **B3.** Within Explore, you can instruct the computer to compute *CI*s around the means of a dependent variable for different subgroups. Run Explore for the variable *bmi* again, but on the opening dialog box, in the slot labeled "Factor List," enter the variable for the woman's poverty status (*poverty*). This will yield information about the mean BMIs of two groups of women: those whose families were above poverty, and those whose families were below poverty. Instruct the computer to compute 95% *CI*s. Then answer the following questions: (a) What was the mean BMI for women below poverty? (b) What was the mean BMI for women above poverty? (c) What are the standard errors for the two groups? Why do you think they are different? (d) What are the 95% *CI*s around the mean BMI for the two groups of women?

† **B4.** Create a graph that presents the statistics from Exercise B3. Click on Graphs ➜ Legacy Dialogs ➜ Error Bar. The dialog box that pops up is set to a default for type of graph (Simple) that you should run. Click the pushbutton Define. In the next dialog box, move *bmi* into the slot for Variable and *poverty* into the slot for Category axis. There are options for whether the graph uses error bars to show *CI*s around the mean (which is the default, with a 95% *CI*), the standard error of the mean, or standard deviations. Run the procedure with both *CI*s and *SEM*s. For the run with the *SEM*, designate a multiplier of 1—this will yield a graph that shows the mean with error bars set at 1 *SEM* around the mean. In which of the two graphs do the error bars encompass a narrower range?

† **B5.** In Chapter 4, we used two variables that are standardized scores on the Short-Form Health Survey or SF12, a widely used 12-item health status measure. This scale yields two subscales scores: a physical health component subscale score (*sf12phys*) and a mental health component subscale score (*sf12ment*). As noted in the previous chapter, the data values for the women in this sample are standardized T scores that were created using national norms with a mean of 50.0 and an *SD* of 10.0. Because there are national norms, we can use a one-sample *t* test to test the null hypothesis that the means for women in this sample on both subscales are 50.0. To run a one-sample *t* test, click Analyze ➜ Compare Means ➜ One-Sample T Test. In the dialog box that appears, insert the two SF-12 variables, which are at the end of the file, in the Test Variable(s) slot. At the bottom, enter the Test Value as 50.0. Click the Options pushbutton to make sure that you are requesting 95% *CI*s for the analysis. Then click Continue ➜ OK to run the analysis and answer these questions: (a) State the null and alternative hypothesis, using the formulas presented in this chapter, for the physical health component score. (b) What are the values of *t* for the two analyses? (c) Are these values statistically significant? If so, at what level of significance? (d) What are the *CI* values, and what do they mean?

† **B6.** Set up a table to display the results from Exercise B5, using Table 5.3 as a model. Then write a few sentences summarizing the results.

B7. Using the variable *poverty* as the row variable in a Crosstabulation analysis, calculate RRs and ORs between the women's poverty status and four to five other dichotomous outcomes of your choosing in the Polit2SetB dataset. (If you have forgotten the commands for doing this, refer back to Chapter 4.) Create a table presenting the results, and write a brief paragraph summarizing key findings. Be sure that your table and your discussion include information about *CI*s.

CHAPTER 6

t Tests: Testing Two Mean Differences

In Chapter 5, we discussed the one-sample t test, which allows researchers to test a specific hypothesized value for a population mean. A more common situation is a researcher's desire to draw inferences about the *difference* between two population means. For example, a researcher might want to evaluate whether the mean body temperature of a population receiving a special treatment is different from the mean temperature of a control population not receiving the treatment, based on data from a sample. Or, a researcher might want to compare the mean weight of a sample of diabetic patients before and after an innovative weight-loss intervention, to draw conclusions about the effect of the innovation in a population of diabetic patients. In these situations, the **two-sample t test** is an appropriate statistical test. When there are three or more groups, statistics described in other chapters would need to be used.

BASIC CONCEPTS FOR THE TWO-SAMPLE t TEST

Suppose that we wished to evaluate whether drinking caffeinated coffee affects intraocular pressure (IOP) in nonglaucomatous adults. Fifty people are randomly assigned to an experimental group that ingests 40 ounces of caffeinated black coffee, whereas fifty people are randomly assigned to a control group that receives 40 ounces of decaffeinated coffee. Thirty minutes later, the IOP of all 100 people is measured. The mean IOP of those in the experimental group is found to be 15.5 mmHg, while the mean IOP of those in the control group is 13.5 mmHg. Can we conclude that the ingestion of caffeinated versus decaffeinated coffee (the nominal-level independent variable) is related to IOP levels (the dependent variable)?

As we saw in Chapter 5, a sample mean is seldom exactly the same as a population mean because of sampling error. Thus, the two populations in question (a hypothetically infinite number of ingestors of caffeinated coffee and a hypothetically infinite number of ingestors of decaffeinated coffee) *could* have the same mean IOPs, even though the sample means are different by 2.0 mmHg. A mere inspection of the sample means is inadequate for reaching conclusions about the two populations.

The Null and Alternative Hypotheses

In our example, there are two possibilities—the ingestion of caffeinated coffee is either related to IOP in adults, or it is not. The null hypothesis posits that there is no relationship between caffeine and IOP. We can state the null hypothesis formally as:

$$H_0:\ \mu_1 = \mu_2$$

where $\mu_1 =$ the population mean for Group 1 (those receiving caffeinated coffee)
$\mu_2 =$ the population mean for Group 2 (those receiving decaffeinated coffee)

The alternative hypothesis is that there *is* a relationship between the independent and dependent variables—that is, that the two population means are not equal:

$$H_1:\ \mu_1 \neq \mu_2$$

Note that the hypotheses are about the population parameters (μ), not about the statistics ($\overline{X}$). We are using sample data to infer what is true in the population. In this example, the alternative hypothesis is nondirectional: It does not specify whether μ_1 is expected to be greater than μ_2 or vice versa, and so we would use a two-tailed test.

Our next task is to test whether the null hypothesis has a high probability of being incorrect. By showing that the null hypothesis is improbable, we can infer that the population means probably are not equal.

Sampling Distribution of a Mean Difference

A two-sample *t* test follows the same hypothesis-testing logic discussed in Chapter 5. A test statistic for this situation is based on a theoretical sampling distribution called the *sampling distribution of the difference between two means*. This distribution allows researchers to conclude whether an observed difference between two sample means is "probable" or "improbable," given the null hypothesis.

A sampling distribution, as we have already seen, is a theoretical distribution of an infinite number of sample values drawn from a population. This distribution is based not on individual sample means, but rather on differences between the means of samples drawn from two different populations. That is, the sampling distribution plots the distribution of an infinite number of mean differences for samples of a specified size, where mean differences are $\overline{X}_1 - \overline{X}_2$. In the example of the IOP, our mean difference value would be: $15.5 - 13.5 = 2.0$.

If we measured the IOPs of a new sample of 50 people drinking caffeinated coffee and 50 drinking decaf coffee, new means—and a new difference value—would be obtained. If an infinite number of mean difference scores were computed and graphed in a frequency polygon, the result would be a sampling distribution of the difference between two means. Just as the mean of a sampling distribution of the mean always equals the population mean, so too *the mean of a sampling distribution of the difference between two means always equals the difference between two population means.* By knowing the standard deviation of such a distribution, we can identify differences that are in the tail and that are, therefore, improbable when the null hypothesis is true.

The standard deviation of such a sampling distribution is called the standard error of the difference between two means or, more commonly, the **standard error of the difference**, which we abbreviate as SE_D. The SE_D summarizes how much sampling error occurs, on average, when a mean difference score is computed, for samples of a given size.

Large standard errors of the difference make it difficult for researchers to reject the null hypothesis, even when it is false. When the SE_D is small, by contrast, it is easier to have confidence in a sample difference as an estimate of the population difference. Similar to the standard error of the mean, the SE_D is influenced by two factors: the size of the two samples (n_1 and n_2), and the variability of scores in the populations. The standard error becomes smaller as the sample size increases and the variability of scores in the populations decreases.

> **TIP:** *By convention, the symbol* **N** *is used to designate total sample size and* **n** *is used to represent the size of a subgroup. In our example,* $n_{caffeinated}$ = 50, $n_{decaffeinated}$ = 50, *and* N = 100.

The *t* statistic for testing the difference between two sample means uses an estimate of the SE_D in its formula, as we discuss in a subsequent section. Let us first consider the underlying requirements for the two-sample *t* test.

Assumptions and Requirements for the *t* test

The *t* test for comparing group means is appropriate when the independent variable is a dichotomous nominal-level variable indicating a person's status in one of two groups, and when the dependent variable approximates interval-scale characteristics or higher. In our example about intraocular pressure, there were two groups—those getting caffeinated coffee and those getting decaffeinated coffee—and a ratio-level dependent variable, IOP measures.

Use of a *t* test is, strictly speaking, justified only if several assumptions are met. First, participants are presumed to be randomly sampled. This assumption is true of virtually all statistical tests, as previously discussed. Second, the dependent variable is presumed to be normally distributed within each of the two populations. The *t* test is fairly robust with regard to the assumption of normality when the sample size is large. Indeed, it has been found that *t* tests yield accurate results even with severe departures from normality, if the number of cases in each group is greater than 40 and group size is roughly comparable.

> **TIP:** *When doing a computer analysis, it is easy to test the assumption of normality. Within SPSS, this can be accomplished within the Explore procedure (within Descriptive Statistics). Two tests for normality can be performed by selecting "Normality plots with tests" within the dialog box for options under "Plots."*

A third assumption for *t* tests is the **assumption of the homogeneity of variance**. That is, the following is assumed:

$$\sigma_1^2 = \sigma_2^2$$

It is usually safe to ignore this assumption when sample sizes are approximately equal. If the sample sizes are markedly dissimilar (e.g., if one group is more than 1.5 times greater than the second group) and if there is reason to suspect that the population variances are unequal, the standard formula for the *t* test may produce erroneous results. More specifically, the risk of a Type II error (incorrectly accepting the null hypothesis) tends to be inflated when larger variation is associated with the larger group size, and the risk of a Type I error (incorrectly rejecting the null hypothesis) tends to be inflated when larger variation is associated with the smaller group size (Zimmerman, 2001). As we will see later in this chapter, there is an alternative formula that you can apply when you suspect that the assumption of homogeneous variances has been violated.

> **TIP:** *When there is reason to suspect in advance that population variances are unequal, it is advisable to design the study in such a way that the two groups are of approximately equal size.*

t TESTS FOR INDEPENDENT AND DEPENDENT GROUPS

A *t* test for comparing group means is appropriate in two types of situation. The **independent groups *t* test** is used when the participants in the two groups are not the same people, nor connected to one another in a systematic way. The independent groups *t* test would be used in our example of the people randomly assigned to either the caffeinated group *or* the decaffeinated coffee group. No one in the caffeinated group received the decaffeinated coffee, and vice versa.

A different formula must be used when the people in the groups are not independent. For example, when the weight of diabetics going through a weight reduction program is measured before and after the intervention, the two groups are made up of the *same* individuals, and so the two samples are not independent. In such a situation, the **dependent groups *t* test** is required. In this section we present computational formulas for both situations.

Independent Groups *t* Test

Suppose that we developed an intervention to reduce the distress of preschool children who are about to undergo the fingerstick procedure for a hematocrit determination. Twenty children will be used to evaluate the effectiveness of the special intervention, with 10 randomly assigned to an experimental (intervention) group and 10 assigned to a control group that receives no special preparation. The dependent variable is the child's pulse rate just prior to the fingerstick. The hypotheses being tested are as follows:

$$\text{H}_0: \mu_1 = \mu_2 \qquad \text{H}_1: \mu_1 \neq \mu_2$$

where μ_1 = the population mean for the experimental group
μ_2 = the population mean for the control group

To test these hypotheses, we compute a *t* statistic. In this example, we would use the formula for the independent groups *t* test, because membership in the experimental group is independent of membership in the control group. A simplified formula for *t* is as follows:

$$t = \frac{\overline{X}_1 - \overline{X}_2}{SE_D}$$

The numerator is the difference in means between the two sample groups, and the denominator is the estimated standard error of the difference. This formula is similar to the formula for the one-sample *t* test presented in Chapter 5, where we saw that the numerator was the mean minus the hypothesized population mean, and the denominator was the standard error of the mean (*SEM*).

POOLED VARIANCE *t* TEST   The standard error of the difference between means, which we need to compute the *t* statistic, is estimated based on the variances of the two samples. If we assume that the variances of the two populations of children (those receiving and those not receiving the special intervention) are equal, we can compute the *t* statistic using the **pooled variance** *estimate* of the SE_D in the denominator. The basic (pooled variance) formula for the independent groups *t* test is as follows:

$$t = \frac{\overline{X}_1 - \overline{X}_2}{\sqrt{\left[\dfrac{(n_1 - 1)SD^2_1 + (n_2 - 1)SD^2_2}{n_1 + n_2 - 2}\right]\left[\dfrac{1}{n_1} + \dfrac{1}{n_2}\right]}}$$

where $\overline{X}_1$ = sample mean of Group 1

$\overline{X}_2$ = sample mean of Group 2

SD^2_1 = Variance of Group 1

SD^2_2 = Variance of Group 2

n_1 = number of cases in Group 1

n_2 = number of cases in Group 2

Although this formula looks complex, it simply boils down to the computation of means and variances for the two groups, and then plugging these values into the equation along with information on the size of the groups.

Some data for our fictitious example about an intervention for the fingerstick are shown in Table 6.1. According to this table, the mean pulse rate of the children in the intervention group was 10.0 bpm lower than that of the children in the control group (95.0 versus 105.0). Does this difference reflect real differences in the populations, or is it merely the result of random fluctuation? The *t* test will enable us to draw a conclusion, at a specified probability level.

All components for the *t* test are shown at the bottom of Table 6.1. (The calculation of the variances—the squared *SD*s—is not shown in the table; *SD* and variance formulas were presented in Chapter 3.) According to the calculation, the value of the *t* statistic is -1.85. To evaluate whether this is statistically significant (i.e., improbable if the null hypothesis is true), we need to compute degrees of freedom. The *df* formula for the independent groups *t* test is as follows:

$$df = n_1 + n_2 - 2$$

Thus, in this example, $df = (10 + 10 - 2) = 18$. Assume that we set $\alpha = .05$ for a two-tailed test. Table A.2 in Appendix A for the *t* distribution indicates that the tabled

TABLE 6.1 Example of Calculation of Pooled Variance Independent Groups t Test

Experimental Group Pulse Rate in bpm (Group 1) X_1	Control Group Pulse Rate in bpm (Group 2) X_2
100	105
86	95
112	120
80	85
115	110
83	100
90	115
94	93
85	107
105	120
$\Sigma X_1 = 950$	$\Sigma X_2 = 1050$
$\overline{X}_1 = 950 \div 10 = 95.0$	$\overline{X}_2 = 1050 \div 10 = 105.0$
$SD^2_1 = 154.46$	$SD^2_2 = 138.67$
$n_1 = 10$	$n_2 = 10$

$$t = \frac{\overline{X}_1 - \overline{X}_2}{\sqrt{\left[\frac{(n_1 - 1)SD^2_1 + (n_2 - 1)SD^2_2}{n_1 + n_2 - 2}\right]\left[\frac{1}{n_1} + \frac{1}{n_2}\right]}}$$

$$t = \frac{95.0 - 105.0}{\sqrt{\left[\frac{(9)154.46 + (9)138.67}{18}\right]\left[\frac{1}{10} + \frac{1}{10}\right]}} = \frac{-10.0}{5.41}$$

$$t = -1.85$$

value of t with df = 18 is 2.10. This tabled value is greater than the absolute value of the calculated t statistic ($|-1.85| = 1.85$), and so we retain the null hypothesis that the two population means are equal. We cannot conclude that the group difference of 10.0 bpm in the children's pulse rates is attributable to the special intervention, given our decision rule.

Of course, we might have tested a different hypothesis, such as the following:

$$\text{H}_0: \mu_1 = \mu_2 \qquad \text{H}_1: \mu_1 < \mu_2$$

This alternative hypothesis is directional: It predicts not only that the two groups will have unequal means, but that the mean pulse rate for the intervention group will be lower than that for the control group. We do not expect that the intervention would *increase* the preprocedure pulse rate of children, and so we may be justified in using a one-tailed test. Returning to Table A.2, we find that with $\alpha = .05$ and df = 18, the tabled t value for a one-tailed test is 1.73. The absolute value of the calculated t statistic, 1.85, is greater than this tabled value, and so the null hypothesis can be rejected. With a one-tailed test, the mean pulse rate of the intervention group is significantly lower than that of the control group for $\alpha = .05$. This example provides an opportunity to re-emphasize the caveat that decisions to use a one-tailed or a two-tailed test should be made *before* the t statistic is computed, not after its value is known.

SEPARATE VARIANCE *t* TEST   We were able to use the standard pooled variance formula for the *t* test in this example because the sample sizes of the two groups were identical. Moreover, we can see in Table 6.1 that the variances of the two groups were reasonably similar (154.5 for the intervention group and 138.7 for the control group). When the assumption of equal population variances is untenable and when sample sizes are unequal, a different formula for the *t* statistic must be used. The **separate variance** formula is

$$t = \frac{\overline{X}_1 - \overline{X}_2}{\sqrt{\dfrac{SD_1^2}{n_1} + \dfrac{SD_2^2}{n_2}}}$$

When analyses are done by computer, as they usually are, you usually do not have to decide which of the two formulas to use, because (at least in SPSS) *t* is computed using both of them. Moreover, SPSS automatically performs a test (called **Levene's test for equality of variances**) that helps you decide which test statistic to report. Levene's test calculates a statistic (called an *F* statistic) that tests the null hypothesis that the two variances are equal ($H_0: \sigma_1 = \sigma_2$). If this *F* statistic is significant, then this null hypothesis must be rejected, and the *t* from the separate variance formula should be reported.

Figure 6.1 shows a computer printout for the present example, which we created in SPSS using the Analyze ➜ Compare Means ➜ Independent Samples T Test commands. The top panel shows basic descriptive information—the *n*, mean, *SD*, and the *SEM* for the dependent variable, children's pulse rate—for the experimental and the control groups. In the bottom panel, reading from left to right, we see first that the *F* for Levene's test equals .134. This statistic is not significant ($p = .719$), and so we

T-Test

Group Statistics

	Group Status	N	Mean	Std. Deviation	Std. Error Mean
Child's pulse rate	Experimental group	10	95.00	12.428	3.930
	Control group	10	105.00	11.776	3.724

Independent Samples Test

		Levene's Test for Equality of Variances		*t*-test for Equality of Means						
									95% Confidence Interval of the Difference	
		F	Sig.	t	df	Sig. (2-tailed)	Mean Difference	Std. Error Difference	Lower	Upper
Child's pulse rate	Equal variances assumed	.134	.719	−1.847	18	.081	−10.000	5.414	−21.374	1.374
	Equal variances not assumed			−1.847	17.948	.081	−10.000	5.414	−21.377	1.377

FIGURE 6.1   Computer printout for independent groups *t* test: testing mean differences in children's pulse rates.

can accept the null hypothesis that the variances of the two groups are equal. In other words, the variance of the experimental group (12.43^2) is not significantly different from the variance of the control group (11.78^2).

The remainder of this panel shows the results of the *t* test, with the first row presenting information on the pooled variance estimate (i.e., for the equal variance assumption) and the second row showing information for the separate variance estimate (for the unequal variance assumption). If the test for homogeneity of variance *had* been statistically significant, the separate variance estimate would have been the appropriate test. In the present case, the value of *t* is -1.85 for both estimates, and the two-tailed significance (*p*) is .081. With $\alpha = .05$ for a two-tailed test, this *p* value is not statistically significant. For the one-tailed test, the printed value of *p* would have to be halved: The one-tailed significance would be .0405, which is statistically significant when α is .05. The next column shows that the estimated standard error of the difference is 5.41. The final column shows the 95% confidence interval (*CI*) for the population mean difference, with the limits of -21.37 and $+1.37$ for the equal variance assumption. All of this information corresponds to the manual calculations previously shown in Table 6.1 and in the text. Clearly, using the computer removed the drudgery of performing the calculations.

We should also note that, because of the small sample size, we began the analysis by testing the assumption that children's pulse rates were normally distributed. One such test is called the **Kolmogorov-Smirnov test**, which can be performed in SPSS through the Explore procedure. This test yielded a $p = .20$, which indicates that departures of the distribution from normality are not statistically significant.

Example of an independent-groups *t* test:

Cho, Holditch-Davis, and Miles (2008) studied maternal depression among mothers with medically at-risk infants. They used *t* tests to examine whether mothers' scores on a depression scale differed for those with male versus female infants, and for mothers with infants in different risk groups (e.g., premature versus medically fragile).

Dependent Groups *t* Test

Sometimes an independent groups *t* test is inappropriate. One such situation occurs when means are computed for the same group of people at two points in time (for example, before and after an intervention). In this within-subjects design, the "groups" are not independent: They comprise the same people. Sampling fluctuation is lower in a within-subject design because the various attributes of individuals that affect sampling variation (e.g., their health, age, motivation, and so on) have a similar effect on both means. The *t* test for independent groups is, therefore, overly conservative or insensitive for testing dependent group differences, since a major source of inter-participant variation is controlled.

Other situations also require a dependent groups *t* test. When participants in one group are paired to those in the second group on the basis of some attribute, the dependent groups *t* test is appropriate. Here are some examples:

- Group 1 = husbands, Group 2 = their wives
- Group 1 = twin A, Group 2 = twin B
- Group 1 = mothers, Group 2 = their daughters

In another relevant situation, researchers sometimes deliberately pair-match participants in one group with unrelated people in another group to enhance group similarity. For instance, people with lung cancer might be pair matched to people without lung cancer on the basis of age and education, and then smoking behaviors in the two groups might be compared. In all of these instances, the selection of people in the second group is constrained by which people are in the first group—their selection is not independent. These situations all call for a dependent groups t test, which is sometimes called a **paired t test** or a **correlated groups t test**.

To illustrate, suppose we wanted to compare direct and indirect methods of blood pressure measurement in a sample of trauma patients. Blood pressure values are obtained from 10 patients via both radial arterial catheter (direct) and the bell component of the stethoscope (indirect). In this example, the hypotheses being tested are as follows:

$$H_0: \mu_1 = \mu_2 \qquad H_1: \mu_1 \neq \mu_2$$

where μ_1 = the population mean for the direct method
μ_2 = the population mean for the indirect method

To test these hypotheses, we need to perform a dependent groups t test, because the same people are in both groups. The formula for the t statistic for dependent groups is as follows:

$$t = \frac{\overline{X}_D}{\sqrt{\dfrac{SD^2_D}{n}}}$$

where $\overline{X}_D$ = the mean difference between pairs of values
SD^2_D = the variance of the difference
n = total number of pairs

In this formula, the $\overline{X}_D$ in the numerator is the average difference between all pairs of individual scores—i.e., the mean of all the $(\overline{X}_1 - \overline{X}_2)$s. The expression in the denominator is the estimate of the standard error of difference. The following equivalent formula can be more readily used for actual calculations:

$$t = \frac{\Sigma D}{\sqrt{\dfrac{(n\Sigma D^2) - (\Sigma D)^2}{n - 1}}}$$

where D = difference scores between the pairs
n = total number of pairs

Again, although the formula looks complex, the components are not hard to compute. The main calculation involves computing difference scores between all pairs, and then either squaring each difference score and summing (ΣD^2), or summing the difference scores and then squaring ($(\Sigma D)^2$).

Some systolic blood pressure (SBP) data for our fictitious example are presented in Table 6.2. As the calculations at the bottom of this table show, the mean systolic blood pressure of the 10 patients is 129.3 mmHg by the direct method and 128.0 mmHg by the indirect method. We can use the t test for dependent groups to determine if the difference of 1.3 mmHg is statistically significant, or likely to reflect sampling error.

TABLE 6.2 Example of the Calculation of Dependent Groups *t* Test

Direct SBP in mmHg X_1	Indirect SBP in mmHg X_2	Difference $(X_1 - X_2)$ D	D^2
130	128	2	4
102	100	2	4
154	155	−1	1
113	110	3	9
139	140	−1	1
125	120	5	25
156	155	1	1
108	105	3	9
161	160	1	1
105	107	−2	4
$\Sigma X_1 = 1293$	$\Sigma X_2 = 1280$	$\Sigma D = 13$	$\Sigma D^2 = 59$
$\overline{X}_1 = 1293/10$	$\overline{X}_2 = 1280/10$	$(\Sigma D)^2 = 169$	
$\overline{X}_1 = 129.3$	$\overline{X}_2 = 128.0$		

$$t = \frac{\Sigma D}{\sqrt{\dfrac{(n\Sigma D^2) - (\Sigma D)^2}{n - 1}}}$$

$$t = \frac{13}{\sqrt{\dfrac{(10)59 - 169}{9}}} = \frac{13}{6.84}$$

$$t = 1.90$$

Table 6.2 shows that the calculated value of *t* is 1.90. We can consult Table A.2 for the tabled *t* value once we know degrees of freedom. For the dependent groups *t* test, the formula is as follows:

$$df = n - 1$$

where *n* = total number of pairs

In this example, $df = 9$ and, with $\alpha = .05$ for a two-tailed test, the tabled value of *t* is 2.26. The tabled value is larger than the computed value of *t*, and so our decision is to accept the null hypothesis. Given our decision rule, we cannot conclude that the mean for the direct blood pressure measurement is different from the mean for the indirect method. Nor, however, can we conclude that the means are the same, because a Type II error might have occurred. Statistical testing is designed to test whether the null hypothesis is probably false, but failure to reject the null does not "prove" that the null is true, only that there is insufficient evidence to reject it.

Computer analysis for the dependent groups *t* test is straightforward. In SPSS, we would use the commands Analyze ➔ Compare Means ➔ Paired-Samples T Test. Figure 6.2 presents an SPSS printout for such a *t* test, using the fictitious data for the direct and indirect blood pressure measurements for 10 people (Table 6.2). The top panel (A) provides basic descriptive information for SBP values for the two measurement methods, direct and indirect. Panel B indicates that the correlation between the two sets of SBP measures was strong ($r = .996$). Panel C shows, reading from regions for rejecting the null hypothesis for α = .05 and .01, respectively. As was true for the t statistic, tables have been created to indicate the minimum value of F needed to reject the null hypothesis.

ANOVA PROCEDURES

Analysis of variance can be used in several situations. Although each requires different calculations, the underlying logic is similar. We present a detailed computational example for the simplest form of ANOVA, and subsequently discuss on a more limited basis two other applications.

One-Way ANOVA

The simplest ANOVA situation involves comparing group means for three or more independent groups, such as in our examples of the effect of body positions on systolic blood pressure, and of the effect of different therapies on stress scores. These situations call for a **one-way analysis of variance**. The phrase "one-way" signifies that there is a single independent variable whose effect on a dependent variable is under study.

> **TIP:** *ANOVA can actually be used when there are only two groups, although the* t *test is usually used in such situations. In fact, for two independent groups, the* F *and the* t *distributions are mathematically related such that* F = t².

The calculation of the F statistic for one-way ANOVA involves computing several deviation scores that are then squared—similar to procedures for computing the variance and SD. We will work through one computational example, using the data on stress scores from Table 7.1.

Table 7.2 shows all the computations required for ANOVA. The formula for the F statistic involves a concept called the **sum of squares**, which is the sum of the squared deviations around a mean. The **sum of squares-within** or SS_W (shown in panel A of Table 7.2) captures the variation of each patient relative to his or her group mean—that is, within-group variability. To find the value of SS_W, we first compute a group mean ($\overline{X}$), subtract this value from each individual score to obtain deviation scores (x), square the deviation scores (x^2), and then sum the squares within each group (Σx^2). In our example, the sum of the squared within-group deviation scores is 20.0 for Group 1, 10.0 for Group 2, and 16.0 for Group 3. Then, the summed, squared deviations for each group are added to yield the value for SS_W. Here, SS_W = 46.0 (20.0 + 10.0 + 16.0).

The **sum of squares-between** or SS_B (shown in panel B of Table 7.2) captures variation of the group means relative to the grand mean—that is, between-groups variability. SS_B is obtained by subtracting the value of the grand mean ($\overline{X}_G$) from each group mean ($\overline{X}$) and then squaring this deviation score (x_G^2). In our example, the mean of 3.0 for Group 1 is subtracted from the grand mean of 4.0, and then the deviation score (-1.0) is squared to yield 1.0. We need a between-group value for each person, so this value must be multiplied by group size (here n = 5), to yield 5.0. When the same process is carried out for each group, the values are added together to obtain the sum of squares—between. In this example, SS_B = 70.0 (5.0 + 20.0 + 45.0).

Although the **total sum of squares** (SS_T) is not needed to compute the F statistic, it is useful to see that SS_W and SS_B, when added, comprise total variability in the

TABLE 7.2 Stress Scores in Three Groups: Computation of the F Statistic

A. Deviations from Group Means (Within-Groups Variation)

Group 1 Music Therapy			Group 2 Relaxation Therapy			Group 3 Controls		
X	$X - \bar{X}_1$	x_1^2	X	$X - \bar{X}_2$	x_2^2	X	$X - \bar{X}_3$	x_3^2
0	−3	9	1	−1	1	5	−2	4
6	3	9	4	2	4	6	−1	1
2	−1	1	3	1	1	10	3	9
4	1	1	2	0	0	8	1	1
3	0	0	0	−2	4	6	−1	1
$\bar{X} = 3.0$			2.0			7.0		

$\Sigma x^2 =$ 20.0   10.0   16.0

Grand Mean $(\bar{X}_G) = 4.0$

$SS_W = 46.0$

B. Deviation of Group Means from Grand Mean (Between-Groups Variation)

$\bar{X}$	$\bar{X} - \bar{X}_G$	x_G^2	n	$(x_G^2 \times n)$
3.0	−1	1	5	5.0
2.0	−2	4	5	20.0
7.0	3	9	5	45.0
$\bar{X}_G = 4.0$				$SS_B = 70.0$

C. Deviations from Grand Mean (Total Variation)

X	$X - \bar{X}_G$	x_G^2
0	−4	16
6	2	4
2	−2	4
4	0	0
3	−1	1
1	−3	9
4	0	0
3	−1	1
2	−2	4
0	−4	16
5	1	1
6	2	4
10	6	36
8	4	16
6	2	4
$\bar{X}_G = 4.0$		$SS_T = 116.0$

D. F Ratio

$SS_B = 70.0$ $df_B = 2$ $MS_B = 35.0$
$SS_W = 46.0$ $df_W = 12$ $MS_W = 3.83$
$SS_T = 116.0$

$F = 35.0 \div 3.83 = 9.13$

distribution of sample scores. Panel C of Table 7.2 shows the calculation of SS_T, which captures the variation of all individual scores relative to the grand mean. The grand mean $(\bar{X}_G)$ is first subtracted from each of the 15 scores, these deviation scores are squared, and then the sum across participants is computed. In our example, $SS_T = 116.0$. Total variability has been partitioned into a between component and a within component, as follows:

$$SS_W + SS_B = SS_T$$
$$46.0 + 70.0 = 116.0$$

We now have almost everything needed to compute the F statistic. The formula for F is as follows:

$$F = \frac{SS_B/df_B}{SS_W/df_W}$$

General Linear Model

A

Tests of Within-Subjects Effects

Measure: Heart Rate

Source		Type III Sum of Squares	df	Mean Square	F	Sig.
Factor1	Sphericity assumed	1896.000	2	948.000	56.674	.000
	Greenhouse-Geisser	1896.000	1.371	1383.060	56.674	.000
	Huynh-Feldt	1896.000	1.501	1263.406	56.674	.000
	Lower-bound	1896.000	1.000	1896.000	56.674	.000
Error (Factor1)	Sphericity assumed	368.000	22	16.727		
	Greenhouse-Geisser	368.000	15.080	24.404		
	Huynh-Feldt	368.000	16.508	22.293		
	Lower-bound	368.000	11.000	33.455		

Estimated Marginal Means

B

1. Grand Mean

Measure: Heart Rate

Mean	Std. Error	95% CI	
		Lower Bound	Upper Bound
160.000	4.388	150.343	169.657

2. Factor1

Measure: Heart Rate

Factor1	Mean	Std. Error	95% CI	
			Lower Bound	Upper Bound
1	153.000	3.776	144.689	161.311
2	157.000	4.187	147.785	166.215
3	170.000	5.363	158.197	181.803

FIGURE 7.5   Selected portions of an SPSS printout for a one-way RM-ANOVA.

grand mean ($\overline{X}_G = 160.000$) with its standard error and 95% CI, followed by the same information for the mean heart rates for the three treatment conditions.

Example of a one-way RM-ANOVA:

Skybo and Buck (2007) gathered data on children's stress and coping four times over the course of a school year (October, February, March, and April) to examine patterns of change in relation to standardized testing. The researchers used repeated measures ANOVA to test changes in mean scores over time, and found numerous significant changes. For example, number of stress symptoms increased from October to 1 month before testing (February), but then declined in March.

OTHER STATISTICAL ISSUES RELATING TO ANOVA

As with *t*-tests, ANOVA addresses the very important question of whether or not a relationship exists between the independent and dependent variables. In this section, we discuss other related analyses that address questions about the nature of the relationship, precision of estimates, magnitude of effects, and the power of the statistical test.

The Nature of the Relationship: Multiple Comparisons

The *F* test for analysis of variance considers the null hypothesis of equality of means against the alternative that not all the population means are equal. The rejection of the null indicates the probability that there is a relationship between the independent and dependent variable—that is, that the population means are unequal. A significant *F* test does not, however, tell us which pairs of means are significantly different from one another. To determine the exact nature of the relationship between the independent and dependent variables, additional analyses are necessary.

A number of alternative tests—called **multiple comparison procedures**—can be used to compare pairs of means. These procedures are preferable to using multiple *t* tests because they offer better protection against the risk of a Type I error (i.e., an incorrect inference that differences between pairs of means are significant). Among the most widely-used multiple comparison tests are the **Scheffé test, Tukey's honestly significant difference (HSD) test, Duncan's multiple-range test**, and **Fisher's least significant difference (LSD) test.** There is some controversy among statisticians regarding which test has the greatest accuracy, but a full discussion of the merits and shortcomings of the alternatives is beyond the scope of this book. A frequent choice among nurse researchers, and the one that Jaccard and Becker (2001) recommend, is Tukey's HSD test.

TIP: *The multiple comparison procedures discussed here are called* **post hoc tests** *or* **a posteriori comparisons,** *which are comparisons completed after a full ANOVA. Researchers sometimes decide in advance which specific pairs of means they want to compare—they have a substantive interest in comparing certain groups, prior to learning what the data look like. In this situation, they might use* **a priori comparisons,** *which are also called* **planned comparisons.** *The advantage of planned comparisons is that they increase the power and precision of the data analysis. Planned comparisons can be performed in SPSS within the Oneway and GLM procedures.*

For manual computations, however, the simplest multiple comparison method is Fisher's LSD test, also called the **protected *t* test.** When an ANOVA *F* test is statistically significant, pairs of means can be compared by *t* tests that use the MS_W term from ANOVA as the estimate of the population variance. To illustrate, we will use our earlier example for one-way ANOVA, which compared mean stress scores for three groups of MI patients (a music therapy group, relaxation therapy group, and a control group). In this example, we rejected the null hypothesis that all the population means were equal, so we can proceed to compare the three pairs of means using protected t tests. The following are the three null and alternative hypotheses being tested via the multiple comparisons:

$$H_0: \mu_1 = \mu_2 \quad H_1: \mu_1 \neq \mu_2$$
$$H_0: \mu_1 = \mu_3 \quad H_1: \mu_1 \neq \mu_3$$
$$H_0: \mu_2 = \mu_3 \quad H_1: \mu_2 \neq \mu_3$$

The formula for Fisher's LSD test (here, using notation for the first null hypothesis) is as follows:

$$t = \frac{\overline{X}_1 - \overline{X}_2}{\sqrt{MS_W \left(\dfrac{1}{n_1} + \dfrac{1}{n_2} \right)}}$$

where $\overline{X}_1, \overline{X}_2$ = means for Groups 1 and 2

MS_W = mean square within, from ANOVA

n_1, n_2 = number of cases for Groups 1 and 2

We can illustrate with the calculation of a protected t for one of the three pairs of means in our stress intervention example—the music therapy group ($\overline{X}_1 = 3.0$) and the control group ($\overline{X}_3 = 7.0$). Using the value of MS_W computed earlier (3.83), we find that the value of the protected t is as follows:

$$t = \frac{3.0 - 7.0}{\sqrt{3.83 \left(\dfrac{1}{5} + \dfrac{1}{5} \right)}} = -3.23$$

Although we do not show the other calculations, the computed values of protected t for the other two pairs are 0.81 ($\overline{X}_1$ versus $\overline{X}_2$), and -4.04 ($\overline{X}_2$ versus $\overline{X}_3$). To find the critical value in the t table, we need to compute the degrees of freedom, which is: $df_W = N - k$. In our present example, then, $df = 12$ (15 − 3). Consulting Table A.2 of Appendix A, we find that the critical value of t for $df = 12$ and $\alpha = .05$ is 2.18. Thus, the difference between the means of Groups 1 and 3, *and* the difference between the means of Groups 2 and 3, are statistically significant. Both therapies resulted in significantly lower stress scores than the absence of a therapy (i.e., the control condition). The means for the two types of therapy were not significantly different.

When group sample sizes are equal, as they are in this example, it is possible to determine what least significant difference (*LSD*) between means is needed for significance, using the following formula:

$$LSD = t_{\text{tabled}} \sqrt{MS_W (2 \div n)}$$

Thus, in our example:

$$LSD = 2.18 \sqrt{3.83(.40)} = 2.70$$

All pairs of means differing by at least 2.70 points on the stress scale would be significantly different from one another at $\alpha = .05$.

Protected t tests can also be used in factorial designs when there are significant F tests that require clarification. Of course, when the design is 2×2, such as the example we presented in this chapter (type of treatment × time of treatment), there is no need to clarify the nature of effect for the two factors: if the F test for a factor is significant, then the two levels of the factor are significantly different. A significant interaction such as we observed in our example *does,* however, require clarification. The issue is determining significant differences between the cell means (combinations of the two factors). We can use the previously presented formula to compute the *LSD*. Although we do not show the computations, the value for MS_W is 2.63, and, for $df = 16$ (20 subjects minus 4 cells) and $\alpha = .05$, the critical (tabled) value of t is 2.12. Thus:

$$LSD = 2.12\sqrt{2.63(.40)} = 2.17$$

The *LSD* indicates that all differences between cell means that are greater than or equal to 2.17 are significant at the .05 level. Referring back to Table 7.3, we find that only one pair of cell means is significantly different: In the evening only, music therapy is significantly different from relaxation therapy. The mean difference of 3.0 between these two cell means $(4.0 - 1.0)$ exceeds the *LSD* of 2.17.

When computers are used to perform the multiple comparisons, researchers can run several alternative multiple comparison tests. Within SPSS, there are over 10 options, including some that can be used when the homogeneity of variance assumption is violated. Figure 7.6 shows the SPSS printout (created within the Oneway procedure) for two tests, Tukey's HSD and the LSD tests. Both tests resulted in the same conclusions: Mean stress scores in both the music therapy and the relaxation therapy were significantly different from those in the control group, but were not significantly different from each other. Note, however, that the actual p values do differ. For example, for the music therapy–control comparison, $p = .018$ for the Tukey test, but $p = .007$ for the LSD test. Tukey's HSD test is more conservative

Multiple Comparisons

Dependent Variable: Stress Scores

	(I) Experimental Group	(J) Experimental Group	Mean Difference (I-J)	Std. Error	Sig.	95% Confidence Interval Lower Bound	95% Confidence Interval Upper Bound
Tukey HSD	Music Therapy	Relaxation Therapy	1.000	1.238	.706	−2.30	4.30
		Control Group	−4.000*	1.238	.018	−7.30	−.70
	Relaxation Therapy	Music Therapy	−1.000	1.238	.706	−4.30	2.30
		Control Group	−5.000*	1.238	.004	−8.30	−1.70
	Control Group	Music Therapy	4.000*	1.238	.018	.70	7.30
		Relaxation Therapy	5.000*	1.238	.004	1.70	8.30
LSD	Music Therapy	Relaxation Therapy	1.000	1.238	.435	−1.70	3.70
		Control Group	−4.000*	1.238	.007	−6.70	−1.30
	Relaxation Therapy	Music Therapy	−1.000	1.238	.435	−3.70	1.70
		Control Group	−5.000*	1.238	.002	−7.70	−2.30
	Control Group	Music Therapy	4.000*	1.238	.007	1.30	6.70
		Relaxation Therapy	5.000*	1.238	.002	2.30	7.70

* The mean difference is significant at the 0.05 level.

FIGURE 7.6 SPSS printout for two multiple comparison tests.

in that probability values are higher, making it more difficult to reject the null hypothesis than when LSD is used, but the HSD test has more desirable statistical properties.

> **TIP:** *A useful concept in statistical analysis is called* **sensitivity testing.** *These are analyses designed to assess the impact of different assumptions or different analytic approaches, to see if conclusions are altered—that is, to see whether decisions are* sensitive *to different approaches. So, for example, one could use different post hoc procedures to see if results are robust to alternative methods.*

Example of multiple comparisons:

Park, Jarrett, Cain, and Heitkemper (2008) compared three groups of women with irritable bowel syndrome who differed in terms of severity of bloating (minimal, mild, and moderate-severe). The groups were compared in terms of symptoms of psychological distress, using one-way ANOVAs. When significant *F*s were obtained, Tukey's HSD test was used for pair-wise comparisons.

Precision of Estimates: Confidence Intervals

When multiple means are being compared, as is the case in ANOVA, confidence intervals can be built around individual means, as shown in the SPSS printout in Figures 7.2, 7.4, and 7.5. More useful information about precision, however, is obtained by constructing *CI*s around the mean differences for pairs of means. Figure 7.6 shows that when multiple comparison tests are performed within SPSS, *CI*s are constructed around differences in means, with a 95% *CI* being the default. As with *t* tests, an interval that includes 0.0 is not statistically significant at the corresponding α level— here at .05. Note that the confidence limits vary depending on which test is used. The 95% *CI* around the mean difference between music and relaxation therapy was -2.30 to 4.30 for the Tukey HSD test, but from -1.70 to 3.70 for the LSD test. Therefore, if *CI*s are reported, you need to indicate the underlying test used to calculate the confidence limits.

The Magnitude of the Relationship: Eta-Squared

As noted in Chapter 6, statistical significance does not necessarily mean a powerful relationship between the independent and dependent variables. When researchers wish to determine the magnitude of a relationship in the context of an ANOVA situation, the effect size index most often used for the overall effect is **eta-squared.** Although Greek letters are typically used in statistics to designate population parameters, an exception is eta-squared, which is most often indicated in research reports as η^2.

Eta-squared can be computed from the components for the *F* formula. For a one-way analysis of variance:

$$\eta^2 = \frac{SS_B}{SS_T}$$

From this formula, we can see that η^2 represents the proportion of the total variability in a set of scores that is attributable to the independent variable (i.e., variability between groups). It may be recalled from Chapter 4 that the correlation coefficient *r*, when squared, represents the proportion of variability in the dependent variable explained by the independent variable, and thus r^2 and η^2 are conceptually equivalent.

For our example that compared stress scores for three groups of MI patients (music therapy, relaxation therapy, controls), we can compute the following:

$$\eta^2 = \frac{70.0}{116.0} = .60$$

This is a powerful relationship: 60% of the variability in stress scores is attributable to the different treatments. It is unusual to find a value of η^2 this high in actual intervention studies, but our example was deliberately contrived to yield significant results. With a small N (again, deliberately small to minimize computational complexity), a strong relationship was needed to achieve statistical significance. (In SPSS, η^2 is computed when one-way ANOVA is performed using the "Compare Means" procedure, but not in the "Oneway" procedure.)

Computing eta-squared for a multifactor ANOVA is similar to procedures just described: The sum of squares attributable to the factor (or interaction) of interest is contrasted with the total sum of squares. Eta^2 can be calculated by SPSS within a multifactor ANOVA using the general linear model (GLM) routine, which was used to create Figure 7.4. In the example that compared stress scores for music versus relaxation therapies administered in the morning or evening, η^2 for the type of therapy factor was .106, that for time of therapy administration was .000, while that for the interaction was .323 (not shown in Figure 7.4).

For a one-way repeated measures ANOVA, the formula for computing eta-squared is as follows:

$$\eta^2 = \frac{S_{treatments}}{SS_{treatments} + SS_{error}}$$

Eta-squared in the context of a one-way RM-ANOVA represents the proportion of variability in the dependent variable attributable to the independent variable *after variability associated with individual differences has been removed.* In our example of the one-way RM-ANOVA, which involved assigning infants to different ordering of three different interventions (Table 7.3), we find that:

$$\eta^2 = \frac{1896.0}{1896.0 + 368.0} = .84$$

This tells us that 84% of the variability in the infants' heart rates is attributable to the different conditions, after the influence of individual differences in heart rates is removed.

As was true in the *t*-test situation, Cohen (1988) has established some guidelines for qualitatively describing effect sizes in an ANOVA context. Cohen's conventional values for small, medium, and large effects correspond to values of eta-squared of .01, .06, and .14, respectively.

Information about the magnitude of the relationship provides valuable information for interpreting the results of an ANOVA. However, the eta-squared index is almost never used in meta-analyses. The problem with eta-squared in the context of a meta-analysis is that this effect size index tells us nothing about the *nature* of the group differences—that is, which pairs of means are different. A more usual procedure is to calculate *d* statistics for the paired comparisons of interest (Cooper, 2010).

Example of eta-squared:

Oostrom and van Mierlo (2008) evaluated an aggression management training program for healthcare workers to help them cope with workplace violence. Participants' scores on various outcomes, including ability to cope with adverse working situations, were obtained before training, after training, and 5 weeks later. Using RM-ANOVA, improvement over time was found to be significant, and η^2 was .67.

Power Analysis for ANOVA

As discussed in Chapter 6, power analysis is used to estimate the probability of correctly rejecting the null hypothesis. When used during the design phase of a study, power analysis helps researchers to make sample size decisions to minimize the risk of a Type II error. When applied after a study is completed, power analysis can sometimes help in interpreting results, particularly if group differences were not statistically significant.

There are alternative methods of doing a power analysis in an ANOVA context. The simplest approach involves estimating the population effect size η^2 (e.g., from prior research or a pilot study). In this situation, with effect size estimated, and the desired power (usually .80) and alpha (usually .05) specified, power analysis solves for the fourth component, sample size. When power analysis is performed following ANOVA for interpretive purposes, the η^2 from the study itself is used as the population estimate of effect size, and the power analysis solves for power.

To illustrate a post hoc power analysis to estimate power for a one-way ANOVA, let us use our example of stress scores in three treatment groups. The η^2 (effect size) for the data shown in Table 7.2 was found to be .60, and the number of participants per group was five. Table 7.5, which is appropriate when $\alpha = .05$ and the number of groups is 3, allows us to estimate power. The top row presents estimates of the population eta^2. Reading down in the column headed by .60, we look for the group size of five, and then read across to the left to find the estimate of power in the first column. Although the group size of five does not appear in the table, we can interpolate: five falls between four and six, so power is between the corresponding power values of .95 and .99. The power analysis suggests, then, that the estimated risk of having committed a Type II error in this study was less than 5%—well below the standardly acceptable risk of 20%.

TABLE 7.5 Power Table for One-Way Between-Groups ANOVA, for $\alpha = .05$—Three Groups

Power	Population Eta-Squared													
	.01	.03	.05	.07	.10	.15	.20	.25	.30	.40	.50	.60	.70	.80
.10	22	8	5	4	3	2	2	2	—	—	—	—	—	—
.25	76	26	16	9	7	5	4	3	—	—	—	—	—	—
.50	165	55	32	23	16	10	8	6	5	3	3	2	2	—
.70	255	84	50	35	24	16	11	9	7	5	4	3	2	2
.80	319	105	62	44	30	19	14	11	9	6	4	3	2	2
.90	417	137	81	57	39	25	18	14	11	7	5	4	3	2
.95	511	168	99	69	47	30	22	16	13	9	6	4	3	2
.99	708	232	137	96	65	41	29	22	18	12	8	6	4	3

NOTE: Entries in body of table are for *n*, the number of participants *per group*.

To use Table 7.5 to estimate sample size needs, you would enter the table at the row for the desired power (usually .80, which is shaded) and the column for the estimated value of η^2. The value at the intersection indicates the needed sample size per group. For example, if the estimated η^2 were .10, 30 people per group would be needed to achieve a power of .80.

When there is limited evidence about effect size values, researchers sometimes use Cohen's guidelines for small, medium, and large effect sizes as a last resort. As was true in the *t*-test situation, we think it is prudent to expect no larger than a small-to-moderate effect size in nursing studies, unless there is good evidence to suggest a larger effect. A small-to-moderate effect would correspond to an η^2 between .01 and .06, i.e., about .04. Our effect size of .60 in the stress-reduction intervention example, as noted, resulted from contrived data values that were designed to yield a significant result with small *n*s. In real situations, an effect size this large would be extremely unlikely.

When there are 4, 5, or 6 independent groups, the power tables in Appendix B, Table B.2 should be used, and power tables for RM-ANOVA for 3, 4, or 5 measurements of the same people are presented in Table B.3. In other situations (e.g., when alpha is not .05, or when the design calls for a two-way ANOVA), the power tables in Cohen (1988) or Jaccard and Becker (2001) can be consulted, or you can use specialized power software or interactive Internet sites to perform the calculations.

RESEARCH APPLICATIONS OF ANOVA

This section briefly reviews some of the major applications of ANOVA, and presents methods of reporting ANOVA results in research reports.

The Uses of ANOVA

The main uses of ANOVA are, not surprisingly, analogous to those of the *t* test, as reviewed in the previous chapter. We briefly illustrate these applications here.

1. *Answering research questions*   Many substantive research questions can be directly answered using ANOVA, as we have shown in the actual examples in this chapter. Research applications for ANOVA are diverse both substantively and methodologically. ANOVA can be used to test differences in means for individuals allocated to different treatments (i.e., in RCTs or quasi-experimental studies), as well as in studies with three or more groups formed nonexperimentally. It can also be used for both within-subjects and between-subjects designs.

2. *Testing biases*   As noted in Chapter 6, researchers often make group comparisons to determine the existence and extent of any biases that could affect the interpretation of the results. Selection biases—group differences resulting from extraneous characteristics rather than from the effect of the independent variable—are among the most worrisome and most frequently tested. For example, Webb (2008) studied the effect of participation in focus groups on low-income African-American's smokers' willingness to participate in smoking intervention studies. She compared participants in the 10 focus groups in terms of such baseline characteristics as number of years smoking and number of cigarettes smoked per day, using one-way ANOVA. Whenever there are more than two groups to compare, ANOVA can also be used to test for other biases discussed in Chapter 6.

3. *Assessing the construct validity of instruments*   ANOVA can be used in conjunction with the known-groups technique to examine the construct validity of instruments, if three or more known groups are being compared. For example,

Salamonson, Everett, Koch, Andrew, and Davidson (2008) undertook a validation study of the English Language Acculturation Scale (ELAS), which is a measure of English-language acculturation. They created three groups of nursing students based on ELAS scores (low, moderate, and high scores), and used ANOVA to test differences in mean grades in four academic subjects among the three groups. The F tests were significant, and Tukey's HSD test revealed that grade differences were especially pronounced among those with low versus high scores on the ELAS. These hypothesis-confirming analyses supported the construct validity of the ELAS.

The Presentation of ANOVA Results in Research Reports

As with t tests, ANOVA results are usually reported in the text alone if there are only one or two F tests. Within the text, it is usual to report the name of the test (F), degrees of freedom, the calculated value of F, and the p value, as in the following example from our one-way ANOVA: $F(2, 12) = 9.13, p < .001$. If there are numerous tests—or if the test is for a complex multifactor design—a table is an efficient way to summarize the results. The text can then be used to highlight the most important features of the table.

Two alternative table styles are often used for reporting ANOVAs. One approach is similar to the table style used for t tests: The table reports the means, SDs, and ns for the groups being compared, as well as the value of F for each group comparison with the associated probability level. Values for η^2 can also be shown, as shown in the example of an ANOVA table in Table 7.6. This table summarizes the results of an experimental study in which three treatment groups were compared with respect to pain control procedures following coronary surgery. The table shows means and SDs for the three groups, F statistics, p values, and η^2 for three pain-related procedure outcomes. According to this table, two of the three ANOVAs were statistically significant beyond the .05 level, but the F value for the first outcome (number of turns) was not significant.

An alternative is to present a full ANOVA summary table such as the one in Table 7.7, which summarizes the results of our 2×2 ANOVA example on stress scores. We have added a fictitious second outcome measure (coping scale scores) to illustrate how information for two outcomes can be presented in the same table. The summary table shows values for sums of squares, degrees of freedom, mean squares, and F statistics for main effects and interactions for both dependent variables. This approach is especially likely to be used in a multifactor ANOVA, because it is a convenient presentation of F tests for all factors and interactions. When such a table is used to summarize ANOVAs, however, a separate table is needed to show means and

TABLE 7.6 Example of a Table for One-Way ANOVA Results

Pain-related Outcomes	Air Mattress Group ($n = 50$)		Mattress + Exercise Group ($n = 50$)		Control Group ($n = 50$)		F	p	η^2
	M	SD	M	SD	M	SD			
Number of turns	7.0	3.2	5.9	3.9	6.9	3.4	1.96	.23	.003
Number of times acetaminophen given	1.6	1.1	0.7	0.6	1.5	1.4	5.01	.007	.024
Number of times other medications given	0.6	1.6	0.6	1.1	1.4	1.7	3.27	.04	.014

Pain Control Procedures for Coronary Surgery Patients, by Treatment Group: ANOVA Results

TABLE 7.7 Example of an ANOVA Summary Table for a Two-Way ANOVA

Outcome and Source of Variation	Sum of Squares	df	Mean Square	F	p
Stress Scale Scores					
Between groups	5.00	1	5.00	1.91	.19
Type of Treatment	0.00	1	0.00	0.00	1.00
Time of Treatment	20.00	1	20.00	7.62	.01
Type % Time Interaction	42.00	16	2.63		
Within	67.00	19	3.53		
Total					
Coping Scale Scores					
Between groups					
Type of Treatment	54.00	1	54.00	6.08	.03
Time of Treatment	27.00	1	27.00	3.04	.23
Type % Time Interaction	35.00	1	35.00	3.94	.20
Within	142.00	16	8.88		
Total	258.00	19	13.58		

*SD*s. In Table 7.7, for example, there is a significant group difference for treatment type on the Coping Scale, but we cannot tell from the table whether the coping scores were better in the Music Therapy or the Relaxation Therapy group.

When ANOVA information is presented in tables, the text can be used to emphasize the main features. Here is an example of how the results from Table 7.7 could be presented in the body of the report (we have added some information about the direction of differences for the Coping Scale):

> A two-way ANOVA was used to examine differences in the effects of the two treatments and two administration times on patients' self-reported stress levels and ability to cope. ANOVA results, shown in Table 7.7, indicated that the time factor had no independent effect on scores on either the Stress or Coping scales. There was, however, a significant type-by-time of treatment interaction for the Stress Scale: In the evening only, Music Therapy resulted in significantly lower stress scores than Relaxation Therapy, $F(1, 16) = 7.62$, $p = .01$. Type of treatment, by itself, had no significant effect on stress scores. With respect to coping, it was found that, across both time periods, patients in the Music Therapy group scored significantly more favorably than those in the Relaxation Therapy group, $F(1,16) = 6.08$, $p < .05$. Time of treatment was unrelated to coping scores.

The text can also be used to expand on information that is less conveniently presented in tables. For example, the results of multiple comparison tests that isolate the group comparisons responsible for a significant F are often presented in the text, although tables may also be used, as we shall see in the next section. If a power analysis has been performed to help interpret nonsignificant results, information on the estimated power usually is reported in the Discussion section of the report.

Graphs are a good way to call attention to significant interactions in multifactor ANOVA. Figure 7.7, created within SPSS in the General Linear Model procedure, presents a graph showing the type-of-treatment by time interaction from our two-way ANOVA example. Graphic displays can also be effective in displaying

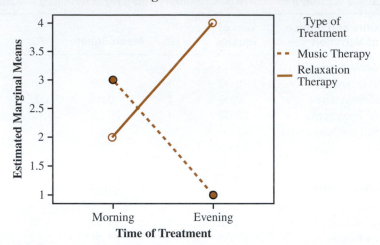

FIGURE 7.7   Graphic display for a two-way ANOVA: SPSS output.

means from an RM-ANOVA, especially for highlighting time trends if the same people have been measured at three or more points in time.

TIP: *Be sure to include sufficient information in your report so that future researchers can include your results in a meta-analysis. Even if you include information about eta-squared, be sure to report means and SDs for key outcomes so that estimated values for* d *can be computed.*

Research Example

The results of a nursing study that used ANOVAs and multiple comparison procedures are summarized here to further illustrate the use of ANOVA to address research questions.

Study: "Association of adolescent physical and emotional health with perceived severity of parental substance abuse" (Gance-Cleveland, Mays, & Steffen, 2008).

Study Purpose: The purpose of this study was to examine the relationship between indicators of adolescent health, and the adolescents' perception of the severity of parental substance abuse.

Methods: The study used data collected at baseline from a group of high school students who were participating in an intervention study for students with one or more substance-abusing family member. A sample of 121 students was recruited from a school-based health center. The data collected at baseline included scores on a 30-item scale (CAST) that measures existence and severity of substance-abuse problems in the family. Students were divided into three groups on the basis of total CAST scores, and this grouping variable was the independent variable in the ANOVA: Low severity ($n = 11$), moderate severity ($n = 35$), and high severity ($n = 75$). Students also completed the Health and Daily Living Inventory for Youth (HDLI-Y) scale, which provided information about the students' health in the prior 3 months. The inventory yields scores on nine subscales, including medical conditions, physical symptoms, positive and negative mood, and five social adjustment scales (e.g., health risk behavior, social integration).

TABLE 7.8 Self-Reported Health of High School Students, by Perceived Severity of Parental Substance Abuse

Health & Daily Living Inventory-Youth (HDLI-Y) Subscale	Severity of Parental Substance Abuse					Paired Comparisons[a]		
	Low M (SD) $n = 11$	Moderate M (SD) $n = 35$	High M (SD) $n = 75$	F	p	L-M	L-H	M-H
Medical conditions	1.27 (1.10)	1.80 (1.02)	2.43 (1.20)	7.08	.001	—	**	*
Physical symptoms	7.45 (3.42)	11.23 (3.56)	14.24 (4.19)	17.80	<.001	***	***	*
Negative mood	5.91 (2.12)	7.74 (3.33)	10.99 (3.50)	18.39	<.001	—	***	***
Positive mood	13.55 (3.01)	12.71 (3.04)	11.23 (3.60)	3.75	.03	—	—	—

[a]Significance levels for Tukey's HSD test comparing low-moderate (L-M), low-high (L-H), and moderate-high (M-H) paired comparisons: * $p < .05$, ** $p < .01$, *** $p < .001$

Adapted from information in Table 2 and in the report text of Gance-Cleveland et al., 2008.

Analysis: One-way ANOVA was used to compare the three student groups with regard to means on the nine subscales of the HDLI-Y. Significant F tests were followed by pairwise comparisons using Tukey's test, with α set at .05. The researchers noted that the test for equality of variances was nonsignificant, which is important given the unequal sizes of the three groups.

Results: The ANOVAs indicated significant group differences for four of the HDLI-Y subscales: medical conditions, physical symptoms, negative mood, and positive mood. Table 7.8 summarizes the ANOVA results (to conserve space, we show only the subscales with significant results—in the report the table summarized all F tests).

For all four outcomes, adolescents in the high severity group had the least favorable outcomes. Table 7.8 also summarizes results from Tukey's HSD test, displaying significance levels comparing low-moderate, low-high, and moderate-high pairings. It shows that the high severity group differed significantly from both the low severity and moderate severity groups on all but the positive mood scale. The low and moderate severity groups differed from each other only with regard to physical symptoms. The table also shows a seemingly anomalous result: Despite the overall significant F for the positive mood subscale, no paired comparisons were significantly different. This likely reflects the smaller ns in the paired comparisons.

Summary Points

- **Analysis of variance (ANOVA)** is used to draw inferences about population means when there are more than two means being compared. Assumptions for basic ANOVA are analogous to those for the t test—i.e., random sampling from the population, a normal distribution for the dependent variables in the population, and equality of group variances.
- ANOVA tests the null hypothesis that the population means are equal against the alternative hypothesis that an inequality of population means exists.
- ANOVA involves the **partitioning of variance** of the dependent variable into the components that contribute to score variability.

- In its most basic form, ANOVA contrasts **between-group variance** (variability from group differences) to **within-group variance** (variability among participants within groups).
- The ratio of the two sources of variation yields a statistic—the **F ratio**—that can be compared to tabled values for F distributions.
- To compute an F ratio, the **sum of squares** (sum of squared deviations about a mean) for each source of variation is divided by its respective degrees of freedom, to yield a **mean square,** which is essentially a variance. Then, the mean square between groups (MS_B) is divided by the mean square within groups (MS_W) to arrive at the F ratio.

- Analysis of variance can be used in a variety of circumstances. A **one-way ANOVA** is used to compare means for three or more independent groups.
- A **multifactor ANOVA** is used when there are two or more independent variables, called **factors** in this context. The most common multifactor ANOVA is a **two-way ANOVA.** Multifactor ANOVA tests for both **main effects** (i.e., the effects of the independent variables on the dependent variable) and **interaction effects** (i.e., the effects of the independent variables in combination).
- **Repeated measures analysis of variance (RM-ANOVA)** is used for within-subjects designs, when means are computed for the *same* people three or more times. Additional assumptions for RM-ANOVA include **compound symmetry** and **sphericity.** These assumptions are usually tested with **Mauchly's test for sphericity.** Adjustments to degrees of freedom are used when sphericity is violated.
- If an ANOVA yields a significant *F,* **multiple comparison procedures** (**post hoc tests**) must be performed to determine the *nature* of the relationship between the independent and dependent variable. There are several alternative procedures, such as **Tukey's HSD test** and **Fisher's *LSD* test** (the **protected *t* test**), that help to identify the group differences that contributed to the significant *F* statistic.
- An effect size statistic called **eta-squared** (η^2) can be computed to estimate the strength of the relationship between the independent and dependent variables in ANOVA. This statistic indicates the proportion of variability in a dependent variable accounted for by the independent variable.
- Eta-squared is used as the estimate of effect size in power analyses for an ANOVA situation.

Exercises

The following exercises cover concepts presented in this chapter. Appendix C provides answers to Part A exercises that are indicated with a dagger (†). Exercises in Part B involve computer analyses using the datasets provided with this textbook, and answers and comments are offered on this book's Web site.

PART A EXERCISES

† **A1.** For each of the following situations, indicate whether ANOVA is appropriate; if not appropriate, the reason why not; and, if appropriate, the type of ANOVA that would be used (i.e., one-way, repeated measures, etc.):

    (a) The independent variable (IV) is age group—people in their 60s, 70s, and 80s; the dependent variable (DV) is health-related hardiness, as measured on a 20-item scale.

    (b) The IVs are ethnicity (white, African American, Hispanic, Asian) and birthweight status (< 2,500 grams versus 2,500 grams); the DV is serum bilirubin levels.

    (c) The IV is maternal breastfeeding status (breastfeeds versus does not breastfeed); the DV is maternal bonding with infant, as measured on a 10-item self-report scale.

    (d) The IV is exposure to a special intervention (before versus after exposure); the DV is myocardial oxygen consumption.

    (e) The IV is length of gestation (preterm versus term versus postterm birth); the DV is epidural anesthesia during labor (yes versus no).

    (f) The IV is time since diagnosis of multiple sclerosis (1 month versus 6 months versus 2 years); the DV is psychological adaptation to the disease, as measure by the Purpose-in-Life test.

† **A2.** Suppose we wanted to compare the somatic complaints (as measured on a scale known as the Physical Symptom Survey or PSS) of three groups of people: nonsmokers, smokers, and people who recently quit smoking. Using the following data for PSS scores, do a one-way ANOVA to test the hypothesis that the population means are equal:

Nonsmokers	Smokers	Quitters
19	26	37
23	29	32
17	22	27
20	30	41
26	23	38

What are the means for the three groups? Compute the sums of squares, degrees of freedom, and mean squares for these data. What is the value of *F*? Using an alpha of .05, is the *F* statistically significant?

† **A3.** Using the data from question A2, compute three protected *t* tests to compare all possible pairs of means. Also, for $\alpha = .05$, what is the value of *LSD*? Which pairs are significantly different from one another, using this multiple comparison procedure?

† **A4.** For the data in question A2, what is the value of η^2? What is the *approximate* estimated power for this ANOVA? Explain what the η^2 and estimated power indicate.

A5. Write a few sentences that could be used to describe the results of the analyses from questions 2–4.

† **A6.** For each of the following F values, indicate whether the F is statistically significant, at the specified alpha level:
  (a) $F = 2.80$, $df = 4, 40$, $\alpha = .01$
  (b) $F = 5.02$, $df = 3, 60$, $\alpha = .001$
  (c) $F = 3.45$, $df = 3, 27$, $\alpha = .05$
  (d) $F = 4.99$, $df = 2, 150$, $\alpha = .01$
  (e) $F = 2.09$, $df = 2, 250$, $\alpha = .05$

† **A7.** Suppose we were interested in studying the self-esteem of men versus women (Factor A) in two exercise status groups—nonexercisers versus exercisers, Factor B—with 20 people in each of the four groups. Use the following information to compute three F tests, and determine which, if any, is statistically significant at the .05 level:

Means: Male
  exercisers: 39.0   Male nonexercisers: 37.0
  Female
  exercisers: 34.0   Female nonexercisers: 29.0
  All exercisers: 36.5   All nonexercisers: 33.0
  All males: 38.0   All females: 31.5

Sums of Squares: $SS_T = 1,190.50$ $SS_W = 1,025.0$
  $SS_A = 74.50$ $SS_B = 37.0$ $SS_{AB} = 54.00$

A8. Interpret the meaning of the F tests from question A7. (Note: higher scores on the self-esteem scale mean higher self-esteem.) Write a few sentences summarizing the results.

† **A9.** Suppose we used a crossover design to test for differences in bruising from subcutaneous sodium heparin injections at three sites (arm, leg, and abdomen) in a sample of 15 medical–surgical patients. Surface area of the bruises (in mm^2) is measured 72 hours after each injection, which are administered to sites in random order at 8-hour intervals. Use the following information to compute the F statistic to determine if there were significant differences in bruising by site, at the .05 level:

Means: Arm: 212.0 mm^2 Leg: 99.0 mm^2
  Abdomen: 93.0 mm^2

Sums of Squares: $SS_{site} = 17,993.00$ $SS_{error} = 48,349.00$

† **A10.** Using Table 7.5 and Appendix Table B.2, estimate the sample sizes per group that would be estimated to achieve a power of .80 and an alpha of .05 for each of the following situations:
  (a) $\eta^2 = .25$, number of groups = 4
  (b) $\eta^2 = .10$, number of groups = 6
  (c) $\eta^2 = .04$, number of groups = 4
  (d) $\eta^2 = .15$, number of groups = 5
  (e) $\eta^2 = .40$, number of groups = 3

PART B EXERCISES

† **B1.** For these exercises, you will be using the SPSS dataset Polit2SetA, which contains a number of variables relating to material hardships and social–environmental health risks. Eight variables in this file (from *utilcut* to *badstove*, which are Variables #25–32) are responses to a series of questions about current housing problems for the women in this sample—for example, whether or not they had their utilities cut off, had vermin in the household, had unreliable heat, and so forth. The variable *housprob* (Variable #33) is a count of the total number of times the women said "yes" to these eight questions. We will use this variable to create groups of women with different numbers of housing problems, so begin by running basic descriptive statistics on *housprob,* using the SPSS Frequencies program with Descriptive Statistics, as described in previous chapters. Then answer these questions: (a) What is the range on this variable, and what is the minimum and maximum value? (b) What is the mean, median, and mode? (c) Comment on the symmetry/skewness of the distribution. (d) What percentage of women had zero problems? One problem? What does the frequency distribution suggest about forming groups on the basis of number of housing problems?

† **B2.** In this exercise, you will create a new variable (call it *hprobgrp*) that divides the sample into three groups based on number of housing problems. The new variable will be coded 1 for no housing problems, 2 for one housing problem, and 3 for two or more housing problems. Click Transform (upper tool bar) ➔ Recode ➔ Into Different Variables. This opens a dialog box where you can enter the variable *housprob* into the field for Numeric Variable. Then, on the right, type in the name of the new variable *hprobgrp,* and then click the pushbutton Change, which will insert the new variable into the first field. Now click on Old and New Values, which brings up a new dialog box. In the field for Old Value, enter 0 (zero problems), then on the right under New Value, type in 1 (for code 1 in the new variable), and click Add. Repeat this process, this time using the code of 1 for *housprob* and 2 for *hprobgrp,* and the click Add again. Finally, on the left click Range (for range of values), and enter 2 and 8—all codes between 2 and 8 for the variable *housprob*. Then enter 3 for New Variable, and click Add and then Continue. Then click OK, and the process is complete. The new variable will be added as the last variable in the file. Add labels for the codes to make reading output easier by clicking on the Variable View tab at the bottom of the screen. Then run Frequencies for *hprobgrp,* and determine how many women are in each of your three housing problems groups. Check to make sure you have correctly created the new variable by comparing the output with output from Exercise B1. Comment on how the distribution of values could affect decisions relating to the homogeneity of variance assumption for ANOVA.

† **B3.** Now run a one-way ANOVA with *hprobgrp* as the independent (group) variable, using the variable *satovrl* (overall satisfaction with material well-being, Variable #43) as the outcome variable. This variable is a summated rating scale variable for women's responses to their degree of satisfaction with four aspects of their material well-being—their housing, food, furniture, and clothing for themselves and

their children. Each item was coded from 1 (very dissatisfied) to 4 (very satisfied), so the overall score for the four items could range from a low of 4 (4 × 1) to 16 (4 × 4). To run the one-way analysis, click Analyze ➡ Compare Means ➡ Oneway. In the opening dialog box, move *satovrl* into the Dependent List, and *hprobgrp* into the slot for Factor. Click the Options pushbutton, and click Descriptives and Homogeneity of Variance, then Continue. Next, click the Post Hoc pushbutton and select LSD, Scheffe, and Tukey. Click Continue, then OK, and answer these questions: (a) What are the mean levels of satisfaction in the three groups? Which group is most dissatisfied? (b) Can the null hypothesis regarding equality of variances in the three populations be rejected? (c) What was the value of the F statistic that tested the equality of mean levels of satisfaction in the three groups? (d) What were the degrees of freedom? (e) What was the probability level for the F statistic? Can the null hypothesis for equality of means be rejected? (f) According to Tukey's HSD test, were any group means significantly different from any others? If yes, which ones? (g) Were our statistical decisions *sensitive* to the particular multiple comparison test we used? In other words, would we have come to different conclusions if we had used the Scheffe or LSD test?

† **B4.** Do another one-way ANOVA for the same independent variable (*hprobgrp*) and dependent variable (*satovrl*), this time using Analyze ➡ Compare Means ➡ Means. On the second dialog box, click the box for ANOVA table and eta. What is the value of eta-squared for this analysis? Would this be considered a small, moderate, or large effect? How would you interpret this effect size index?

† **B5.** For the next analysis, run a two-way ANOVA in which the dependent variable will again be *satovrl*, the women's overall degree of satisfaction with their material well-being. The two dichotomous independent variables will be whether or not the woman was working at the time of the interview (*worknow*, Variable #8) and whether or not she was receiving cash welfare assistance (*cashwelf*, Variable #19), both coded 1 for "yes" and 0 for "no." Run two-way ANOVA

through Analyze ➡ General Linear Model ➡ Univariate. In the opening dialog box, move *satovrl* into the Dependent List, and move *worknow* and *cashwelf* into the Fixed Factors list. Click the pushbutton for Model and unclick "Include intercept in model" at the bottom of the next dialog box. Then click Continue. Next, click the pushbutton Plots on the initial dialog box. Move *worknow* into the Horizontal Axis slot, and then move *cashwelf* into the Separate Lines slot. Click the Add pushbutton, then Continue. Next, click the Options pushbutton on the original dialog box and select the following options: Descriptives, Estimates of Effect Size, and Homogeneity Tests. Click Continue, then OK, and answer the following questions: (a) What are the null hypotheses being tested? (b) Which of the four groups created by the 2 × 2 design was, on average, least satisfied with their housing? How many women were in that group? (c) Which group was most satisfied? How many women were in that group? (d) Are the variances homogeneous? (e) In the ANOVA, which (if either) main effect was statistically significant? What were the probability levels? (f) What were the values of eta-squared for the main effects? How would you describe these effect sizes? (g) Was the interaction effect significant? What was the probability level for the interaction? Describe interaction effects as displayed on the Profile Plot.

† **B6.** Run one-way ANOVAs for two outcomes in the Polit2SetA dataset: overall satisfaction with material well-being, which is already completed if you did Exercise B1 (*satovrl*), and rating of neighborhood as a good place to live and raise children (*nabrqual*, Variable #18). Be sure to look in the codebook or in the file itself to see how *nabrqual* was coded. Use the variable created earlier for groups based on number of housing problems as the independent variable (i.e., *hprobgrp*). In the One-Way ANOVA procedure in SPSS, insert the two outcome variables in the list of Dependent Variables, and *hprobgrp* in the Factor slot. Use the SPSS Means procedure to determine values of eta-squared. When you have run these analyses, create a table to present your results, using Table 7.6 as a model. Then write a paragraph summarizing the results.

Chi-Square
and Nonparametric Tests

Thus far, we have discussed inferential statistical tests that are parametric. In this chapter we examine several nonparametric tests.

THE CHI-SQUARE TEST

The nonparametric test that researchers most often use is the **chi-square test**. The chi-square statistic is used in several applications, but we focus primarily on the most widely-used application known as the **chi-square test of independence** or **Pearson's chi-square**. This test is designed to make inferences about the existence of a relationship between two categorical variables that are crosstabulated in a contingency table (see Chapter 4).

    Suppose we wanted to examine whether there were differences in the rate of complications for patients receiving intravenous medications with a heparin lock in place, without changing it, for 72 hours versus 96 hours. Patients are randomly assigned to the two groups, and then the incidence of any complication (e.g., blocking, leaking, purulence, phlebitis, etc.) is recorded. Table 8.1 presents fictitious data for 100 patients (50 in each group), arrayed in a 2 × 2 contingency table. The table shows that there was a higher rate of complications in the 96-hour group (22%) than in the 72-hour group (18%). The research question is whether the observed group differences in the proportion of people with complications (the dependent variable) reflects the effect of length of time the heparin locks were in place (the independent variable), or whether differences reflect random sampling fluctuations. The chi-square test would be used to address this question.

TABLE 8.1 Hypothetical Data for Heparin Lock Chi-Square Example

Complication Incidence	Heparin Lock Placement Time Group		
	72 Hours	96 Hours	Total
Had Complications	9 (18.0%)	11 (22.0%)	20 (20.0%)
Had No Complications	41 (82.0%)	39 (78.0%)	80 (80.0%)
Total	50	50	100

The Null and Alternative Hypotheses for the Chi-Square Test

The null hypothesis for the chi-square test stipulates the absence of a relationship between the independent and dependent variable. The null hypothesis is stated in terms of the independence of the two variables. For our current example, the null and alternate hypotheses may be stated as follows:

H_0: Complication incidence and length of heparin lock placement are independent (not related)

H_1: Complication incidence and length of heparin lock placement are *not* independent (they *are* related)

Assumptions and Requirements for the Chi-Square Test

The chi-square test is used when both the independent and the dependent variable are measured on a nominal scale—that is, when variables can best be described through percentages, rather than means. Chi-square can also be used for ordinal-level variables if there are only a few categories (e.g., very low birthweight, low birthweight, normal birthweight). The chi-square test could also be applied to interval or ratio data that have been grouped into categories. For example, the variable age (a ratio-level variable) could be recoded as an ordinal-level variable with three categories: under 30, 30–39, and 40 or older. When researchers have interval-level or ratio-level data, however, it is often preferable to use more powerful parametric tests, such as ANOVA or a *t* test, with the raw ungrouped data.

Like parametric tests for between-subjects designs, the chi-square test assumes that the observations are randomly and independently sampled from the population of interest. Each participant must qualify for one and only one cell of the contingency table.

Unlike tests discussed in preceding chapters, the chi-square test does not make any assumption about the distribution of values in the population, nor about the homogeneity of group variances. One further issue, however, concerns sample size: Chi-square requires that the *expected frequency* of each cell in the contingency table be greater than zero. (Expected frequencies are explained later.) In fact, it is often recommended that the expected frequency of each cell be at least 5, especially if the number of cells is small, as in a 2×2 contingency table. When there are a large number of cells, the chi-square test will yield valid results if no more than 20% of the cells have expected frequencies under 5—so long as all cells have an expected frequency greater than 0. For example, in a 5×4 contingency table, four cells ($20\% \times 20$) could have expected frequencies between 1 and 4. Note that the cell size requirement involves *expected* frequencies, not observed ones. However, as the size of the overall sample increases, so do expected frequencies.

TIP: *If chi-square is invalid for a 2 × 2 table because of low expected frequencies, an alternative test known as* **Fisher's exact test** *can be used. The computations for this test are complex, but most computer programs for chi-square analysis compute Fisher's exact test automatically.*

General Logic of the Chi-Square Test

The chi-square test contrasts **observed frequencies** in each cell of a contingency table (i.e., the frequencies observed within the actual data) with expected frequencies. **Expected frequencies** are the number of cases that would be found in each cell if the null hypothesis were true—that is, if the two variables were totally unrelated. In our example, if the length of heparin lock placement had no effect on the rate of complications, the percentages should be identical in the two groups. Because 20% of the overall sample of patients had complications, we would expect that 20% in both groups (20% × 50 = 10 patients) would experience complications if the null hypothesis were true. Similarly, 80% of the patients did not have complications, so the expected frequency for the two bottom cells of Table 8.1 would be 40 (80% × 50).

If the actual, observed frequencies in a crosstabs table are *identical* to the expected frequencies, the value of the chi-square statistic will equal 0, which is the population value of chi-square for two unrelated variables. A chi-square based on sample data will often not equal exactly 0, even when the variables are not related, because of sampling error. Thus, as with other statistics, the computed value of the chi-square statistic must be compared to a critical value in a table, to determine if the value of the statistic is "improbable" at a specified significance criterion. The critical tabled values are based on **sampling distributions of the chi-square statistic**.

There are different chi-square distributions depending on degrees of freedom, which in turn depends on the number of categories for each variable. (We discuss the calculation of degrees of freedom subsequently.) Figure 8.1 presents examples of two chi-square distributions, for tests involving a 2 × 2 (4-cell) contingency table

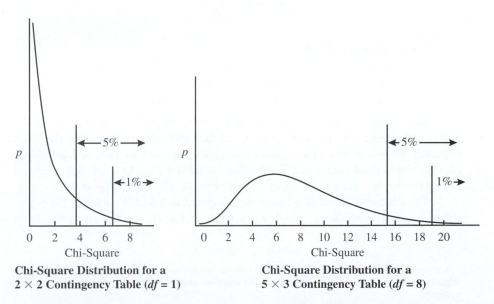

**Chi-Square Distribution for a
2 × 2 Contingency Table (*df* = 1)**

**Chi-Square Distribution for a
5 × 3 Contingency Table (*df* = 8)**

FIGURE 8.1 Example of chi-square distributions with different degrees of freedom.

and a 5×3 (15-cell) contingency table. The figure shows the areas corresponding to 5% and 1% of these distributions, which constitute the critical regions for the rejection of the null hypothesis with $\alpha = .05$ and $.01$, respectively.

Calculation of the Chi-Square Statistic

The chi-square statistic is relatively easy to compute manually. The first step is to calculate the expected frequencies for each cell of the contingency table. The following formula can be used:

$$E = \frac{R_f \times C_f}{N}$$

where E = expected frequency for a cell
   R_f = observed frequency for the entire row the cell is in
   C_f = observed frequency for the entire column the cell is in
   N = total sample size

Let us apply this formula to the first cell in our example of heparin lock placement groups (Table 8.1):

$$E = \frac{50 \times 20}{100} = \frac{1000}{100} = 10$$

This is consistent with our earlier discussion, in which we noted that 20% of the sample had complications, so 20% of each group ($n = 10$) would be expected to have complications if the null hypothesis were true. Thus, the expected frequency for the two upper cells is 10, while that for the two bottom cells is 40.

We can now compute the chi-square statistic, which involves comparing expected and observed frequencies in each cell. The formula for chi-square is:

$$\chi^2 = \Sigma \frac{(O - E)^2}{E}$$

where χ^2 = chi-square
   O = observed frequency for a cell
   E = expected frequency for a cell
   Σ = the sum of the $(O - E)^2/E$ ratios for all cells

To compute χ^2, the expected frequency for each cell is subtracted from the observed frequency, the result is squared, and then this value is divided by the cell's expected frequency. When these calculations are performed for each cell, all values are summed to yield a value of χ^2 (chi-square[1]). Table 8.2 works through the computations for our heparin lock example. In this example, the value of χ^2 is 0.25.

The computed value of χ^2 must be compared to a tabled value for the established level of significance, which we will set at .05. To use the chi-square table

---

[1] Although widely referred to as the chi-square test, the test is sometimes called chi-squared, which is actually more appropriate because the symbolic representation for the test is the Greek letter chi, squared.

TABLE 8.2 Calculation of the Chi-Square Statistic for Heparin Lock Data

Cell	Observed Frequency O	Expected Frequency E	$(O - E)$	$(O - E)^2$	$(O - E)^2/E$
Complication, 72 Hr.	9	10	−1	1	0.100
Complication, 96 Hr.	11	10	1	1	0.100
No Complication, 72 Hr.	41	40	1	1	0.025
No Complication, 96 Hr.	39	40	−1	1	0.025
					$\chi^2 = 0.250$

(Table A.4 of Appendix A), we must first compute degrees of freedom. For the chi-square test, the formula is:

$$df = (R - 1)(C - 1)$$

where R = number of rows
       C = number of columns

In our example, both R and C are equal to 2, so degrees of freedom is $(2 - 1)$ $(2 - 1)$, which equals 1. We find in Table A.4 that with $\alpha = .05$ and $df = 1$, the tabled value of χ^2 is 3.84. Since our calculated value of chi-square is considerably less than 3.84, we accept the null hypothesis that complication rates are unrelated to heparin lock placement time.

Like most statistics, chi-square analysis is most often done by computer. Figure 8.2 presents output from an SPSS run using Analyze ➜ Descriptive statistics ➜ Crosstabs with the fictitious heparin lock data from Table 8.1. Panel A of this printout shows the descriptive crosstab table. Each cell of this 2 × 2 table contains information on the frequency (count) and column percentage (% within placement time) for that cell. (A more detailed discussion of how to read contingency tables was presented in Chapter 4.) We also instructed the computer to print the expected count for each cell. Thus, for the first cell there were nine patients with complications in the 72-hour heparin lock group, the expected frequency was 10, and the percentage with complications in the 72-hour group was 18.0%.

Panel B of Figure 8.2 presents the results of the chi-square tests. The basic chi-square statistic (Pearson chi-square) is shown in the first row, with a computed value of .250, which is the value we obtained with manual calculation. With 1 df, the probability of obtaining this value of chi-square is .617, which is not statistically significant.

Some of the other entries in Panel B will be mentioned briefly, although they are not often used in nursing studies. When both variables in a contingency table have only two levels (i.e., when there is a 2 × 2 analysis, as in our example), the sampling distribution of the chi-square statistic corresponds less closely to a chi-square distribution than when there are more levels for at least one variable. Because of this, a correction factor known as **Yates' continuity correction** is sometimes used in computing chi-square for a 2 × 2 table. There is some disagreement regarding the use of Yates' correction (see Jaccard & Becker, 2001), but it is routinely calculated in SPSS for 2 × 2 tables. The correction involves subtracting 0.5 from the absolute value of $O-E$ for each cell before this value is squared, thus making the value of the statistic smaller. Thus, one reason this correction is controversial is that it reduces power.

Crosstabs

A   **Had complications? * Heparin lock placement time crosstabulation**

			Heparin Lock Placement Time		
			72 Hours	96 Hours	Total
Had Complications?	Yes	Count	9	11	20
		Expected count	10.0	10.0	20.0
		% within Heparin lock placement time	18.0%	22.0%	20.0%
	No	Count	41	39	80
		Expected count	40.0	40.0	80.0
		% within Heparin lock placement time	82.0%	78.0%	80.0%
	Total	Count	50	50	100
		Expected count	50.0	50.0	100.0
		% within Heparin lock placement time	100.0%	100.0%	100.0%

B   **Chi-Square Tests**

	Value	df	Asymp. Sig. (two-sided)	Exact Sig. (two-sided)	Exact Sig. (one-sided)
Pearson Chi-Square	.250[a]	1	.617		
Continuity Correction[b]	.062	1	.803		
Likelihood Ratio	.250	1	.617		
Fisher's Exact Test				.803	.402
Linear-by-Linear Association	.248	1	.619		
N of Valid Cases	100				

a. 0 cells (.0%) have expected count less than 5. The minimum expected count is 10.00.
b. Computed only for a 2 x 2 table

C   **Symmetric Measures**

		Value	Approx. Sig.
Nominal by Nominal	Phi	−.050	.617
	Cramer's V	.050	.617
	N of Valid Cases	100	

FIGURE 8.2   SPSS printout of a chi-square analysis.

When the continuity correction is applied to the data in our heparin lock example, the value of χ^2 is reduced from 0.25 to 0.063, as shown in Panel B of Figure 8.2. In both cases, the null hypothesis would be accepted, but sometimes the application of Yates' correction alters a decision from rejection to acceptance of the null. If expected frequencies are large, the correction factor should probably not be applied.

When SPSS executes a command to produce the chi-square statistic, it also computes other similar statistics. For example, one is called the **likelihood ratio chi-square**, which is an alternative method of testing the null hypothesis of lack of relationship between rows and columns of a crosstab table. It is computed differently than the Pearson chi-square, but it is interpreted the same way and usually yields the same results—as is the case with our heparin lock example. This and the other statistics that are generated along with Pearson's chi-square statistic are explained in SPSS manuals (e.g., Norušis, 2008), but they are rarely reported. (Likelihood ratio tests are discussed at greater length in Chapter 12.)

Example of a chi-square analysis:

Park and colleagues (2008) studied factors related to lymphoedema among patients with breast cancer. They used chi-square tests to test associations with risk factors measured on a nominal scale. For example, they found that patients with lymphoedema were significantly more likely than those without it to be overweight or obese ($\chi^2 = 10.77$, $df = 2$, $p = .001$).

Nature of the Relationship

When the contingency table is 2×2 and a chi-square test has led to the rejection of the null hypothesis, the direction of the relationship between the two variables can be determined by inspecting the percentages. For instance, if our heparin lock example *had* yielded a significant chi-square value, we would conclude that complications were greater when the heparin locks were left in place for 96 hours than when they were in place only 72 hours because the complication rate was higher in the 96-hour group.

Like ANOVA, the chi-square test applies to data for the two variables taken as a whole. For tables larger than 2×2, a significant chi-square provides no information regarding which cells are responsible for rejecting the null hypothesis. There are multiple comparison procedures for chi-square tests just as for ANOVA, but the mathematics are complex and these procedures are not usually available in widely used statistical software packages. We can, however, gain descriptive insight into the nature of the relationship by examining the components contributing to the value of χ^2—i.e., the values shown in the last column of Table 8.2. In a 4×2 table, for example, there would be eight such components, and those with the greatest values are the ones disproportionately contributing to a high χ^2. These components would help us to better understand which cells are most responsible for the rejection of the null hypothesis.

Magnitude of Effects in Contingency Tables

The chi-square statistic provides information about the existence of a relationship between two nominal-level variables, but not about the magnitude of the relationship. It may be useful, in interpreting the results, to have a measure of the strength of the association.

Several alternative indexes have been proposed. In a 2×2 table, one alternative is the **phi coefficient** (ϕ). The formula for φ is based directly on the computed chi-square statistic:

$$\phi = \sqrt{\frac{\chi^2}{N}}$$

In our heparin lock example, the phi coefficient would be:

$$\phi = \sqrt{\frac{0.25}{100}} = \sqrt{.0025} = .05$$

This same value for phi is shown in Panel C of Figure 8.2, which shows the SPSS output for the heparin lock data.

The phi coefficient usually ranges from 0 to 1, and can be interpreted similar to a Pearson r. The larger the value of φ, the stronger the relationship between the variables. Thus, a φ of .05 indicates a weak relationship between placement time groups and incidence of complications.[2]

When a crosstabs table is larger than 2 × 2, phi is not appropriate for measuring the strength of the relationship between the two variables, but a statistic called **Cramér's** V can be used. The formula for V is as follows:

$$V = \sqrt{\frac{\chi^2}{N(k-1)}}$$

In this formula, k is the smaller of either R (number of rows) or C (number of columns). In our heparin lock example, $k = 2$, so that the formula for V in this case is identical to the formula for φ—and, as shown in Panel C of Figure 8.2, the value of V as calculated in SPSS is .05 for both indexes. As with φ, the V statistic can range from 0 to 1, and larger values indicate a stronger relationship between the variables. For tables that are bigger than 2 × 2, a large value for the V statistic means that there is a tendency for particular categories of the independent variable to be associated with particular categories of the dependent variable.

Increasingly, risk indexes such as those discussed in Chapter 4 are being used to communicate magnitude of effects, especially for outcomes that are dichotomous. In a 2 × 2 situation, the odds ratio (OR) and relative risk (RR) are most often used, and these are both popular as effect size indexes in meta-analysis. As noted in Chapter 4, the odds ratio can be computed within SPSS as part of the Crosstabs procedure. In our present example, the OR for complications with a 96-hour placement (versus 72-hour placement) is 1.285, and the relative risk index is 1.222 (calculations not shown).

We described in Chapter 5 how confidence intervals can (and should) be constructed around proportions and risk indexes to provide information about precision of estimates. In the present example, the 95% CI around the OR of 1.285 ranged from .480 to 3.437. This interval includes the OR of 1.0, which indicates the possibility that placement time and complications were unrelated—consistent with the decision to retain the null hypothesis.

TIP: *Within the context of an odds ratio, the null hypothesis being tested is that the odds ratio is 1.0. The 95%* CI *around the odds ratio thus provides information about the likelihood that the null hypothesis is correct. The null hypothesis regarding the lack of relationship between a risk factor and an event (outcome) can also be tested with* **tests of conditional independence,** *such as* **Cochran's chi-square** *and* **Mantel-Haenszel's chi square,** *both of which can be run within the Crosstabs procedure in SPSS. In our present example, both tests were nonsignificant.*

Power Analysis

Cramér's V statistic can be used as the effect size index in a power analysis for contingency tables of any size. As noted in earlier chapters, power analysis is most often used in planning a study to estimate how large a sample is needed. For this

---

[2] In SPSS, a minus sign is added to phi in 2 × 2 tables if the value of a Pearson correlation between the two variables would be negative. This occurred in this example (Figure 8.2). Phi can, in theory, be greater than 1 but usually is not.

application, researchers need to have an estimate of Cramér's V. Post hoc power analysis is also used sometimes to interpret results, especially when the chi square statistic is nonsignificant.

Tables for estimating power and sample size needs using Cramér's V are presented in Table B.4 of Appendix B. Different tables are needed for contingency tables of different dimensions and for different levels of alpha, and so this appendix covers only the most common situations—that is, for $\alpha = .05$, and for contingency tables no greater than 4×4. Let us use the heparin lock example to illustrate, using the table A for a 2×2 design at the top of Table B.4. The left-hand column presents different power levels, and the top row presents population values for Cramér's V. In our example, the value of V was .05, which is not represented in the table. We can see, however, that even if V were estimated to be .10, we would need a sample of 785 participants to detect the effect with a .05 risk of a Type I error and a .20 risk of a Type II error. Clearly, our sample of 100 patients was inadequate to detect a small effect of $V = .05$, if the relationship were real.

In terms of post hoc power estimation, we can see that with a sample of 100 patients and a V less than .10 (the lowest V shown in the table), the power of the chi-square test was substantially less than .25—in fact, power was actually only .06. In other words, the risk of a Type II error was about 94%, if the null hypothesis was really false. With such a risk, we would likely want to replicate the study with a larger sample of patients.

A more convenient way to estimate sample size needs for a 2×2 design is to use Table 8.3 or one of the many interactive power analysis calculators on the Internet (e.g., *http://statpages.org/proppowr.html* or *http://www.stat.uiowa.edu/~rlenth/Power/*). Table 8.3 can be used when you estimate the proportions in the two populations, and when you use the standard criteria of $\alpha = .05$ and power = .80. For example, if we estimated complication rates for the 72-hour placement population to be .15 and the complication rate for the 96-hour placement population to be .20, this table indicates at the intersection of these two proportions that we would need 945 patients per group. (Although not shown in this table, for the actual obtained proportions of .18 and .22, we would need 1,618 patients per group.)

As Table 8.3 shows, sample size needs for testing differences between two proportions is influenced not only by expected differences in proportions (e.g., .60 in one group versus .40 in another, a .difference of .20), but also by the absolute values of the proportions. For any given difference in proportions, sample size needs are smaller at the extremes than near the midpoint. A .20 difference is easier to detect if the proportions are .10 and .30 than if they are near the middle, such as .40 and .60. Table 8.3 tells us that we would need 71 participants per group in the first situation, compared to 107 per group in the second. Because of this fact, it is difficult to offer guidelines for small, medium, and large effects in a chi-square context. We can, however, give *examples* of differences in proportions that conform to the conventions in a 2×2 situation:

Small: .05 versus .10, .20 versus .29, .40 versus .50, .60 versus .70, .80 versus .87

Medium: .05 versus .21, .20 versus .43, .40 versus .65, .60 versus .82, .80 versus .96

Large: .05 versus .34, .20 versus .58, .40 versus .78, .60 versus .92, .80 versus .96

If, for example, the expected proportion for a control group were .40, we would need about 385, 70, and 24 per group if an intervention group was expected to have higher proportions, and the effect was expected to be small, medium, and large, respectively. Researchers are, as always, encouraged to avoid using these "tee-shirt-size"

TABLE 8.3 Sample Size Estimates[a] for Each Group, Testing Differences in Two Proportions, for α = .05 and Power = .80

Proportion for: →	Group 2[b] (P_2)										
Group 1 (P_1) ↓	.00	.05	.10	.15	.20	.25	.30	.35	.40	.45	.50
.05	190	—									
.10	92	474	—								
.15	60	159	725	—							
.20	44	88	219	945	—						
.25	34	58	112	270	1133	—					
.30	27	43	71	133	313	1290	—				
.35	23	33	50	82	151	348	1416	—			
.40	19	27	38	57	91	165	376	1510	—		
.45	16	22	30	42	62	98	175	395	1573	—	
.50	14	18	24	32	45	65	103	182	407	1604	—
.55	12	16	20	26	34	47	68	106	186	411	1604
.60	11	14	17	21	27	36	48	69	107	186	407
.65	10	12	14	18	22	28	36	49	69	106	182
.70	9	10	12	15	18	22	28	36	48	68	103
.75	8	9	11	13	15	18	22	28	36	47	65
.80	7	8	9	11	13	15	18	22	27	34	45
.85	6	7	8	9	11	13	15	18	21	26	32
.90	5	6	7	8	9	11	12	14	17	20	24
.95	5	5	6	7	8	9	10	12	14	16	18
1.00	4	5	5	6	7	8	9	10	11	12	14

[a]Sample sizes are for each group, and assume equal ns for the two groups being compared.

[b]For Group 2 proportions (P_2) greater than .50, use the row corresponding to $1.0 - P_2$ and the column corresponding to $1 - P_1$. For example, if P_1 = .85 and P_2 = .75, use the column for .15 and the row for .25.

conventions, if possible, in favor of more precise estimates from prior studies. If reliance on these conventions cannot be avoided, conservative estimates should be used to minimize the risk of wrongly retaining the null hypothesis.

TIP: *The chi-square test of independence, just discussed, is the most commonly used application of the chi-square statistic. Another situation calls for the* **chi-square goodness-of-fit test,** *which is used to draw inferences when there is one nominal-level variable and we had theoretical or other reasons for hypothesizing a specific population proportion. In other words, this goodness-of-fit test is similar to a one-sample* t *test.*

OTHER NONPARAMETRIC TESTS

Nonparametric tests are generally used either when the dependent variable is measured on a nominal or ordinal scale or when the assumptions for more powerful parametric tests cannot be met, especially when sample sizes are small. There are dozens of nonparametric tests for different situations, only a handful of which are covered here. Those interested in a fuller coverage of nonparametric tests, or in more

TABLE 8.4 Decision Matrix for Selected Nonparametric and Parametric Tests

Type of Design	Number of Groups	Measurement Level of Dependent Variable		
		Nominal	Ordinal	Interval or Ratio
Independent Groups (Between-subjects)	2	Chi-square test	Mann-Whitney U test	t test
	3	Chi-square test	Kruskal-Wallis test	ANOVA
Dependent Groups (Within-subjects)	2	McNemar test	Wilcoxon signed-ranks test	Paired t test
	3	Cochran's Q	Friedman test	RM-ANOVA

comprehensive statistical tables for the tests covered, should consult such textbooks as those by Sprent and Smeeton (2007) or Conover (1999).

Table 8.4 summarizes the tests covered in this chapter, and indicates situations in which these tests are appropriate. For situations in which a parametric test such as the t test or ANOVA cannot be used because underlying assumptions are presumed to be violated, the nonparametric ordinal-level test in the same row as the parametric test (listed in the last column of this table) would usually be used. For example, if an independent groups t test is inappropriate because the distribution of the dependent variable is markedly nonnormal and N is small, the Mann-Whitney U test would probably be used to test group differences.

Most nonparametric tests described in this section are **rank tests**. Whereas parametric tests focus on group differences in population means, rank tests deal with group differences in *location* (distributions of scores) between populations, based on ranks. Significance tests for rank tests are used either when the original data are in the form of rankings or, more typically, when a set of scores have been converted into ranks for the purpose of performing the test. To illustrate the basic ranking process, consider the following five heart rate values and their corresponding ranks:

Heart Rate	Rank
130	5
93	2
112	4
89	1
101	3

In this example, the person with the lowest heart rate is ranked 1, and the person with the highest heart rate is ranked 5. When a tie occurs, the scores are assigned the average of the ranks. Thus, if the fifth person in the above list had a heart rate of 112, both scores of 112 (participants 3 and 5) would be ranked 3.5.

TIP: *We could have reversed the ranking so that the lowest heart rate had the highest ranking, and so on—the computational procedures for rank tests would be the same either way. It is usually easier to interpret the results if low ranks are associated with low data values and high ranks are associated with high values.*

The Mann-Whitney *U* Test

The **Mann-Whitney *U* test** is a nonparametric analog of the independent groups *t* test. This statistic tests the null hypothesis that two population distributions are identical against the alternative hypothesis that the distributions are *not* identical.

Suppose we had two groups of burn patients (Group A and Group B) who obtained the following scores on a scale measuring positive body image:

Group A: 14,   19,   11,   22,   17
Group B: 10,   16,   15,   18,   13

To perform the Mann-Whitney *U* test, we must arrange the scores in order and rank them, while maintaining information about group affiliation:

Score:	10	11	13	14	15	16	17	18	19	22
Group:	B	A	B	A	B	B	A	B	A	A
Rank:	1	2	3	4	5	6	7	8	9	10

The ranks associated with each group are then separately summed to yield R_A and R_B:

$$R_A = 2 + 4 + 7 + 9 + 10 = 32$$
$$R_B = 1 + 3 + 5 + 6 + 8 = 23$$

The formula for computing the *U*-statistic for group A is as follows:

$$U_A = n_A n_B + \left[\frac{n_A(n_A + 1)}{2} \right] - R_A$$

where n_A = number of observations in Group A
n_B = number of observations in Group B
R_A = summed ranks for Group A

The formula for computing U_B would be analogous, except that the *n* for group B would be used in the numerator of the second term, and the *R* for group B would be used in the third term of the formula. Using this equation, we would obtain the following:

$$U_A = (5)(5) + \left[\frac{(5)(6)}{2} \right] - 32 = 8$$

$$U_B = (5)(5) + \left[\frac{(5)(6)}{2} \right] - 23 = 17$$

The *U* value that is used as the test statistic is the smaller of the two *U*s, which in this case is $U_A = 8$. The critical values for *U* (for $\alpha = .05$) for a non-directional test are presented in Table A.5 of Appendix A. To use the table, we look for the number at the intersection of the appropriate row and column for n_A and n_B. In our present example, with $n_A = 5$ and $n_B = 5$, the critical value is 2. One must be very careful in using this table, because it is different from other tables of critical values we have described thus far: To be statistically significant, the observed *U* must be *equal to or less than* the tabled value. Our obtained value of 8 is greater than the tabled value of 2, and so we must retain the null hypothesis that the two distributions are identical.

TIP: *Table A.5 should be used only when the sample size of each group is 20 or fewer. When the n for either group is greater than 20, the value of U approaches a normal distribution. A transformation (described in nonparametric textbooks) can be applied to the obtained U statistic to yield a z statistic, which can then be compared to the critical values for the normal distribution.*

Figure 8.3 shows the SPSS printout for a Mann-Whitney U test using the same data, which was run in the Analyze → Nonparametric Tests → Two Independent Samples analysis. The printout shows in Panel A that the mean rank for Group A was 6.40, while that for Group B was 4.60, and the sum of ranks was 32.0 and 23.0 for these groups, respectively. The value of the U statistic is 8.0. Wilcoxon W is the sum of ranks for the group with the smallest n. In this case, since both ns were 5, the value of $W = 23.0$, the sum of ranks for the group with the smallest U value. Using the binomial distribution, the exact probability value for $U = 8.0$ is .421, which is nonsignificant. The value for z was also computed ($-.940$) and the associated probability is shown (.347). In this example, since the n for both groups was under 20, the exact probability rather than the probability based on the normal distribution should be used. In either case, however, group differences were not statistically significant.

Mann-Whitney *U*-Test

A   **Ranks**

	Burn Patient Group	N	Mean Rank	Sum of Ranks
Positive Body Image	Group A	5	6.40	32.00
	Group B	5	4.60	23.00
	Total	10		

B   **Test Statistics**[b]

	Positive Body Image
Mann-Whitney U	8.000
Wilcoxon W	23.000
Z	−.940
Asymp. Sig. (2-tailed)	.347
Exact Sig. [2*(1-tailed Sig.)]	.421[a]

a. Not corrected for ties
b. Grouping variable: Burn patient group

FIGURE 8.3 SPSS printout of a Mann-Whitney U test.

Example of a Mann-Whitney *U* test:

Yip and colleagues (2007) tested the effectiveness of an arthritis self-management program on pain and functional ability outcomes, using a two-group experimental design. Because their outcome measures had significant departures from normality, they used nonparametric statistics. For example, change scores in pain ratings and fatigue were compared for the two groups using the Mann-Whitney *U* test. Differences were significant for both pain ratings ($p = .0001$) and fatigue ($p = .008$).

Kruskal-Wallis Test

The **Kruskal-Wallis test** is the nonparametric counterpart of a one-way ANOVA. It is used to analyze the relationship between an ordinal dependent variable and a categorical independent variable that has three or more levels (i.e., when there are three or more groups). The Kruskal-Wallis procedure tests the null hypothesis that the population distributions for the three (or more) groups are identical against the alternative that there are differences in the distributions. This test should be used only if there are five or more cases per group.

Suppose that we measured the life satisfaction of patients in three nursing homes, using a six-item scale and obtained the following scores:

Home A: 6, 12, 18, 14, 17
Home B: 15, 19, 16, 20, 10
Home C: 30, 27, 24, 25, 22

Comparing the three groups involves ranking the scores for the sample as a whole, and then summing the ranks separately for each group:

Score: 6   10   12   14   15   16   17   18   19   20   22   24   25   27   30
Group: A   B   A   A   B   B   A   A   B   B   C   C   C   C   C
Rank: 1   2   3   4   5   6   7   8   9   10   11   12   13   14   15

$R_A = 1 + 3 + 4 + 7 + 8$ $= 23$
$R_B = 2 + 5 + 6 + 9 + 10$ $= 32$
$R_C = 11 + 12 + 13 + 14 + 15$ $= 65$

Kruskal and Wallis proposed the following formula for the test statistic, the **H statistic**:

$$H = \left[\frac{12}{N(N + 1)} \right] \left[\Sigma \frac{R^2}{n} \right] - 3(N + 1)$$

where N = total sample size
  R^2 = summed ranks for a group, squared
  n = number of observations in a group
  Σ = the sum of the R^2/n ratios for all groups

For the data in our example of life satisfaction in three groups of nursing home patients, the value of H using this formula is 9.78 (computation not shown). The H statistic has a sampling distribution that approximates a chi-square distribution with $k - 1$ degrees of freedom, where k is the number of groups. For $\alpha = .05$ with 2 degrees of freedom, the critical value of H from the chi-square table in Table A.4 of

Kruskal-Wallis Test

A   **Ranks**

	Nursing Home	N	Mean Rank
Life Satisfaction Score	Home A	5	4.60
	Home B	5	6.40
	Home C	5	13.00
	Total	15	

B   **Test Statistics[a,b]**

	Life Satisfaction Score
Chi-Square	9.780
df	2
Asymp. Sig.	.008

a. Kruskal-Wallis Test
b. Grouping variable: Nursing home

FIGURE 8.4   SPSS printout of a Kruskal-Wallis test.

Appendix A is 5.99. Since the calculated value of H (9.78) is greater than this critical value, we reject the null hypothesis that the distribution of life satisfaction scores in the three nursing homes is identical.

Figure 8.4 presents the SPSS output for a Kruskal-Wallis test using these same data. (We used the procedure for "K Independent Samples" within the Nonparametric Tests set of SPSS Analysis commands.) The printout shows that the mean ranks for the scores in the three nursing homes were 4.6, 6.4, and 13.0, respectively. The value of the test statistic (shown as "Chi Square") is 9.78, the same value we obtained manually. The actual significance level is .008, indicating a statistically significant difference in the ranks.

As with ANOVA, a significant result does not mean that all groups are significantly different from one another. Post hoc tests are needed to assess the nature of the relationship between nursing homes and life satisfaction. Various procedures have been proposed but the one that is most often recommended is the **Dunn procedure**. This procedure involves using the Mann-Whitney U test to compare the ranks for all possible pairs of groups. To avoid a higher-than-desired risk of a Type I error, a correction factor (often called a **Bonferroni correction**) is used. The correction involves adjusting the significance criterion: The desired alpha is divided by the number of pairs being compared. In the present example, to test for differences between the three pairs at the .05 level, the alpha would be .05 ÷ 3, or .017. This means that for a difference between pairs to be significant at $\alpha = .05$, the computed value for the U statistic would be compared to the critical value for $\alpha = .017$. If we applied the Dunn procedure to our current example, we would find that Home C was significantly different from the other two nursing homes, but that Home A and Home B were not statistically different from each other.[3]

---

[3] According to a computer analysis of these data, the actual significance levels were .42 (Home A vs. Home B); .009 (Home A vs. Home C); and .009 (Home B vs. Home C).

TIP: *The Bonferroni correction is sometimes applied when researchers are testing hypotheses with multiple dependent variables. For example, if a dependent groups t test were used to compare means before and after an intervention for three separate outcomes, a researcher might use .017 as the significance criterion to guard against the risk of a Type I error when multiple tests are performed. Some have argued, however, that the Bonferroni correction in such situations is overly conservative and increases the risk of a Type II error.*

Example of a Kruskal-Wallis test:

Im, Chee, Guevara, Lim, and Shin (2008) studied ethnic differences in cancer patients' needs for help, and used the Kruskal-Wallis test to compare responses about needs for Asian, African-American, White, and Hispanic patients. They found significant ethnic differences, for example, with regard to psychological needs ($p < .01$). Post hoc comparisons using the Mann-Whitney U test with an adjusted alpha using Bonferroni corrections were performed, with alpha adjusted to .0083.

McNemar Test

The **McNemar test** is used to test differences in proportions for dependent groups in a 2×2 within-subjects design. For example, if 50 women were asked before and after a special health-promotion intervention whether or not they practiced breast self-examination (BSE), the McNemar test could be used to test changes in the rates of BSE. The null hypothesis is that there are no pretreatment to posttreatment changes in BSE, and the alternative hypothesis is that there are changes. Suppose that 30% of the women ($n = 15$) practiced BSE before the intervention, while 40% ($n = 20$) did so after the intervention. What is the likelihood that the 10 percentage point increase reflects a true difference in BSE practice?

The data for our example must be arranged in a table that distributes the women based on whether they did or did not practice BSE at the two time points, as in Table 8.5. This table shows that 15 women practiced BSE both before and after the intervention (cell A), 30 women did not practice BSE at either point (cell D), and 5 women who originally did not practice BSE did so after the intervention (cell C). No woman who originally practiced BSE ceased to do so after the intervention (cell B).

It is possible to determine exact probabilities in this situation through the use of the binomial distribution. Unless the sample size is very small, however, it is more convenient to use the chi-square distribution. The following formula can be applied:

$$\chi^2 = \frac{(|C - B| - 1)^2}{C + B}$$

where C = number in cell C (changed from *no* to *yes*)

B = number in cell B (changed from *yes* to *no*)

| | = the absolute value of the difference

If we applied this formula to the data at hand, we would find that $\chi^2 = 3.20$ (computation not shown). For the McNemar test, there is always 1 degree of freedom. If we set $\alpha = .05$, we find in the chi-square table (Table A.4 of Appendix A) that the critical value of chi-square is 3.84. Thus, we must retain the null hypothesis. The change in the percentage of women who practiced BSE was not statistically

TABLE 8.5 Distribution of Data on BSE Practice for McNemar Test Example

		BSE After Intervention?	
		Yes	No
BSE Before Intervention?	Yes	Cell A: 15 women	Cell B: 0 women
	No	Cell C: 5 women	Cell D: 30 women

significant at the .05 level. (When the McNemar analysis was performed in SPSS, we found that the exact probability was .063.)

Wilcoxon Signed-Ranks Test

The **Wilcoxon signed-ranks test** is the nonparametric counterpart of the paired (dependent groups) *t* test when outcomes are measured on an ordinal scale. It is used to test group differences in ordinal-level measures when there are two paired groups or a within-subjects design. The Wilcoxon signed-ranks procedure tests the null hypothesis that the population distributions for the two sets of observations are identical, against the alternative hypothesis that they are not identical.

Suppose we had 10 married couples whose child has undergone surgery. Both the husband and wife have completed a scale designed to measure parental anxiety, resulting in the scores shown in the first two columns of Table 8.6. We are testing the null hypothesis that husbands and wives have comparable anxiety. To perform the signed-ranks test, the score from one set must be subtracted from the corresponding scores in the other set, as shown in column 3. Next, the absolute values of the differences (column 4) are ranked, with the rank of 1 assigned for the smallest difference (column 5). Then, the ranks for the positive differences are separately summed, as are the ranks for the negative differences, as shown in the last two columns of Table 8.6. The table indicates that the positive ranks (which are associated with higher anxiety scores among the wives) totaled 30, while the negative ranks (associated with higher scores for the husbands) totaled 25.

If the null hypothesis that the husbands' and wives' anxiety scores are similarly distributed were true, the sum of the ranks for negative differences should be the

TABLE 8.6 Wilcoxon Signed-Ranks Test Example: Wives' Versus Husbands' Anxiety

(1) Wife	(2) Husband	(3) Difference	(4) |Difference|	(5) Rank	(6) R_+	(7) R_-
17	16	1	1	1	1	
19	14	5	5	5	5	
16	20	−4	4	4		4
18	12	6	6	6	6	
22	24	−2	2	2		2
18	21	−3	3	3		3
15	24	−9	9	9		9
22	11	11	11	10	10	
14	21	−7	7	7		7
23	15	8	8	8	8	
					$R_+ = 30$	$R_- = 25$

same as the sum of ranks for positive differences. In our example, the expected value of the ranks for both groups (R_E) is 27.5 ($(R_+ + R_-) \div 2$) if the null hypothesis were true. Tables for the Wilcoxon signed-ranks test statistic, called the **T statistic**, are available in nonparametric textbooks and are precise when the number of pairs is 50 or fewer. When the number of pairs is 10 or greater, however, the sampling distribution of T approximates a normal distribution, and the following formula[4] can be used to compute a z statistic:

$$z = \frac{R_- - R_E}{\sqrt{\dfrac{(2n + 1)R_E}{6}}}$$

Using the data from Table 8.6 in this formula, we would compute z to be $-.255$ (computations not shown). According to Table A.1 in Appendix A for the normal distribution, the critical value for rejecting the null hypothesis with $\alpha = .05$ is about 1.96. Thus, the null hypothesis is accepted. The data do not justify an inference that husbands and wives in the population differ in their anxiety in relation to their child's surgery.

Figure 8.5 shows the SPSS printout for the Wilcoxon signed-ranks test example, which we created using the Analyze ➜ Nonparametric Tests ➜ Two Related Samples routine. Panel A shows ranking information, and confirms that the sum of

Wilcoxon Signed-Ranks Test

A   **Ranks**

		N	Mean Rank	Sum of Ranks
Husband's Anxiety Score–	Negative ranks	5[a]	6.00	30.00
Wife's Anxiety Score	Positive ranks	5[b]	5.00	25.00
	Ties	0[c]		
	Total	10		

a. Husband's anxiety score < Wife's anxiety score

b. Husband's anxiety score > Wife's anxiety score

c. Husband's anxiety score = Wife's anxiety score

B   **Test Statistics[b]**

	Husband's Anxiety Score – Wife's Anxiety Score
Z	$-.255$[a]
Asymp. Sig. (2-tailed)	.799

a. Based on positive ranks

b. Wilcoxon Signed-Ranks Test

FIGURE 8.5   SPSS printout of a Wilcoxon Signed-Ranks test.

---

[4] It does not matter whether R_+ or R_- is used in the numerator of the formula, since both are equal distances from R_E. The only effect of the substitution would be to change the sign of z.

the negative ranks was 30.0 and the sum of the positive ranks was 25.0, consistent with Table 8.6. The actual probability for a z of $-.255$, shown in Panel B, is .799.

Example of a Wilcoxon signed-ranks test:

Liu (2008) compared patients' satisfaction with their appearance before and after tumor excision among patients with head and neck tumors. Using the Wilcoxon signed-ranks test, Liu found a significant decline in patients' satisfaction ($z = -6.39, p < .001$).

Cochran's Q Test

The **Cochran Q test** can be used to test for population differences in proportions when the dependent variable is dichotomous and when there are three or more repeated observations or correlated groups. For example, suppose a sample of 10 elderly patients with constipation problems was put on a special fiber-rich diet, and bowel movements were recorded for three consecutive days, beginning with the day the treatment was initiated. Table 8.7 presents some hypothetical data for this example, with no bowel movement coded 0 and a bowel movement coded 1. According to this table, three patients had bowel movements on Day 1, while 7 and 8 patients had bowel movements on Days 2 and 3, respectively. The research question is whether the differences reflect true population changes or are the result of sampling fluctuation.

To compute the Q statistic, the number of cases coded 1 must be summed across both columns (S_C) and rows (S_R), as shown in Table 8.7. Then, each summed row value must be squared, and these squared values must be summed (S_R^2). The Q statistic can then be computed using the following formula:

$$Q = \frac{k(k-1) \times \Sigma(S_C - M_R)^2}{k(S_R) - S_R^2}$$

TABLE 8.7 Cochran's Q Test Example: Bowel Movements Following Fiber-Rich Diet

Patient	Day 1	Day 2	Day 3	Row Sum	Row Sum^2
1	1	0	1	2	4
2	0	1	1	2	4
3	0	1	0	1	1
4	0	1	1	2	4
5	1	1	1	3	9
6	0	0	1	1	1
7	0	1	0	1	1
8	1	0	1	2	4
9	0	1	1	2	4
10	0	1	1	2	4
	$S_{C_1} = 3$	$S_{C_2} = 7$	$S_{C_3} = 8$	$S_R = 18$	$S_R^2 = 36$
				Mean (M_R) = 18/3 = 6	

Codes: 0 = no bowel movement
1 = bowel movement

where k = number of groups/times of observation
S_C = sum for each column (i.e., for each k)
S_R = sum of all summed rows
M_R = mean of the summed rows ($S_R \div k$)
Σ = sum of the $(S_C - M_R)^2$ values for the k columns

Although the formula looks complex, it boils down to the insertion of various sums and squares, most of which we have already calculated and are shown in Table 8.7. In our example, we find that Q = 4.67 (computation not shown). When the number of observations per group is 10 or greater, Q is distributed approximately as chi-square with k − 1 *degrees of freedom*. In our example, with df = 2 and α = .05, the critical value of Q from the chi-square distribution (Table A.4 of Appendix A) is 5.99. Our obtained value of Q is less than the tabled value, so we accept the null hypothesis. The differences in the proportions for the three days of observation are not statistically significant (the actual p for these data, using SPSS, is .097).

Friedman Test

Like Cochran's Q test, the **Friedman test** is used when there are three or more correlated groups, or three or more sets of observations for the same subjects, but the Friedman test is used when the dependent variable is measured on an ordinal scale. The Friedman test is the nonparametric analog of the one-way repeated measures ANOVA.

Suppose that nine nurses were asked to read case reports of three patients with Do-Not-Resuscitate orders—an AIDS patient, a cancer patient, and a patient with Alzheimer's disease. The case reports are presented to the nurses in a random order. For each patient, nurses are questioned about the care that they think should be provided, and the responses are used to create an index of aggressiveness of nursing care. Fictitious data for this hypothetical study are presented in Table 8.8. The null hypothesis is that scores on aggressiveness of nursing care are unrelated to the patient's type of illness.

The Friedman test involves ranking the scores for each participant across the different conditions. For example, the first nurse had a score of 15 for the Alzheimer

TABLE 8.8 Friedman's Test Example: Aggressiveness of Nursing Care for DNR Patients with Different Illnesses

Nurse	Score (Rank) AIDS	Cancer	Alzheimer
1	17 (2)	18 (3)	15 (1)
2	15 (2)	20 (3)	11 (1)
3	14 (3)	12 (1)	13 (2)
4	11 (1)	19 (3)	18 (2)
5	18 (2)	20 (3)	17 (1)
6	16 (3)	14 (1)	15 (2)
7	12 (1)	14 (3)	13 (2)
8	9 (1)	13 (3)	12 (2)
9	16 (2)	17 (3)	15 (1)
	R_1 = 17	R_2 = 23	R_3 = 14

patient description, which is assigned the rank of 1 because it is the lowest score for that nurse. The ranks of 2 and 3 are assigned to the AIDS and Cancer patient conditions, respectively, for the first nurse. The ranks for each condition are then summed. For example, the sum of the ranks for the AIDS patient description is 17. If the null hypothesis were true, we would expect the sum of the ranks for each condition to be about equal; any differences in the rankings across nurses would simply reflect sampling error. The formula for the Friedman test, which follows a chi-square distribution, is as follows:

$$\chi^2 = \left[\frac{12(\Sigma R^2)}{Nk(k + 1)} \right] - 3N(k + 1)$$

where k = number of conditions or groups
  R^2 = sum of the ranks for each k condition/group, squared
  Σ = sum of the squared sum of ranks (R^2) for the k conditions
  N = number of participants

If we applied this formula to the data in Table 8.8, we would find that $\chi^2 = 4.67$ (computations not shown). With an alpha level of .05 and $k - 1 = 2$ degrees of freedom, the critical value from the chi-square table (Table A.4 of Appendix A) is 5.99. The computed value does not exceed the tabled value of chi-square, and so the null hypothesis is retained. The nurses' scores for aggressiveness of care are not significantly different for the three patient descriptions.

Figure 8.6 shows the SPSS printout for the Friedman test, created through Analyze ➔ Nonparametric Tests ➔ K Related Samples. Panel A shows the mean ranks for each patient type—i.e., the total ranks shown at the bottom of Table 8.8, divided by 9 (N). Panel B shows that the value of the test statistic is 4.667, and that the probability associated with it is .097.

If we had rejected the null hypothesis in this example, it would have been necessary to conduct additional analyses to determine which comparisons were driving the overall results. The Dunn procedure with Bonferroni correction, described earlier, could be used to isolate the pairs of conditions that were significantly different from one another.

Friedman Test

A   **Ranks**

	Mean Rank
Patients with AIDS	1.89
Patients with Cancer	2.56
Patients with Alzheimer's	1.56

B   **Test Statistics[a]**

N	9.000
Chi-Square	4.667
df	2.000
Asymp. Sig.	.097

a. Friedman Test

FIGURE 8.6 SPSS printout of a Friedman Test.

Example of a Friedman test:

Rungreangkulkij and Wongtakee (2008) evaluated the psychological impact of Buddhist counseling for Thai patients suffering from anxiety. They measured anxiety before the intervention, after it, and then 2 months later using the Friedman test. Anxiety declined over the course of the study, and differences were significant ($\chi^2 = 42.0$, $p < .001$).

TIP: *Each of the nonparametric tests we have described tests the existence of a relationship between an independent and dependent variable. It is beyond the scope of this book to describe indexes for measuring the strength of the relationship for situations in which these nonparametric tests would be used, but such indexes do exist. For further information, you can consult Jaccard and Becker (2001).*

RESEARCH APPLICATIONS OF NONPARAMETRIC TESTS

Except for the chi-square test for independence, nonparametric tests are infrequently used in nursing research. In large part, this is because parametric tests are more powerful than their nonparametric counterparts and are fairly robust to violations of many underlying assumptions. Yet, nonparametric tests are often appropriate, especially if there is evidence that the assumptions for parametric tests cannot possibly be met (e.g., a markedly skewed distribution of the dependent variable). This section examines some of the major applications of nonparametric tests and discusses methods of effectively displaying results from these tests in a research report.

The Uses of Nonparametric Tests

The nonparametric tests we have discussed in this chapter are, for the most part, used in much the same applications as those we discussed for *t* tests and ANOVA in the previous two chapters, except for differences in how the outcome variables were measured. Thus, we provide only a few illustrations.

1. *Answering research questions*   As with most inferential statistics, the primary use of nonparametric tests is substantive—that is, they are used mainly to test hypotheses and to answer research questions. Throughout this chapter we have illustrated the wide array of research questions that have relied on the use of nonparametric tests, using actual examples from the nursing literature.
2. *Testing biases*   Nonparametric tests are also used to examine the nature and extent of any biases that need to be considered in interpreting substantive results. For example, Nyamathi and colleagues (2008) studied the effectiveness of a nurse case-managed intervention for latent tuberculosis among the homeless. First, however, they compared the background characteristics of those in the intervention and control groups to assess selection bias. They used chi-square tests to assess the equivalence of the two groups with respect to such characteristics as ethnicity, marital status, and sex.
3. *Variable selection for multivariate analyses*   As mentioned in Chapter 6, researchers sometimes undertake complex multivariate analyses to assess the contribution of multiple independent variables, taken simultaneously, in predicting an outcome. They often begin by looking at each potential predictor in relation to the outcome of interest in a bivariate fashion, to see if some should be eliminated from further consideration. When outcomes of interest are

dichotomous (e.g., had a fall versus did not have a fall), chi-squared tests or bivariate odds ratios are likely to be used in these preliminary analyses. For example, Certain, Mueller, Jagodzinski, and Fleming (2008) developed a model to identify predictors of domestic abuse in postpartum women. Each possible independent variable or predictor, such as marital status, employment status, and alcohol use, was tested for its relationship to abuse status using chi-square tests. Variables that had a $p < .10$ were placed in the final model.

Presentation of Nonparametric Tests in Research Reports

Like other statistical tests, nonparametric tests usually are summarized in the text of a report when there are only one or two tests, but are presented in a table if there are more. The standard convention is to provide information about the name of the test, the value of the test statistic, degrees of freedom, sample size, and significance level. Here is a fictitious example: "A chi-square test indicated that diabetic patients who had regular inspection of their feet by a nurse or other healthcare professional were significantly more likely than those who did not to regularly inspect their own feet for foot complications and ulcers (χ^2 [1, $N = 653$] = 45.3, $p < .001$)."

For tests with a nominal-level dependent variable, such as the chi-square test of independence, multiple tests can be reported in a table in much the same fashion as a table for t tests, except that the descriptive information is group percentages rather than group means. Table 8.9 presents an example of such a table that elaborates on our earlier example of heparin lock placement time groups. For four separate complication outcomes, the table shows the percent in each group with the complication, the value of the chi-square statistic, and the p-value. The table illustrates how Fisher's exact test was reported for an outcome for which the expected frequency for some cells was less than five.

When a table is used to summarize multiple tests, the text highlights key results. Here is an example of how the text corresponding to Table 8.9 might read:

> The table shows that the rates of various complications in the two heparin lock placement time groups were comparable for every type of complication considered. Overall, 18.0% of the 72-hour group, compared to 22.0% of the 96-hour group, had a complication, a difference that was not statistically significant. Although none of the differences was significant, there was a modestly higher rate of complications in the 96-hour group for every complication. A post hoc power analysis revealed that the power of the statistical tests was quite low, and therefore replication with a larger sample of participants seems warranted.

TABLE 8.9 Example of a Table for Chi-Square Test Results

Complication	Heparin Lock Placement Time Group		χ^2	p
	72 Hours ($n = 50$)	96 Hours ($n = 50$)		
Phlebitis	12.0%	16.0%	.38	.54
Blocking/Leaking	8.0%	12.0%	.44	.51
Purulence/Septicemia	0.0%	2.0%	a	1.00
Any complication	18.0%	22.0%	.25	.62

[a] Fisher's exact test, expected frequency < 5 in two cells

Percentage of Patients with Various Complications, by Length of Time Heparin Lock was in Place

When a chi-square test is applied to contingency tables of fairly large dimensionality—for example, for a 3×4 design—it may be more informative to present the full crosstabulation, particularly if there is a complex pattern of results for individual cells. When a full contingency table is presented, the results of the statistical tests can be placed in a footnote. For example, refer back to Table 4.5 in Chapter 4, which concerned women's cancer screening behaviors. If the relationship between screening status and women's age were tested using a chi-square test for mammography and PAP tests, two footnotes with statistical information could be placed at the bottom of the table.

When information about odds ratios or relative risk is communicated in a report, they are almost always shown with their 95% *CI*s. As we see in the next section, odds ratios and chi-square tests can sometimes be effectively presented in a single table.

TIP: *We urge you to report ORs or RRs when it is appropriate to do so, to facilitate the work of future meta-analysts. If page constraints or other considerations make it difficult to do so, be sure to include sufficient information about absolute risks (the appropriate percentages) so that an OR or RR can be computed with your data by others.*

When dependent variables are measured on an ordinal scale—for example, when Mann-Whitney *U* tests or Kruskal-Wallis tests have been performed—a common strategy for table presentation is to present the medians for the different groups being compared for each dependent variable, followed by information on the statistical test results.

Research Example

In this section we briefly summarize a study that used multiple chi-square tests of independence.

Study: "Health outcomes associated with potentially inappropriate medication use in older adults" (Fick, Mion, Beers, & Waller, 2008)

Study Purpose: The purpose of this study was to examine the prevalence of potentially inappropriate medication use (PIMs) among older community-dwelling adults, and to explore the relationships between PIMs and healthcare outcomes.

Methods: Data were obtained from an administrative database for adults in a managed care organization. The database contained medication information for nearly 17,000 individuals aged 65 and older. The researchers used a list referred to as Beers criteria for identifying high-risk PIMs—drugs that should be avoided in the elderly either because they are ineffective or they pose high risks for the elderly. Any person using at least one such drug was classified as being in the PIMs group, while those not using any PIM were in a comparison group. The analysis involved comparing these two groups with respect to the proportion experiencing a drug-related problem (DRP) within 30 days of a prescription.

Analysis: Chi-square tests and *t* tests were used to assess the demographic comparability of the PIMs and Comparison group. Chi-square and Fisher's exact tests were used to compare the two groups with regard to prevalence of various drug-related problems. Odds ratios were computed to assess the relative risk of the use of a PIM in relation to adverse outcomes.

Results: The two groups differed significantly on several background characteristics. For example, significantly more of the elders in the PIMs group (71.0%) than in the comparison group (54.4%) were female ($\chi^2 = 476.1$, $p < .001$). In terms of DRPs, Table 8.10 highlights some of the results. With only a few exceptions (not shown in this table), elders in the PIMs group were significantly more likely to experience DRPs than those in the

TABLE 8.10 Differences in Prevalence of Selected Drug-Related Problems Among Elders with and without Potentially Inappropriate Medications (PIMs)

Drug-Related Problem	PIMs Group (n = 6,875)		Comparisons (n = 10,002)		χ^2	Odds Ratios	
	n	%	n	%		OR	95% CI
Syncope	246	3.58	122	1.22	106.3*	3.01	2.41–3.74
Malaise and fatigue	237	3.45	106	1.06	116.6*	3.33	2.65–4.20
Dehydration	126	1.83	44	0.44	79.3*	4.23	2.99–5.96
Sleep disturbances	102	1.48	42	0.42	54.5*	3.57	2.49–5.12
Urinary incontinence	61	0.89	24	0.24	34.1*	3.72	2.32–5.97
Alteration of consciousness	35	0.51	14	0.14	19.2*	3.65	1.96–6.79

*All chi-square tests were significant at $p < .001$

Abridged and adapted from Table 3 of Fick et al., 2008

comparison group. By looking at the percentages (the absolute risks), we see that the prevalence of most problems was relatively small. In most cases, fewer than 2% of those in either group experienced any particular problem. The chi-square information communicates that, although rates were relatively low in both groups, many group differences had a high probability of being real

(i.e., not the result of chance fluctuations). The inclusion of OR information adds an important perspective. In most cases, the risk of a DRP was three or more times as high in the PIMs group as in the comparison group. Finally, the 95% *CI*s communicate information about the accuracy of the risk information.

Summary Points

- Nonparametric tests are most often used when the measurement scale of the variables is nominal or ordinal, or when assumptions for parametric tests are presumed to be severely violated, especially when samples are small.
- The **chi-square test of independence** (*Pearson's chi-square*) is a test for making inferences about population differences in proportions between two or more independent groups. It is used when both the independent and dependent variable are measured on the nominal scale (or an ordinal scale with few levels).
- The chi-square statistic (χ^2) is computed by contrasting **expected frequencies** (frequencies expected if the null hypothesis of no relationship between variables were true) and **observed frequencies** for each cell in a contingency table.
- In a 2 × 2 table in which the expected frequency is less than 10, it is sometimes recommended that **Yates' correction for continuity** be applied. When the expected frequency in a cell is less than

5, an alternative test known as **Fisher's exact test** is often used.
- The index used to measure the strength of the relationship is the **phi coefficient** for a 2 × 2 table and **Cramér's** *V* for a larger table. Cramér's *V* can be used as the effect size index in a power analysis in the context of a chi-square situation.
- Although Cramér's *V* is sometimes used as an overall effect size index, the odds ratio and relative risk index are often used, especially for meta-analysis. Power analysis in a chi-square type situation requires estimates of either Cramér's *V* or, in a 2 × 2 design, the two population proportions.
- Numerous nonparametric tests exist, and key issues is selecting such a test is whether the design is between-subjects (independent groups) or within-subjects (dependent groups or repeated measures), and what the measurement scale of the dependent variable is. Many nonparametric tests are **rank tests** that involve assigning ranks to scores.

- For between-subjects designs with an ordinal-level dependent variable, the **Mann-Whitney U test** can be used to test differences in ranks between two groups, and the **Kruskal-Wallis test** can be used to compare ranks when there are three or more groups. These tests are the nonparametric counterparts of the t test and ANOVA, respectively.
- For dependent groups and a dichotomous dependent variable, the **McNemar test** can be used for two sets of observations, and **Cochran's Q test** is appropriate for three or more observations.
- For two dependent groups with ordinal data, the **Wilcoxon signed-ranks test** may be used, and

when there are more than two groups or observations, the **Friedman test** is appropriate. These tests are the nonparametric analogs of the paired t test and repeated measures ANOVA, respectively.
- When either the Kruskal-Wallis or Friedman test is statistically significant, the **Dunn procedure** (ideally with a **Bonferroni correction** to reduce the risk of a Type I error) can be used to determine the nature of the relationship between the independent and dependent variables (i.e., to isolate the pairs of groups or observations responsible for a significant overall test).

Exercises

The following exercises cover concepts presented in this chapter. Appendix C provides answers to Part A exercises that are indicated with a dagger (†). Exercises in Part B involve computer analyses using the datasets provided with this textbook, and answers and comments are offered on this book's Web site.

PART A EXERCISES

† **A1.** Calculate the chi-square statistic and degrees of freedom for the following set of data for 300 elders exposed to different interventions to encourage flu shots:

Flu Shot Status	Group A	Group B	Group C	Total
Had a flu shot	20	45	25	90
Did not have a flu shot	80	55	75	210
Total	100	100	100	300

Is the value of chi-square statistically significant at the .05 level? Based on the $(O - E)^2/E$ components contributing to chi-square, comment on the nature of the relationship between groups and flu shot status.

† **A2.** For the data in Exercise A1, compute Cramér's V statistic. Then estimate the approximate power of the chi-square test, using Table B.4 in Appendix B.

A3. Using the statistical information from the first two exercises, write a paragraph summarizing the results of the analyses.

† **A4.** Given each of the following situations, determine whether the calculated values of chi-square are statistically significant:
(a) $\chi^2 = 3.72$, $df = 1$, $\alpha = .05$
(b) $\chi^2 = 9.59$, $df = 4$, $\alpha = .05$
(c) $\chi^2 = 10.67$, $df = 3$, $\alpha = .01$
(d) $\chi^2 = 9.88$, $df = 2$, $\alpha = .01$

† **A5.** Assume that a researcher has conducted a pilot intervention study and wants to use the pilot results to estimate the

number of participants needed in a full-scale study to achieve a power of .80 with $\alpha = .05$. For each of the hypothetical pilot results presented below, how many study participants in each group would be needed in the larger study? (Note that in using Table 8.3, it makes no difference which of two groups is considered Group 1 or Group 2.)
(a) Experimental group: 45%, Control group: 65%
(b) Experimental group: 15%, Control group: 5%
(c) Experimental group: 20%, Control group: 35%
(d) Experimental group: 60%, Control group: 75%

† **A6.** Match each of the nonparametric tests in Column A with its parametric counterpart in Column B:

A. Nonparametric Test	**B. Parametric Test**
1. Mann-Whitney U Test	a. Paired t test
2. Friedman Test	b. One-way ANOVA
3. Kruskal-Wallis Test	c. Independent groups t test
4. Wilcoxon Signed-Ranks Test	d. Repeated measures ANOVA

† **A7.** Using the information provided, indicate which test you think should be used for each of the following situations:
(a) Independent variable: normal birthweight versus low birthweight infants; dependent variable: 1-minute Apgar scores (0 to 10 scale); sample size: eight infants per group
(b) Independent variable: time of measurement (before, during, and after surgery); dependent variable: heart rate; sample size: 80
(c) Independent variable: time of measurement (before, during, and after intervention); dependent variable: did versus did not exercise daily; sample size: 30
(d) Independent variable: infertility treatment A versus infertility treatment B versus control condition; dependent variable: did versus did not become pregnant; sample size: 180

(e) Independent variable: Drug A versus Drug B versus placebo; dependent variable: pain measured on a 0 to 10 scale; sample size: nine per group

(f) Independent variable: role (elderly parent versus adult child); dependent variable: preference for nursing home placement versus home care for parent

PART B EXERCISES

† **B1.** For Exercises B1 to B5, you will be using the SPSS dataset Polit2SetB. Begin by running a crosstabs (Analyze ➔ Descriptive Statistics ➔ Crosstabs) for the variables *bmicat* and *hlthlimit*. The first is a variable that uses the women's body mass index (BMI), computed from their height and weight, to form four groups: those classified in the normal BMI range (values under 25.0), overweight (values from 25.0 to 29.99), obese (values from 30.0 to 40.0), and morbidly obese (values over 40.0). The second variable is dichotomous responses to whether or not the woman had a health condition that limited her ability to work (yes is coded 1, no is coded 0). In the first dialog box for the Crosstabs, enter *hlthlimit* as the row variable and *bmicat* as the column variable. Click the pushbutton for Cells, and select Observed, Expected, and Row and Column percentages. Click on Continue, then open the dialog box for Statistics. Select Chi-square and also Phi and Cramér's V. Then click Continue and OK to initiate the analysis. Answer the following questions about the output: (a) How many normal-weight women were *expected* to have a health limitation, if BMI and health limitations were unrelated? How many actually did have a limitation? What are the two values for women who were morbidly obese? (b) What percent of all women had a health condition that limited their ability to work? (c) What is the null hypothesis being tested in this analysis? (d) What is the value of the chi-square statistic? (e) How many degrees of freedom are there? (f) Are the results statistically significant for $\alpha = .05$? At what level? (g) Comment on the nature of the relationship. (h) What is the value of Cramér's *V?* (i) Based on this effect size value, approximately how much power was there to correctly reject the null hypothesis in this analysis? (You will need to consult Table B.4.)

† **B2.** Within SPSS, it is possible to introduce a third categorical variable into a Crosstabs analysis, to see if the relationship between two variables is consistent for different levels of a third variable. In this exercise, run the same analysis that you ran in Exercise B1, except this time enter the variable *poverty* as the "Layer" variable in the third slot of the opening dialog box. This will run the crosstab and chi-square analysis between *bmicat* and *hlthlimit* separately for women who were below poverty and those who were not. Then answer the following questions: (a) Among normal-weight women who were below poverty, what is the *expected* frequency of having a health limitation? How many actually did have a limitation? What are the two values for normal-weight women who were *above* poverty? (b) What percent of women below poverty and above poverty had a health condition that limited their ability to work? (c) What were the values of the chi-square statistic in the below poverty and above poverty subgroups? (d) Were both statistics statistically significant for $\alpha = .05$? At what level? (e) What were the values of Cramér's *V* for the below poverty and above poverty groups? (f) Comment on these values of *V* in relation to power in these analyses.

† **B3.** In this exercise, we will be testing the null hypothesis that smoking status (*smoker*) is unrelated to having a health limitation. Because we want "cell a" to be the cell with the risk factor and the unfavorable outcome, we will recode *smoker* (which is coded 1 for smokers and 0 for nonsmokers) so that smokers are coded 2. Similarly, we recode *hlthlimt* so that those without a limitation are coded 2 rather than 0. Click Transform ➔ Recode ➔ Into Different Variables. Select *smoker* and move it into the Numeric Variables slot. Then type in a new variable name (*newsmoke*) in the slot for Output Variable, and click Change. Do the same process for *hlthlimit,* creating a new variable *newlimit*. Now click on the pushbutton for Old and New Values. In the next dialog box, in the Old Value field, enter 1, and also enter 1 for New Value (we are keeping code 1 the same), and then click Add. Next, enter 0 for Old Value and 2 for New Value, and click Add, Continue, and OK. The two new variables are at the end of the data file, and you can label them by clicking the Variable View tab at the bottom of the data editor. Now, run Analyze ➔ Descriptive Statistics ➔ Crosstabs, placing *newsmoke* in the slot for Rows and *newlimit* in the slot for Columns. For Cell options, click Observed, Expected, and Row Percentages. For options in the Statistics dialog box, click Chi-square and Risk. Then click Continue and OK and answer the following questions: (a) What was the absolute risk of having a health limitation among smokers? And among nonsmokers? (b) What is the value of the chi-square statistic in this analysis? (c) Is this statistically significant for $\alpha = .05$? What is the probability level, and what does this mean? (d) What is the odds ratio for this analysis? What does this mean? (e) What is the 95% *CI* around the odds ratio? (f) What is the relative risk of having a health limitation for smokers, relative to nonsmokers?

† **B4.** For this exercise, you will be running a Mann-Whitney *U* test, comparing smokers and nonsmokers on an ordinal-level variable, *drunk*. This variable measures how frequently in the prior month the woman had consumed enough alcohol to get drunk (*drunk*), from never (code 1) to 10+ times (code 5). Begin by running a simple Crosstabs (following steps described previously) so that you can examine the distribution of values for *drunk* for smokers and nonsmokers. Instruct the computer to show observed frequencies and column percentages. Then run the Mann-Whitney *U* test via Analyze ➔ Nonparametric ➔ Two Independent Samples Test. Move *drunk* into the slot

for Test Variable List, and *smoker* (the original smoking variable) into the Grouping Variable slot. Define the smoking groups as code 0 for Group 1 and code 1 for Group 2. Select Mann-Whitney U as the Test Type. Then click OK and answer these questions: (a) What percentage of smokers versus nonsmokers never got drunk in the prior month? (b) For the overall sample, what percentage of women got drunk *at least once* in the month prior to the interview? (c) What is the mean rank of "scores" for smokers versus nonsmokers? (d) What is the value of the *U* statistic? (e) Is this significant for $\alpha = .05$? At what level? (f) What does the result mean? (g) Could we have analyzed these data using a chi-square test? Why or why not?

† **B5.** In this analysis, you will be running a Kruskal-Wallis test, comparing women in the four BMI categories (*bmicat*) with regard to the number of miscarriages they had ever had (*miscarr*). Number of miscarriages in a ratio-level variable, but it is skewed, with most women having had no miscarriages. Begin by running a simple Crosstabs (following steps described previously) to examine the distribution of miscarriages among women in the four BMI groups. Then run the Kruskal-Wallis test via Analyze ➔ Nonparametric ➔ K Independent Samples Test. Move *miscarr* into the slot for Test Variable List, and *bmicat* into the Grouping Variable slot. Define the range for the groups as 1 (Minimum) to 4 (Maximum). Select Kruskal-Wallis as the Test Type. Click the Options pushbutton and request Descriptive Statistics. Then click Continue, then OK, and answer these questions: (a) What percentage of women had had one or more miscarriage in this sample? (b) Which

BMI group had the highest incidence of a miscarriage? Which group had the lowest incidence? (c) What was the range of values for the miscarriage variable? (d) What was the mean number of miscarriages? (e) Based on the mean ranks within the Kruskal-Wallis test, was the relationship between number of miscarriages and BMI linear—that is, was there an incremental progression of ranks for miscarriage as BMI got larger? (f) What is the value of the chi-square statistic for this Kruskal-Wallis analysis? (g) Is this significant for $\alpha = .05$? At what level? (h) What does the result mean? (i) Could we have analyzed these data using a chi-square test? Why or why not? (j) Could we have analyzed these data using ANOVA? Why or why not?

† **B6.** Run Crosstabs for four outcomes in the Polit2SetC dataset. (Note that this is a different file than for the previous exercises.) The four outcomes are responses to a series of questions about whether the women had experienced different forms of abuse in the prior year: verbal abuse, *verbalab* (someone yelling at them and putting them down); control, *controld* (efforts to control their every move); threats, *threatn* (threats of physical harm), and physical abuse, *harmed* (being hit, slapped, kicked, or otherwise physically harmed). We want to test the hypothesis that poverty is a risk factor for these outcomes, and so *poverty* will be used as the independent variable. In the Crosstabs, use *poverty* as the Row variable, and the four abuse variables as the Column variables. Select Chi-square and Risk as the statistics. Use the output to create a table to present your results, using Table 8.10 as a model. (You can choose to report either OR or RR values.) Then write a paragraph summarizing the results.

Correlation and Simple Regression

In Chapter 4, we discussed Pearson's *r* as a descriptive statistic that summarizes the magnitude and direction of a relationship between two variables. Correlation coefficients are also used to draw inferences about relationships in populations. This chapter discusses the inferential aspects of correlation coefficients, and introduces the closely related topic of linear regression.

PEARSON'S *r* AND INFERENTIAL STATISTICS

Suppose we were interested in examining the relationship between widows' grief resolution following their husbands' death (the dependent variable) and the length of their husbands' illness prior to death (the independent variable). We find that, for a sample of 50 widows, the Pearson *r* between scores on a grief resolution scale and length of spouse's illness is .26, indicating a modest tendency among women in the sample for longer spousal illnesses to be associated with more favorable grief resolution. The observed correlation in the sample, however, does not tell us whether the relationship exists in the population. A correlation of .26 could reflect sampling error. We need inferential statistics to assess the probability that there is a population correlation.

The Null and Alternative Hypotheses

The basic and most widely tested correlational null hypothesis is that there is no relationship between the two variables in the population. When there is no relationship, the correlation is zero. The population correlation coefficient is symbolized as ρ—rho (the lowercase Greek r), so we can formally state the null hypothesis as follows:

$$H_0: \rho = .00$$

The alternative hypothesis is that there *is* a relationship between the two variables. The nondirectional alternative hypothesis is:

$$H_1: \rho \neq .00$$

This alternative hypothesis does not predict the nature of the relationship between the two variables—it is nondirectional. If we had an a priori reason for hypothesizing the direction of the relationship, the alternative hypothesis could specify that direction. That is, we could test the hypothesis that ρ is greater than zero (if we had reason to believe that the variables were positively correlated) or that ρ is less than zero (if we expected the variables to be negatively correlated).

In testing the null correlation hypothesis, the sample correlation coefficient r is used as the estimate of ρ. The statistic can be compared to a sampling distribution to determine whether its value is "improbable" if the null hypothesis is true.

A theoretical **sampling distribution of a correlation coefficient** can be constructed in the same fashion as other sampling distributions. One has to imagine drawing an infinite number of samples of a specified size and plotting the values of the correlation coefficients in a frequency distribution. The mean of the sampling distribution of the correlation coefficient is approximately ρ, the true population correlation. When $\rho = 0$ (i.e., when the null hypothesis is true), the sampling distribution is approximately normal with the mean centered on 0.0. Statisticians have developed tabled values of r to test the null hypothesis that a population correlation is zero.

Assumptions and Requirements for Pearson's *r*

Pearson's r is appropriate when both variables are measured on approximately an interval level or on a ratio level. As discussed in Chapter 4, Pearson's r is suitable for detecting *linear* relationships between two variables.

The test of the null hypothesis that $\rho = .00$ is based on several assumptions. First, as with other tests, it is assumed that participants have been randomly and independently sampled from a population. Second, the variables being correlated (X and Y) are assumed to have an underlying distribution that is **bivariate normal**—that is, scores on variable X are assumed to be normally distributed *for each value of variable Y*, and vice versa. Finally, scores are assumed to be **homoscedastic**—that is, for each value of X, the variability of Y scores must be about the same, and vice versa. Bivariate normality is not easy to test, but fortunately failure to meet this assumption typically has only a small effect on the validity of the statistical test, particularly when the sample size is larger than 15.

Testing the Significance of Pearson's r

We discussed computations for Pearson's r in Chapter 4, and also illustrated SPSS output from a correlation analysis. Here we discuss using Pearson's r as an inferential statistic.

Earlier, we presented an example in which the correlation between widows' score on a grief resolution scale and husband's length of illness in a sample of 50 widows was .26. Can we conclude that a correlation exists in the population, or does the correlation of .26 in the sample reflect sampling error? To test the null hypothesis that the population correlation is zero against the alternative hypothesis that it is not, we compare the calculated test statistic (r) against a critical value for r in the appropriate table (Table A.6 of Appendix A). First, however, we must calculate degrees of freedom. For Pearson's r, the formula is as follows:

$$df = N - 2$$

In our example, there are 48 degrees of freedom ($50 - 2 = 48$). For a nondirectional (two-tailed) test with $\alpha = .05$, we find in column 3 of the table that the critical value of r with $df = 48$ is between .273 and .288 (i.e., between the values for 45 and 50 degrees of freedom). The obtained value of r (.26) is smaller than .272, so we must accept the null hypothesis that the population correlation is zero. There is a greater than 5% probability that a correlation coefficient of .26 is the result of sampling error, and thus we cannot conclude that the length of a spouse's illness is related to a widow's grief resolution in the population (the actual p was .07 for a two-tailed test).

If we had tested a directional hypothesis, the outcome would have been different. If theory or prior research had led us to hypothesize in advance that grief resolution would be greater for widows whose husbands were ill for longer periods prior to death, we would find in column 2 of Table A.6 that the critical value for a directional (one-tailed) test with $\alpha = .05$ would be about .233. The computed value of r is greater than this critical value, so the null hypothesis would be rejected. We reiterate that it is inappropriate to use the critical values for a directional test *after* r has been computed if a directional hypothesis was not specified in advance.

Note that when we accept a null hypothesis, we cannot conclude that there is no relationship between the two variables in the population. The possibility of a Type II error—the incorrect acceptance of the null hypothesis—still remains. Moreover, there is also a possibility that the variables are related in the population, but in a nonlinear fashion. The acceptance of the null hypothesis should, as always, be treated conservatively.

Testing Differences Between Two Correlations

Researchers most often want to test the null hypothesis that the population correlation is zero, but other hypotheses can also be tested. The most common alternative involves a test of the equivalence of two independent correlations. In our example of grief resolution, all participants were widows. Suppose we did another study with a sample of 50 widowers, using the same measure of grief resolution, and obtained a correlation coefficient of .45.

The question is whether the difference in observed correlations for men versus women occurred simply as a function of chance, or whether there is a true population difference between men and women in the relationship between grief resolution and length of spouse's illness. In this situation, the null hypothesis being tested is as follows:

$$H_0: \rho_A = \rho_B$$

where ρ_A = population correlation for group A (widows)
ρ_B = population correlation for group B (widowers)

When ρ is not equal to zero—which this null hypothesis assumes—the sampling distribution of the correlation coefficient is skewed rather than approximately normal, and therefore the same table that we used to test the basic hypothesis of no relationship between variables is no longer appropriate. The statistician Fisher, however, developed a logarithmic transformation of r (called the **r-to-z transformation**) that allows us to use the normal distribution for comparing two correlation coefficients.

Table A.7 of Appendix A presents values for transforming correlation coefficients into values of z. To use this table, we must first find the value of r, and then read directly to the right the corresponding value of z. From this table we find that for $r = .26$ (widows), $z_A = .266$. For $r = .45$ (widowers), $z_B = .485$. With these transformed z values, the following formula can be used to compute a test statistic (z_{obs}) for the significance of the difference between the two:

$$z_{obs} = \frac{|z_A - z_B|}{\sqrt{\dfrac{1}{n_A - 3} + \dfrac{1}{n_B - 3}}}$$

In our present example, the computed z_{obs} statistic is 1.06 (computation not shown), which must now be compared to the critical value from the normal distribution (Table A.1). For $\alpha = .05$, that critical value is 1.96. Our value of z_{obs} is less than the critical value, so the null hypothesis is retained. We cannot conclude that the correlation between grief resolution and length of spouse's illness is different for widows and widowers in the populations.

TIP: *A useful interactive Web site for computing the significance of differences between two independent correlations is http://peaks .informatik.uni-erlangen.de/cgi-bin/usignificance.cgi.*

The Magnitude and Nature of Relationships

Unlike most other inferential statistics, Pearson's r directly conveys information about the magnitude and nature of the relationship between variables. The nature of the relationship is indicated by the sign of the correlation coefficient. A negative sign indicates that high values on one variable are associated with low values on the second. A positive sign (or a coefficient without a sign, which by convention is assumed to indicate a positive correlation) indicates that high values on X are associated with high values on Y.

The magnitude of the relationship between variables is directly indicated by the absolute value of Pearson's r. The higher the absolute value of the correlation coefficient, the stronger the relationship. As discussed in Chapter 4, however, magnitude is often expressed in terms of r^2, which is sometimes called the **coefficient of determination.**

As we saw in the chapter on ANOVA, eta^2 is the ratio of explained variance ($SS_{Explained}$) to total variance (SS_{Total}), and r^2 is directly equivalent to eta-squared. Thus:

$$r^2 = eta^2 = \frac{SS_{Explained}}{SS_{Total}}$$

The coefficient of determination, then, tells us the proportion of variance in variable Y that is associated with variable X—the proportion of variance that is *shared* by the two variables. Thus, in the example we have used in this chapter where $r = .26$, we could say that about 7% of the variability in grief resolution is shared by (explained by) variability in spouse's length of illness ($.26^2 = .068$).

When comparing the magnitude of different correlations, it is more appropriate to use r^2 than r. For example, suppose the correlation between widows' grief resolution and their age was .13—half the value of the correlation between grief resolution and spouse's length of illness. Yet, length of illness explains *four* times as much of the variance in grief resolution scores as widow's age (.068 versus .017), and this is a more informative and meaningful comparison.

Precision and Pearson's *r*

It is possible, although cumbersome, to compute a confidence interval around r. The calculation of a *CI* requires converting r to z using the *r*-to-*z* transformation, calculating the standard error for z using a formula ($1 \div \sqrt{N - 3}$), computing confidence limits around z by multiplying the *SE* by 1.96 for a 95% *CI*, then converting the calculated confidence limits back to values of r. This effort can be avoided, however, by using an interactive Web site that does the calculations for you (e.g., *http://faculty.vassar.edu/lowry/rho.html*). In our example of correlating grief resolution with spouse's length of illness for 50 widows, r was .26 and the 95% *CI* is $-.02$ to .50. This is a wide interval that includes the value of .00, which corresponds to the null hypothesis. The benefit of calculating the confidence interval is that it makes apparent how imprecise the point estimate of .26 really is.

Power and Pearson's *r*

As discussed in previous chapters, a primary reason for performing a power analysis when planning a study is to learn how large a sample is needed to minimize the risk of a Type II error. In a situation involving Pearson's r, the effect size for the power analysis is the estimated value of ρ. Thus, we can use the sample correlation coefficient r as the estimate of ρ, the effect size. In meta-analyses involving correlations, r can be used directly as the estimated effect.

For fine determinations of needed sample size, interactive power analysis Web sites on the Internet are helpful (for example, *http://www.quantitativeskills.com/sisa/statistics/correl.htm*). For the sake of convenience, we offer a simple table (Table 9.1) for estimating sample size needs for two-tailed tests with $\alpha = .05$. To use this table to estimate needed sample size, you would find the estimated ρ in the top row (for example, using r from a pilot study or other similar research), select the desired power in the leftmost column (typically .80, the shaded row), and find N at the intersection.

TABLE 9.1 Sample Size and Power as a Function of the Population Correlation Coefficient, for Alpha = .05 (Two-Tailed Test)

Power	Estimated Population Correlation (ρ)												
	.05	.10	.15	.20	.25	.30	.35	.40	.45	.50	.60	.70	.80
.20	499	127	57	32	21	15	12	9	7	6	5	4	3
.30	823	207	92	53	34	24	18	14	11	9	7	5	4
.40	1163	292	130	73	47	32	24	18	15	12	9	6	5
.50	1533	383	171	96	61	42	31	24	18	15	11	8	6
.60	1956	489	217	122	78	54	39	30	24	19	13	9	7
.70	2463	614	272	152	97	67	49	37	29	23	16	11	8
.80	3149	785	347	194	123	85	62	47	36	29	19	13	10
.90	4200	1047	463	258	164	112	81	61	47	37	25	17	12

The entries in the table indicate the sample size required to achieve the specified power, for the given correlation coefficient.

For example, with r = .25, a sample of 123 participants would be needed to keep risks of statistical errors to standard levels.

When estimates of ρ are unavailable from pilot data or prior research, a last resort is to use the small-medium-large conventions of .10, .30, and .50, respectively. This corresponds to estimated sample size needs of 785, 85, and 29 participants, assuming standard criteria for power and alpha. It is probably safest, in the absence any other information, to estimate no more than a small-to-medium effect size of .20, which would require a sample size of 194 participants. (Polit and Sherman [1990] found that the average correlation coefficient across hundreds of nursing studies was about .20; although not recent, these findings are probably still valid.)

For estimating post hoc power for a completed analysis, you would need to find a close approximation to the actual sample size in the column corresponding most closely to the obtained r. For example, in our earlier example in which r was .26, we would use the column for .25. The actual sample size of 50 is between the values of 47 and 61 in that column, and so power was between .40 and .50. Using interactive power calculators, we found that power in this example could be estimated at .453, which translates to an estimated 55% risk of a Type II error.

Factors Affecting Pearson's *r*

Several factors affect the magnitude of Pearson's *r*. These factors should be kept in mind in designing a correlational study and interpreting results of correlational analyses. One of these factors is the existence of a curvilinear, rather than linear, relationship between the two variables, an issue noted in Chapter 4. Several other issues are discussed here.

THE EFFECT OF A RESTRICTED RANGE   If two variables are linearly related, the magnitude of the correlation coefficient is reduced when the range of values on one of the variables is restricted. In Chapter 4 we discussed how the formula for the correlation coefficient involves deviation scores—that is, deviations from the means of the two variables. When the range is restricted, deviations are smaller and thus the magnitude of r is reduced.

This principle can best be illustrated graphically. Suppose we had a sample of 70 smokers and nonsmokers and plotted their weekly number of packs of cigarettes

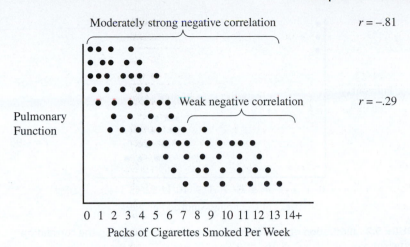

FIGURE 9.1 Illustration of the effect of a restricted range on the correlation coefficient.

smoked against a measure of pulmonary function, as shown in Figure 9.1. For the overall sample, the scatterplot suggests a strong negative correlation between weekly packs of cigarettes and pulmonary function. In fact, the computed r is $-.81$, a correlation that is significantly different from zero at $p < .001$. Now suppose that instead of using the entire group, we restricted the sample to the 25 people who smoked at least one pack of cigarettes per day—i.e., at least 7 packs per week. The figure illustrates that the relationship between cigarette consumption and pulmonary function is now less clear cut. The scatterplot shows a much weaker negative correlation among the regular smokers. Indeed, the computed correlation coefficient is $-.29$, which is not statistically significant from zero for $N = 25$. Note that a similar reduction in the correlation would occur if the range for pulmonary function variable were restricted (e.g., if only those with very high or very low function were included in the sample).

THE EFFECT OF EXTREME GROUPS   When only extreme groups from both ends of a distribution are included in a sample, the magnitude of the correlation coefficient may *increase*. To continue with our example of the correlation between smoking and pulmonary function, suppose our sample included only nonsmokers and people who smoked 10 or more packs of cigarettes per week. In this situation, illustrated in Figure 9.2, the range of values on both variables is the same as originally, but deviations from the mean are exaggerated because no participants were close to the mean on either variable. With this extreme-group sample, the correlation is markedly negative, $r = -.96$. Thus, when extreme groups from a population have been sampled, care must be taken not to interpret correlation coefficients as reflecting relationships for the entire population.

THE EFFECT OF AN OUTLIER   When a sample is relatively small, a person with an extreme value on one or both variables being correlated can have a dramatic effect on the magnitude of the coefficient. An exaggerated illustration is graphed in Figure 9.3. In this example, 11 of the 12 people in the sample had values of 7 or less for both the X and Y variables. The 12th person, labeled A on the scatterplot, had extremely high values on both variables. The smaller ellipse surrounding the values without the outlier suggests a modest correlation—in fact, the actual value of r for these 11 cases is .10.

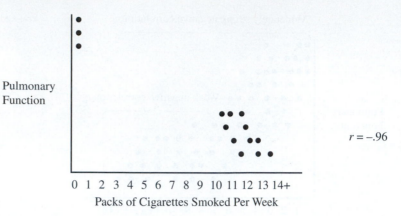

Pulmonary
Function

$r = -.96$

0 1 2 3 4 5 6 7 8 9 10 11 12 13 14+
Packs of Cigarettes Smoked Per Week

FIGURE 9.2 Illustration of the effect of using extreme groups on the correlation coefficient.

When the outlier is included, however, the shape of the outer ellipse indicates a much stronger relationship. The calculated value of r when the outlier is included is .71—a dramatically higher, and misleading, correlation coefficient.

When outliers represent legitimate score values rather than data entry or coding errors, care must be taken in using them in the analysis. Researchers sometimes analyze their data both ways—with and without outliers—and present both sets of results when the disparity is great. Barnett and Lewis (1994) suggest alternative strategies for handling outliers.

Example of outlier effects:

Winkelman, Norman, Maloni, and Kless (2008) did a study of pain measurement during labor and examined correlations between pain measurement via a 100-point visual analog scale and dermatome assessment at multiple points in time after administration of epidural anesthesia. Pearson correlations ranged from .33 at 25 minutes to .55 at 15 minutes. Noting that higher correlations had been found in earlier research, the researchers speculated that correlations could have been affected by the presence of several outliers.

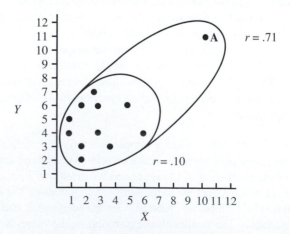

FIGURE 9.3 Illustration of the effect of an outlier on the correlation coefficient.

THE EFFECT OF UNRELIABLE MEASURES   Virtually all quantitative measures of variables contain some measurement error. Psychometricians generally refer to this error as *unreliability*, and they have developed methods to assess degree of **reliability** of measures (a topic we discuss briefly later in this chapter and in Chapter 13). Measurement error reduces the magnitude of correlation coefficients, and this effect is called **attenuation**. Thus, in interpreting modest correlation coefficients, it may be important to consider whether the magnitude might have been diminished by the use of relatively weak instruments. Note, though, that psychometricians have developed a formula for correcting attenuated correlation coefficients. The correction takes the reliability coefficients for one or both variables into account (see Nunnally & Bernstein, 1994, p. 256).

> **TIP:** *Because of the issues discussed in this section, it is wise to examine scatterplots as a first step in doing a correlation analysis—and to know the reliability of any scaled measures. Scatterplots will help you detect any anomalies in the data, such as outliers and extreme values.*

OTHER MEASURES OF ASSOCIATION

In addition to Pearson's r, there are other statistical indexes that describe relationships between two variables and permit inferences about relationships in the population. Indeed, we have already discussed some of these—for example in Chapter 8 we discussed the phi coefficient and Cramér's V as measures of association for two nominal-level variables. In this section we examine other measures of bivariate relationships.

Spearman's Rank-Order Correlation

A statistic known as **Spearman's rank-order correlation** is a nonparametric analog of Pearson's r. A Spearman correlation is typically used when the dependent variable is measured on the ordinal scale, or when one or both variables being correlated is severely skewed or has an outlier. It is also preferred by some researchers when there are fewer than 30 cases.

Suppose that we wanted to examine the correlation between nursing students' class rank at graduation and the students' rating of how likely it is that they would pursue a graduate degree, on a scale from 0 (extremely probable) to 10 (extremely unlikely). A Spearman's correlation coefficient (often called **Spearman's rho**) could be computed in such a situation. We use the symbol r_S for Spearman's rho, to avoid confusion with rho, the population correlation. Some hypothetical data for ten students are presented in Table 9.2.

To compute Spearman's correlation coefficient, both variables must be rank ordered. The class rank variable is inherently rank ordered, but we must also rank order students' ratings of the likelihood of going to graduate school. The rankings for this variable are shown in Column 3 of Table 9.2. As we can see, in Column 2, there was one tie: two students had a rating of 2. When ties occur, the two adjacent ranks (here, the ranks of 3 and 4) are averaged, and the average rank (here, 3.5) is assigned to both people. In the next step, the difference between the ranks for the two variables (D) is taken (column 5), and then the difference is squared (column 6). The sum of the squared differences is then used in the following formula:

$$r_S = 1 - \frac{6(\Sigma D^2)}{N(N^2 - 1)}$$

† **B5.** Run a simple regression between family income (*income*), which we will use as the *Y* or dependent variable, and number of hours worked (*workweek*), which we will use as the *X* or predictor variable. You can do this through Analyze ➡ Regression ➡ Linear. Move *income* into the slot for Dependent Variable and *workweek* into the slot for Independent Variable. Click the Statistics pushbutton and make sure the following options are selected: Estimates, Confidence Intervals, and Model fit; then click Continue. (We do not have to run Descriptives because we already did this earlier in Exercise B1.) Then click OK on the main dialog box and use the output to answer the following questions: (a) What is the value of r^2 and adjusted r^2? (b) What is the *SE* estimate? (c) What is the regression sum of squares and the total sum of squares in this analysis? What is the value of $SS_{Regression}$ divided by SS_{Total}? (d) What is the intercept constant and the slope in this regression?

(e) What is the regression equation for predicting new values of family income? (f) Using the regression equation, what is the predicted monthly family income for women working 35 hours per week?

† **B6.** Run Correlations for the following variables in the Polit2SetB dataset (note that this is a different file than for the previous exercises): the woman's age (*age*); number of children living in the household (*kidshh*); number of ER visits in the past 12 months (*ervisit*); number of doctor visits in the past 12 months (*docvisit*); body mass index (*bmi*); number of miscarriages (*miscarr*); score on the SF-12 physical health component (*sf12phys*); and score on the SF-12 mental health component (*sf12ment*). Use the output to create a table to present the correlations between the two SF-12 scores on the one hand and the other variables on the other. Use Table 9.4 as a model, using the SF-12 variables as column headings. Then write a paragraph summarizing the results.

10

Multiple Regression

This chapter focuses on multiple regression, a useful and versatile statistical procedure. First, however, we briefly discuss the general topic of multivariate statistics.

INTRODUCTION TO MULTIVARIATE STATISTICS

The bivariate inferential statistics we have examined thus far concern the relationship between two variables, typically one independent variable and one dependent variable. Researchers have become aware of the limited ability of bivariate statistics to unravel the complex phenomena in which they are interested. Phenomena such as infection, pain, coping, and blood pressure have multiple determinants. Two-variable analyses cannot adequately capture the multiple influences on, or causes of, these phenomena. Thus, the use of **multivariate statistics**, which involve analyses of three or more variables, is expanding. The widespread availability of computers has made it possible for even novice researchers to use complex statistical procedures.

This chapter and the three that follow describe widely used multivariate statistics. In these chapters, formulas and actual calculations for multivariate procedures are minimized. Multivariate statistics are computationally formidable and are never done by hand, so no attempt is made to present fully worked-out examples. At the same time, these chapters offer more guidance on reading computer printouts.

BASIC CONCEPTS FOR MULTIPLE REGRESSION

When a researcher discovers that the correlation between two variables is, say, .50, it means that 25% ($.50^2$) of the variance in the dependent variable is explained by the independent variable. Yet, a full 75% of the variance is *un*explained. Scientists strive to fully understand—and predict—the phenomena in which they are interested, and so they value statistical techniques that can mirror human complexity.

Multiple regression analysis, an extension of simple linear regression, allows researchers to improve their predictions by using two or more variables to predict a dependent variable. For example, suppose we wanted to predict a person's weight. If we did a regression using a person's sex as the sole predictor variable, the accuracy of our predictions would be modest. We would predict that men would be heavier than women, but we would sometimes be wrong. Moreover, the regression equation would predict men to have the mean weight for males and women to have the mean weight for females, despite the fact that men's and women's weights can range over hundreds of pounds. If, however, we could use information on a person's height *and* sex, our ability to predict weight would be dramatically improved. Multiple regression yields an equation that provides the best prediction possible, given the correlations among all variables in the analysis.

The Basic Multiple Regression Equation

The multiple regression equation is, conceptually, a simple extension of the simple regression equation. The basic equation is as follows:

$$Y' = a + b_1X_1 + b_2X_2 + \ldots + b_kX_k$$

where Y' = predicted value for variable Y
a = intercept constant
k = number of independent (predictor) variables
b_1 to b_k = regression coefficients for the k predictor variables
X_1 to X_k = values for the k predictor variables

This equation, or **model,** stipulates that the predicted value of Y is a linear combination of an intercept constant, plus predictor variables that are weighted by regression coefficients. Regression analysis yields best-fitting values of a and the bs, using the least squares criterion that the squared error terms (the differences between Y and Y') are minimized.

In multiple regression equations, regression coefficients (b-weights) are associated with each predictor variable. The coefficients are the weights associated with a given independent variable *when the other predictors are in the equation*. If predictor variables were added to or removed from the regression equation, the bs would change.

As an example, suppose a graduate nursing program wanted to ensure the selection of the most worthy applicants. The school uses information from current graduate students to develop a regression equation to predict academic performance of prospective students. Table 10.1 shows data for 20 students for the dependent variable, graduate

TABLE 10.1 Fictitious Data for Multiple Regression Analysis Predicting Graduate GPA

| Student | Independent (Predictor) Variables | | | | Dependent Variable |
	Undergrad GPA X_1	GRE-Verbal X_2	GRE-Quant X_3	Motivation X_4	Graduate GPA Y
1	3.4	600	540	75	3.6
2	3.1	510	480	70	3.0
3	3.7	650	710	85	3.9
4	3.2	530	450	60	2.8
5	3.5	610	500	90	3.7
6	2.9	540	620	60	2.6
7	3.3	530	510	75	3.4
8	2.9	540	600	55	2.7
9	3.4	550	580	75	3.3
10	3.2	700	630	65	3.5
11	3.7	630	700	80	3.6
12	3.0	480	490	75	2.8
13	3.1	530	520	60	3.0
14	3.7	580	610	65	3.5
15	3.9	710	660	80	3.8
16	3.5	500	480	75	3.2
17	3.1	490	510	60	2.4
18	2.9	560	540	55	2.7
19	3.2	550	590	65	3.1
20	3.6	600	550	60	3.6
Mean	3.32	569.50	563.50	69.25	3.21
SD	.30	65.09	74.92	10.17	.44

grade point average (GPA) and four independent variables—undergraduate GPA (X_1); scores on the standardized test called the Graduate Record Exam (GRE) Verbal Test (X_2); scores on the GRE Quantitative Test (X_3); and scores on an achievement motivation scale (X_4). Although we do not show actual computations, the regression equation using these data is as follows:

$$Y' = -1.215 + .672X_1 + .0031X_2 - .00067X_3 + .0117X_4$$

This equation specifies that graduate grade point average can be predicted by *subtracting* (because the value of the intercept constant is negative) 1.215 from the sum of applicants' raw scores on the four predictors, multiplied by their respective regression coefficients. In this equation, the *b*-weight for GRE Quantitative is negative, so this term would be subtracted rather than added.

To examine the equation's accuracy, suppose we used this equation to "predict" the graduate grade point average of the first student in Table 10.1:

$$Y' = -1.215 + .672(3.4) + .0031(600) - .00067(540) + .0117(75)$$
$$Y' = 3.446$$

For this first student we "predict" a graduate grade point average of 3.446, but the actual value is 3.6. The error of prediction $(Y' - Y)$ is $-.154$ ($3.446 - 3.6$), and the squared error term is .024 ($-.154^2$). In the aggregate, the sum of the squared error terms is minimized in the analysis. Any values for the regression coefficients and intercept constant other than those in the regression equation would yield a larger sum of squared residuals.

The Standardized Multiple Regression Equation

In multiple regression, the independent variables are typically in different measurement units. In our example, GRE scores are on a scale that can range from 200 to 800, while undergraduate GPA can range from 0.0 to 4.0. Regression coefficients necessarily incorporate differences in the measurement units, and so b-weights cannot directly be compared.

To address this issue, the regression equation is often presented in the following standardized form:

$$Z_{Y'} = \beta_1 z_{x_1} + \beta_2 z_{x_2} + \ldots \beta_k z_{x_2}$$

where
$z_{Y'}$ = predicted value of the standard score for Y
β_1 to β_k = standardized regression weights for k predictor variables
z_{x_1} to z_{x_k} = standard scores for k predictor variables

In standardized form, the raw values of the predictor variables are converted to z scores, each of which has a mean of 0.0 and an SD of 1.0. The z scores are weighted by standardized regression coefficients that are usually referred to as **beta weights** (βs). In the standardized regression equation, there is no intercept constant because the intercept is always 0.0. In our example, the standardized regression equation is as follows:

$$z_{Y'} = .46z_{x_1} + .46z_{x_2} - .11z_{x_3} + .27z_{x_4}$$

This equation indicates that the predicted standard score (z score) for graduate GPA equals the sum of the standard scores for the four predictors multiplied by their respective beta weights. Note that, as in the original regression equation, the regression coefficient for GRE Quantitative is negative and so the third term is subtracted from, rather than added to, the others.

TIP: *Beta weights in regression analysis should not be confused with β, the risk of a Type II error, as in a power analysis.*

Multiple Correlation

Multiple regression analysis allows researchers to address several important questions about the relationships among variables. One key question is how well the independent variables, taken together, predict a dependent variable. In our example, this question is: How well do undergraduate GPA, GRE Verbal and Quantitative scores, and motivation scores predict graduate GPA?

This question is addressed through the **multiple correlation** of the dependent and the predictor variables. Just as simple linear regression is closely linked to bivariate correlation, so multiple regression is closely related to multiple correlation. The **multiple correlation coefficient**, symbolized as R, summarizes the magnitude of the

TABLE 10.2 Correlation Matrix for Multiple Regression Example

	Undergrad GPA X_1	GRE Verbal X_2	GRE Quant X_3	Motivation X_4	Graduate GPA Y
Undergrad GPA X_1	1.00				
GRE Verbal X_2	.62	1.00			
GRE Quant X_3	.44	.71	1.00		
Motivation X_4	.64	.37	.20	1.00	
Graduate GPA Y	.87	.76	.47	.71	1.00

relationship between a dependent variable and several independent variables, considered simultaneously.

Unlike Pearson's r, R cannot be a negative value. R ranges from a low of .00 to a high of 1.00, with higher values indicating a stronger relationship between several independent variables and a dependent variable. R conveys no information about the *direction* of relationship, which is sensible when you consider that some independent variables could be negatively correlated with the dependent variable, while others could be positively correlated.

R, when squared, indicates the proportion of variance in the dependent variable accounted for by the predictors. R^2 thus provides a direct means of evaluating the accuracy of the multiple regression equation. When R^2 is 1.0, perfect prediction can be achieved. When R^2 is, say, 0.10, prediction errors will be large.

Researchers can also use R^2 to determine how much the accuracy of their predictions is *improved* by adding independent variables. In our example of predicting graduate GPA, the multiple correlation coefficient is .94, and so the proportion of explained variance in graduate GPA is .88 ($.94^2$). Table 10.2 presents the full correlation matrix for the four predictors and the dependent variable. This matrix shows that the bivariate correlation (sometimes called the **zero-order correlation**) between undergraduate GPA and graduate GPA is .87, so $r^2 = .76$ ($.87^2$). Thus, the inclusion of three additional predictors in the regression increased the proportion of variance explained by .12 (i.e., from .76 to .88).

An important point is that R cannot be less than the highest bivariate correlation between Y and the Xs. Table 10.2 shows that the independent variable that is correlated most strongly with graduate GPA is X_1 (undergraduate GPA), $r = .87$. Thus, R could not have been less than .87.

A second point is that as predictors are added to the equation, R tends to increase most when the predictors are not themselves highly correlated with each other. If all the independent variables were perfectly correlated, the value of R would be the same as the r between any X and Y—all rs would be identical, and additional independent variables beyond the first one would contribute no new information. By contrast, if two independent variables (X_1 and X_2) are totally *un*correlated (i.e., $r_{12} = .00$), the rs between Y and the Xs could be added together to determine the value of R (i.e., $R = r_{y1} + r_{y2}$). When the bivariate correlations among the independent variables are between .00 and 1.00, as they usually are, the increment to R as variables are added to the equation tends to be relatively small. Thus, R in our example is not substantially higher than the r between Y and X_1 alone (.94 versus .87). This is because there is redundancy of information among correlated predictors. When the correlations among the independent variables are high, each predictor adds little new information.

When correlations among predictors are low, each variable can potentially explain a unique portion of the variability in the dependent variable.

A third and related point is that increments to R tend to decrease as additional predictors are included in the regression equation. Redundancy among predictors is the rule, not the exception, and redundancy increases as the number of predictors increases. In our example, Table 10.2 shows that the correlations among the independent variables are moderate to strong. We can see a decline in the increment to R as predictors are added:

$$r_{y1} = .87$$
$$R_{y12} = .91$$
$$R_{y123} = .92$$
$$R_{y1234} = .94$$

The coefficient increases from .87 for X_1 and Y alone, to .91 (an increment of .04) when X_2 is added to X_1 for predicting Y. The increment is smaller at subsequent additions of predictors. Typically, the inclusion of independent variables beyond the first three or four does little to improve the value of R.

Adjustments to R^2

In bivariate correlation, coefficients from samples are expected to fluctuate above and below the population value. In multiple correlation, however, the value of R cannot be negative, so that all chance fluctuations are in a direction that inflates the magnitude of R. Sampling fluctuation tends to be more severe in small samples, so overestimation of R is usually greatest in small samples. For this reason, R^2 is often adjusted to yield a better estimation of the population value, and sample size is taken into account in the adjustment. In some textbooks, the result is called **adjusted R^2**, while others referred to it as **shrunken R^2**.

The formula for the adjusted value (which we label $\tilde{R}^2$) is straightforward:

$$\tilde{R}^2 = 1 - (1 - R^2)\left[\frac{N - 1}{N - k - 1}\right]$$

In our example of predicting graduate GPA with all four independent variables, R^2 was .88. Applying the adjustment formula, with $N = 20$ and $k = 4$, we would calculate $\tilde{R}^2$ to be .85 (calculations not shown). Most computer programs routinely calculate both R^2 and $\tilde{R}^2$.

Statistical Control: Partial and Semipartial Correlation

Regression coefficients in multiple regression must be interpreted somewhat differently than coefficients in bivariate regression. In simple regression, the value of b indicates the amount of change in the predicted value of Y for a specified rate of change in X. In multiple regression, the coefficients represent the number of units the dependent variable is predicted to change for each unit change in a given predictor *when the effects of the other predictors are held constant*. In the example we have been using, the coefficient of .672 associated with undergraduate GPA in our equation means that, holding constant the two GRE scores and motivation scores, graduate GPA is predicted to increase by .672 units for every change of 1.0 (1 unit) in undergraduate GPA.

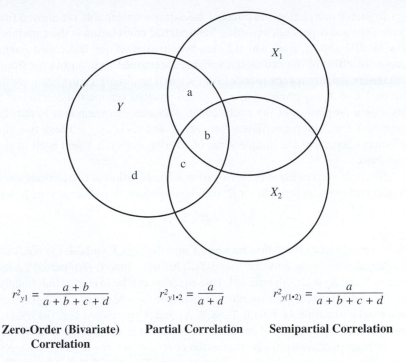

$$r^2_{y1} = \frac{a + b}{a + b + c + d} \qquad r^2_{y1\cdot2} = \frac{a}{a + d} \qquad r^2_{y(1\cdot2)} = \frac{a}{a + b + c + d}$$

Zero-Order (Bivariate)   Partial Correlation   Semipartial Correlation
Correlation

FIGURE 10.1 Venn diagram illustrating partial and semipartial correlation.

The concept of "holding constant" other predictor variables is important and relates to a key issue of research design and analysis: control. In a research context, **control** means the control of variance in the dependent variable. Control can be achieved in a number of ways (see Polit & Beck, 2008), but here we focus on statistical control. **Statistical control** uses statistical methods to isolate or nullify variance in a dependent variable that is associated with variables that are extraneous to the relationship under study. For example, in a study of the association between teenagers' self-esteem and their use of drugs, researchers would want to control potentially confounding factors that are known to be related to drug use (e.g., family income, academic performance). Multiple regression and other multivariate analyses provide a mechanism for achieving such control. The process can best be explained through visual representations of partial and semipartial correlation.

Partial correlation provides a measure of the relationship between a dependent variable (Y) and an independent variable (X_1) while controlling for the effect of a third variable (X_2). Figure 10.1 presents a diagram that portrays relationships among variables. As explained earlier, the circles represent total variability in the variables, and the degree to which circles overlap indicates the magnitude of the correlation between them—i.e., how much variance is shared. Figure 10.1 illustrates a situation in which Y is correlated with both X_1 and X_2, which in turn are correlated with each other. Y's variability has four components—variability uniquely shared with X_1 (labeled a); variability uniquely shared with X_2 (labeled c); variability common to all three variables (labeled b); and variability that Y does not share with the other two variables (d). With partial correlation, the influence of X_2 on Y (areas b and c) is removed statistically. The partial correlation between X_1 and Y (symbolized as $r_{y1\cdot2}$) indicates the degree to which these two variables are correlated *after* the influence of X_2 is partialled out. Thus, the squared partial correlation reflects a as a proportion of $a + d$, not as a proportion of the entire circle.

In partial correlation, the effect of the extraneous variable is removed from the independent and dependent variables. **Semipartial correlation** is the correlation between *all* of Y and X_1, from which X_2 has been partialled out. It is called *semi*partial because the effect of the extraneous variable is removed from X_1 but not from Y. In the diagram, the area *a* corresponds to the squared semipartial correlation coefficient between Y and X_1 (symbolized as $r_{y(1\cdot2)}$); this squared semipartial coefficient represents *a* as a proportion of the entire circle. The area *c* corresponds to the squared semipartial correlation coefficient between Y and X_2 ($r_{y(2\cdot1)}$). These two squared coefficients represent the unique areas of overlap between Y and each of the two X variables.

Multiple correlation may be viewed as a combination of correlations and semipartial correlations. A formula for R^2 that demonstrates this concept is as follows:

$$R^2_{y12} = r^2_{y1} + r^2_{y(2\cdot1)}$$

That is, the squared correlation between Y and the two X variables is equivalent to the squared correlation between Y and X_1, plus the squared semipartial correlation between Y and X_2 with X_1 partialled. This equation can be extended indefinitely. The term for a third predictor variable, for example, would be $r^2_{y(3\cdot12)}$—the squared semipartial correlation of Y with X_3, with X_1 and X_2 partialled out. (In research reports, the squared semipartial correlation coefficient is sometimes symbolized **sr^2**.)

In regression analysis, the regression coefficients—the *b* weights—are sometimes referred to as *partial regression coefficients*. This signifies that the coefficients are the weights associated with a given predictor when partialling out or controlling for the effects of the other predictors in the equation.

TESTS OF SIGNIFICANCE FOR MULTIPLE REGRESSION

Thus far we have considered multiple regression in a descriptive sense: The regression equation and R are specific to the sample being used. However, researchers are usually interested in generalizing results to a population, and tests of significance are needed to facilitate the required inferences. There are several relevant tests of significance, each used to address a different research question. Assumptions that underlie the statistical tests are discussed in a later section.

Test of the Overall Equation and R

The most basic statistical test in multiple regression is a test of the null hypothesis that the population value of R is zero. This is equivalent to testing the null hypothesis that all the regression coefficients in the multiple regression equation are zero.

The test for the significance of R is based on principles analogous to those discussed for analysis of variance in Chapter 7. Total variability in the dependent variable is partitioned into contributing components, and an F ratio is constructed. The computed F statistic is then compared to tabled values for the F distribution.

In ANOVA, the F ratio is composed of two sums of squared deviations for the dependent variable—the sum-of-squares between (the numerator) and the sum-of-squares within (the denominator). For multiple regression, the general form of the F ratio is similar:

$$F = \frac{SS_{regression}/df_{regression}}{SS_{residuals}/df_{residuals}}$$

The underlying principle for the overall test in multiple regression is the same as in ANOVA: Variability in the dependent variable that is attributable to the independent variables ($SS_{regression}$) is contrasted with variability attributable to other factors or error ($SS_{residuals}$).

There are several formulas for computing the multiple regression F statistic, but the most convenient is as follows:

$$F = \frac{R^2/k}{(1 - R^2)/(N - k - 1)}$$

where k = number of predictor (independent) variables
N = total number of cases (sample size)

We can use this formula to test the significance of the regression for predicting graduate GPA, for which the value of R^2 with four predictor variables is .88 (more precisely, .883). Therefore, the value of the F-statistic would be as follows:

$$F = \frac{.883/4}{.117/15} = \frac{.2208}{.0078} = 28.31$$

In regression, $df_{regression}$ is equal to k, the number of predictors, and $df_{residuals}$ is $(N - k - 1)$, so in this example there are 4 and 15 degrees of freedom. In Table A.3 of Appendix A we find that the critical value of F with 4 and 15 df for $\alpha = .05$ is 3.06. Our calculated value of F is larger than the critical value, so we can reject the null hypothesis that the population value of R is zero.

Tests for Regression Coefficients

T statistics associated with each regression coefficient can be used to test the significance of each independent variable. A significant t value indicates that the regression coefficient is significantly different from zero. This means that the variable associated with the regression coefficient contributes significantly to the regression, once the other predictors are taken into account.

In our example of predicting graduate GPA, the t statistic associated with the regression coefficient for undergraduate GPA ($b = .672$ for X_1) is 3.36. (The calculations, not shown here, involve dividing each b by its standard error; later we present computer output for this analysis.) For individual regression coefficients, the appropriate degrees of freedom is $df_{residual}$, which in this case is 15. For $df = 15$ and $\alpha = .05$, the critical value of t (Table A.2) is 2.13. Thus, the regression coefficient associated with undergraduate GPA is statistically significant. Each coefficient in the equation would be evaluated in a similar fashion.

Tests for Added Predictors

Another question of interest is whether adding predictors significantly improves the predictive power of the regression equation. That is, does adding X_{k+1} to the regression equation significantly increase R over that which was achieved with X_k predictors?

In the graduate GPA example, we might ask a question such as: Does adding the two GRE scores and the motivation scores to the regression equation increase our ability to predict graduate GPA over what we obtained using undergraduate GPA alone? As noted earlier, the bivariate correlation between undergraduate and graduate GPA (r_{y1}) is .87, and thus $r_{y1}^2 = .76$. The multiple correlation between Y and all four predictors (R_{y1234}) is .94, so $R_{y1234}^2 = .88$. We can see that the inclusion of three predictors improved R^2 by .12—but is this increase statistically significant? In other words, does the added predictive power reflect chance fluctuations for this sample only, or is the increase likely to be true in the population?

An F statistic is computed to answer this question. Although we do not show the actual computations, the calculated F statistic for testing whether the addition of the three predictors results in a significant improvement in predicting graduate GPA over predictions using undergraduate GPA alone is 4.50. Degrees of freedom for this F test are 3 and 15. Consulting Table A.3, we find that the critical value of F for $\alpha = .05$ with 3 and 15 degrees of freedom is 3.29. Our calculated value of F is larger, so we can conclude that the addition of X_2, X_3, and X_4 as a set significantly improved the accuracy of predictions of Y over what could be achieved using X_1 alone.

STRATEGIES FOR ENTERING PREDICTORS IN MULTIPLE REGRESSION

Several strategies can be used to enter independent variables in regression equations. Differences among the alternative strategies involve what happens to overlapping variability among correlated independent variables, and how the order of entry of predictors into the equation is determined.

Venn diagrams help to illustrate how three strategies allocate overlapping variability differently. Figure 10.2 shows a schematic diagram of the relationship between four variables—a dependent variable, Y, and three independent variables, X_1, X_2, and X_3. In this example, all three predictors are correlated with the dependent variable. Based on the extent of overlap between the X and Y variables, we can see that Y is most strongly correlated with X_1, and least strongly correlated with X_3. The diagram also indicates that X_2 is correlated with both X_1 and X_3. Yet, X_1 and X_3 do not overlap at all—they are uncorrelated. What is at issue is how to allocate the variability that the three predictor variables have in common with Y—the areas designated as m and o in Figure 10.2.

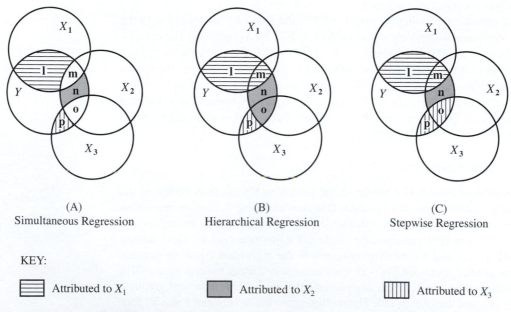

(A)
Simultaneous Regression

(B)
Hierarchical Regression

(C)
Stepwise Regression

KEY:

▤ Attributed to X_1 ▨ Attributed to X_2 ▥ Attributed to X_3

FIGURE 10.2   Venn diagrams illustrating alternative regression strategies.

Simultaneous Multiple Regression

The standard multiple regression strategy, **simultaneous multiple regression**, enters all independent variables into the equation simultaneously. One regression equation is developed, and the regression coefficients indicate the relationship between each predictor when all other predictors have been taken into account. The regression equation presented earlier for predicting graduate GPA used simultaneous multiple regression.

Figure 10.2(A) illustrates this strategy. The shaded areas of the circles (labeled l, n, and p) indicate the variability allocated to X_1, X_2, and X_3, respectively, with this procedure. As this figure shows, each independent variable is assigned only the portion of Y's variability that it contributes uniquely—the portions we described as corresponding to the squared semipartial correlations. The areas of overlap—areas m and o—contribute to the prediction of Y and to the magnitude of R, but these areas are not attributed to any particular independent variable.

Thus, in standard multiple regression, all independent variables are dealt with on an equal footing. This strategy is most appropriate when there is no theoretical basis for considering any particular independent variable as causally prior to another, and when all independent variables are of equal importance to the research problem.

Example of simultaneous regression:

Groth (2008) studied the long-term impact of adolescent gestational weight gain on the mothers' weight, as measured by the body mass index (BMI). She used simultaneous regression to regress the mothers' changes in BMI 6 and 9 years after giving birth on four predictors: gestational weight gain, age, prepregnant BMI, and number of additional children.

Hierarchical Multiple Regression

In **hierarchical multiple regression,** independent variables are entered into the model in a series of steps, with the order of entry controlled by the researcher. Hierarchical regression allows researchers to observe what an independent variable (or block of independent variables) adds to the equation at the point that it is entered.

The order of entering predictors should be based on logical or theoretical considerations. For example, some independent variables may be conceptualized as being causally or temporally prior to other independent variables, and these could be entered early in the analysis. Suppose, for instance, that we wanted to predict breast self-examination practices on the basis of women's health beliefs and age. It could be argued that age should be entered into the equation first, because age (or, to think of it another way, year of birth) is temporally and perhaps even causally prior to health beliefs.

Another reason for using hierarchical regression is to examine the effect of key independent variables after the effect of other variables has been controlled. For example, suppose our main research interest was in examining the relationship between a woman's alcohol consumption during pregnancy and infant birthweight. Hierarchical regression could be used to first control (remove the effect of) confounding variables that also influence infant birthweight (e.g., length of gestation, maternal age, and so on). With these variables entered in an early step, it would be possible to determine what alcohol consumption *adds* to the regression.

Figure 10.2(B) illustrates hierarchical or *sequential* regression. In this example, the researcher has entered X_1, X_2, and X_3 in three successive steps. The *process* of variable entry is shown in Figure 10.3. Panel A shows that in the first step, all of the

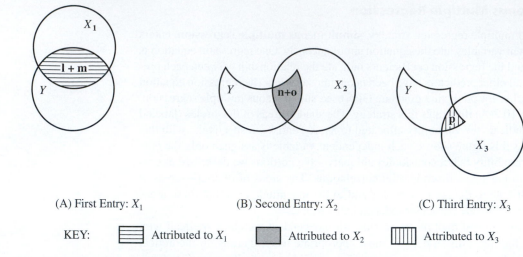

(A) First Entry: X_1 (B) Second Entry: X_2 (C) Third Entry: X_3

KEY: ▤ Attributed to X_1 ▨ Attributed to X_2 ▥ Attributed to X_3

FIGURE 10.3   Illustration of hierarchical regression.

variability that is shared between X_1 and the dependent variable is attributed to X_1, and this variability is removed from further consideration. Thus, referring back to Figure 10.2, the overlapping area between X_1 and X_2 (the area labeled m) is assigned to X_1. In the next step of the analysis (panel B of Figure 10.3), only a portion of Y's variability remains to be explained: Variability associated with X_1 has been "controlled" or held constant. When X_2 is entered into the equation, the variability that remains between Y and X_2 is assigned to X_2, and this is the area labeled o in Figure 10.2. In the third phase, only variability that is unique to X_3 is attributed to this predictor because all overlapping variability has already been taken into account.

In hierarchical regression, the researcher determines the number of steps and the variables included at each step. When several variables are added as a block, the analysis is a simultaneous regression for those variables at that stage. Thus, hierarchical regression can be viewed as an ordered series of simultaneous regressions.

Example of hierarchical regression:

Bekhet, Zauszniewski, and Wykle (2008) used hierarchical multiple regression in their study of relocation adjustment among elders who relocated to retirement communities. With relocation adjustment as their dependent variable, they examined the effect of relocation controllability—the degree of external pressure to move—after first controlling background characteristics (e.g., age, marital status, education) and relocation factors (e.g., type of facility, time since relocation).

Stepwise Multiple Regression

A third strategy, **stepwise multiple regression**, is controversial because variables are entered into the regression equation based on statistical rather than theoretical criteria. Basic stepwise regression involves successive steps in which predictors are entered, one at a time, in the order in which the increment to R is greatest. The computer, rather than the researcher, determines the order of entry of predictors.

The first independent variable entered in stepwise regression is the variable that has the highest bivariate correlation with the dependent variable. In Figure 10.2, X_1 has the highest correlation, and so X_1 is the first variable included in the equation. As shown in panel C of this figure, all of the shared variability between X_1 and Y (areas l and m) is attributed to this first predictor, as was true in hierarchical regression.

The predictor variable selected to enter in the second step is not necessarily the one with the second highest correlation with Y. The selected variable is the independent variable that accounts for the largest portion of what *remains* of Y's variability after the first variable entered has been taken into account. In our example, X_2 is more strongly correlated with Y than is X_3. Yet, much of the predictive power of X_2 has already been accounted for by X_1 because these two predictors are correlated. By contrast, X_3 is not correlated with X_1, and thus X_3 can account for a greater proportion of what remains of Y's variability—and thus contribute more to R. Thus, X_3 is entered in step 2 of the stepwise regression. Panel C of Figure 10.2 shows that all of the variability shared between X_3 and Y is attributed to X_3, including the area labeled o that represents overlap between X_2 and X_3. In the third step, X_2 is finally entered, but X_2 accounts for only a small portion of Y's variability (area n).

Stepwise regression is most often used when there are more than three variables. At each step, the predictor entered into the equation is the one that accounts for the greatest proportion of variability in Y *after removing the effect of previous variables*. The analysis proceeds so long as there are predictors that contribute significantly to R. When no more independent variables result in a significant increment to R, the analysis stops.

Stepwise regression offers several options for evaluating predictors. The one just described is called **forward selection**. The equation starts from scratch and is built forward, a step at a time, with the addition of variables that meet statistical criteria. A second option is **backward deletion**, which starts out with *all* independent variables in the equation, as in simultaneous regression. Then, in successive steps, variables that fail to contribute to the regression are deleted. A third alternative is a **true stepwise solution**, which proceeds in a similar fashion to forward selection, except that variables already in the equation are re-evaluated and dropped in later steps if they fail to contribute significantly to the regression once later-added variables are in the equation.

Stepwise regression is controversial because there is no underlying theoretical rationale to the entry or inclusion of variables in the equation. The selection of the next variable to be entered may be based on relatively minor differences between remaining variables, and differences could reflect sampling error. The regression equation from any single sample may not be the best reflection of population values. Stepwise regression is perhaps best suited to exploratory work. Even then, caution is needed when using stepwise regression, and replication with a second sample is strongly advised. If a single sample is sufficiently large, **cross-validation** can be accomplished by dividing the sample in half (preferably at random) to determine if a similar regression equation results from both subsets of data.

Example of stepwise regression:

Eastwood, Doering, Roper, and Hays (2008) used stepwise multiple regression to explore factors that affected health-related quality of life one year after coronary angiography. They found that baseline health-related quality of life, degree of illness-related uncertainty, and life stress were strong predictors of postangiography health-related quality of life, even after controlling for angiographic outcome.

NATURE OF THE INDEPENDENT VARIABLES

Multiple regression is used to predict a dependent variable that is measured on an interval or ratio-level scale. There is, however, flexibility with regard to the independent variables. This section reviews major options for properties of independent variables used in regression analysis.

Interval and Ratio-Level Independent Variables

Independent variables used in multiple regression are often variables measured on an interval or ratio scale, or on a scale that approximates interval characteristics. In our example of predicting graduate GPA, the four predictors were measured on scales that are reasonably close approximations to interval-level measurement. The use of variables measured on interval and ratio scales is straightforward. The values typically do not have to be transformed or manipulated—the raw data values are used directly in the analysis.

TIP: *Ordinal-level variables can also be used in regression analyses, if there are a sufficiently large number of categories and the distribution is reasonably close to being normal, as long as the ordinal variable has a linear relationship with other variables. If an ordinal-level variable has only a few categories (e.g., assistant professor, associate professor, and full professor), it should be treated like a nominal-level variable.*

Nominal-Level Independent Variables

Nominal-level variables can also be included in regression analysis, but care must be taken regarding how they are represented. Nominal-level variables must be **coded** in a manner that allows for appropriate interpretation of the regression coefficients. Let us take as an example the variable race/ethnicity. Suppose that we originally assigned four codes to this variable: 1 = White, 2 = African American, 3 = Hispanic, and 4 = Asian. The raw data for this variable could not meaningfully be used in regression analysis because the analysis assumes that 4 means "more of" the variable than 3, and so on. The original codes have no inherent quantitative meaning, so regression coefficients for this variable could not be sensibly interpreted. Nominal-level variables typically have to be recoded for regression analysis.

Several alternative systems can be used to code nominal variables. Whichever option is chosen, the value of R remains the same, but the values of the regression coefficients and intercept constant are affected. The coding options share one feature in common: they involve creating $c - 1$ newly coded variables to represent the original variable, where c is the number of original categories. Thus, for sex (male/female), there would be one newly coded variable ($2 - 1 = 1$), but for our four-category race/ethnicity variable, there need to be three new variables ($4 - 1 = 3$).

DUMMY CODING   The most widely used coding scheme for regression analysis is **dummy coding**, which involves creating a series of dichotomous variables that contrast members in one category with everyone else. The code of 1 designates membership in the specified category, and 0 designates nonmembership. For example, if we were coding sex, the code of 1 could be assigned to all females, and the code of 0 could be assigned to all males, or vice versa.

When there are more than two categories, there needs to be $c - 1$ variables, all of which are coded either 1 or 0. Table 10.3 shows how race/ethnicity would be dummy coded. The original four-category codes are shown in the second column. In the next three columns are three new variables, which are descriptively named as they might be for a computer analysis: *white, afroamer,* and *hispanic.* Any participant whose code on the original variable was 1 would be coded 1 for *white,* and any participant whose original code was 2, 3, or 4 (i.e., those who were non-White) would be

TABLE 10.3 Dummy Coding of Race/Ethnicity Variable

Race/Ethnicity	Original Code	white X_1	afroamer X_2	hispanic X_3
White	1	1	0	0
African American	2	0	1	0
Hispanic	3	0	0	1
Asian	4	0	0	0

coded 0. In effect, the new variable represents "whiteness" and the codes indicate yes or no for each person's status on this variable. For the variable *afroamer,* only people with an original code of 2 would be coded 1 and all others would be coded 0, while for *hispanic,* those originally coded 3 would be coded 1 and all others would be 0.

There need to be $c - 1$ new variables, and so the one category that is omitted serves as a **reference group**. In this case, the reference group is Asian. Asian partic- ipants in the sample, who were coded 4 on the original race/ethnicity variable, would be coded 0 on *white, afroamer,* and *hispanic.* A fourth variable is not necessary because the information would be redundant: An Asian person is non-White, non–African American, and non-Hispanic, and can be designated by having all 0s for these three variables. It does not matter which group is omitted, but the reference group is often the one that has the smallest membership.

The new variables can then be used as predictors in a multiple regression analysis. Suppose we wanted to predict infant birthweight based on mothers' race/ ethnicity. The multiple regression equation would be as follows:

$$birthwt = a + b_1 white + b_2 afroamer + b_3 hispanic$$

In this analysis, the intercept term is the mean on the dependent variable (*birthwt*) for the reference group; for this group (Asians) all the dummy variables are equal to zero, and therefore all other expressions after a in the equation would also equal zero. The regression coefficient on each dummy variable is the estimate of the difference in the dependent variable between the designated group and the reference group. Thus, the coefficient for *white* estimates the difference in infant birthweight between White mothers and Asian mothers. The t test associated with the coefficient for a particular dummy-coded predictor tests whether that group differs significantly from the reference group.

EFFECT CODING **Effect coding** is similar to dummy coding, except that the refer- ence group is assigned -1 rather than 0 for each newly-created variable. Thus, if effect coding were used for the race/ethnicity variable, people who were originally coded 4 (Asian) would be assigned -1 on the *white, afroamer,* and *hispanic* variables. All others would be coded with 1s and 0s as for dummy coding, as shown in Table 10.4.

TABLE 10.4 Effect Coding of Race/Ethnicity Variable

Race/Ethnicity	Original Code	white X_1	afroamer X_2	hispanic X_3
White	1	1	0	0
African American	2	0	1	0
Hispanic	3	0	0	1
Asian	4	-1	-1	-1

With effect coding, the *a* in the equation is the grand mean—the mean of the entire sample—on the dependent variable rather than the mean of the reference group. The regression coefficient associated with each predictor now indicates the group's mean on the dependent variable relative to the grand mean, and the *t* test associated with each coefficient tests the significance of the group's difference from the grand mean.

Using effect coding in our example, we could compare the mean birthweights for White, African-American, and Hispanic mothers against the overall grand mean. To find the mean for Asian mothers, we would have to perform a calculation. All *b*s—including that for the omitted group—must total zero, since the *b*-weights reflect deviations from the mean. Thus, if the regression coefficients for White, African-American, and Hispanic mothers were $+4$, -3, and $+1$, respectively, the coefficient for the Asian group would be -2 (i.e., $4 - 3 + 1 - 2 = 0$).

ORTHOGONAL CODING   If dummy or effect coding is used, the researcher cannot draw conclusions about differences between all pairs of group means. In our above example, the regression analysis would not enable us to conclude that the birthweights of African-American and White babies differed significantly. When researchers have specific hypotheses about group differences, they sometimes use **orthogonal coding** to test these differences. Orthogonal coding provides a means of performing planned (a priori) comparisons that yield a more powerful statistical test than post hoc comparisons.

> **TIP:** *The term* **orthogonal** *refers to a perfect nonrelationship between variables. If variable* X *and variable* Y *are orthogonal (r = .00), knowledge of the value of* X *tells us nothing about the value of* Y*. Orthogonal coding sets up group contrasts that are independent.*

In our example of four racial/ethnic groups, suppose that 40% of the population was White, 40% was African American, 10% was Hispanic, and 10% was Asian. We might, therefore, want to contrast the two "majority" groups (Whites and African Americans) with the two "minority" groups (Hispanics and Asians). We can do this by assigning codes of ½ and ½ (that is, .5 and .5) to participants in these categories, as we show for the first contrast in Table 10.5. This contrast compares the combined mean for Whites and African Americans with the combined mean for Hispanics and Asians. Next, suppose that we wanted to test the hypothesis that Whites and African Americans were different. This contrast is represented with a code of 1 for Whites and a code of -1 for African Americans; the other two groups that are not being compared are coded 0 (contrast 2 in the table). Our final hypothesis (contrast 3 in the table) concerns differences between Hispanics and Asians.

TABLE 10.5 Orthogonal Coding of Race/Ethnicity Variable

Race/Ethnicity	Original Code	Contrast 1 X_1	Contrast 2 X_2	Contrast 3 X_3
White	1	½	1	0
African American	2	½	-1	0
Hispanic	3	$-½$	0	1
Asian	4	$-½$	0	-1

There are three requirements for orthogonal codes. First, there must be $c - 1$ contrasts. Second, the codes established *within* a contrast must add up to 0. In Table 10.5, the sum of codes for contrast 1 is zero ($\frac{1}{2} + \frac{1}{2} - \frac{1}{2} - \frac{1}{2} = 0$), as is the sum of codes for contrast 2 ($1 - 1 + 0 + 0 = 0$) and contrast 3 ($0 + 0 + 1 - 1 = 0$). Finally, the sum of cross products must also equal zero. For example, the summed cross products for the first two contrasts are $[(\frac{1}{2})(1) + (\frac{1}{2})(1) + (\frac{1}{2})(0) + (\frac{1}{2})(0) = 0]$. The summed cross products for contrasts 1 with 3 and contrasts 2 with 3 must also equal zero, as they do in this example.

When orthogonal coding is used, a is the grand mean of the dependent variable. Each regression coefficient (b) represents one of the hypothesized contrasts.

Interaction Terms

In addition to predictors that are continuous variables and coded nominal-level variables, interactions between variables can be represented in the multiple regression equation. As explained in Chapter 7, an interaction refers to the combined effect of two variables—e.g., the effect of a specific "cell" when two independent variables are crossed, as in a factorial design. In multiple regression, interaction terms can be constructed between nominal-level and continuous variables and used as variables in the equation.

It is beyond the scope of this book to explain interaction within multiple regression in detail and to fully discuss how interaction terms should be interpreted. However, we briefly illustrate the use of interaction terms with a simple example that involves two nominal-level variables that have been dummy coded. Suppose we designed a randomized controlled trial to test the effectiveness of an intervention to alleviate pain for male versus female cancer patients, using a randomized block design. As shown in Table 10.6, the first independent variable (X_1) is *group*; those in the intervention group are coded 1, and controls are coded 0 on this variable. For *sex* (X_2), females are coded 1 and males are coded 0. The interaction term for the interaction between *group* and *sex* (X_3) is constructed by multiplying the two codes for X_1 and X_2 together, as shown in the right-hand column of Table 10.6. In this example, females in the experimental group are coded 1 on the X_3 variable (*interact*) as a result of the multiplication of codes, while all others are coded 0. Conceptually, it makes sense to multiply: The interaction term represents the joint effect of two variables over and above any additive combination of their separate effects. The regression coefficient for the interaction term (b_3) equals the difference between the regression coefficient of X_1 for males and females in the two groups. If the regression coefficient for the interaction is significant, we can conclude that the regression of the pain measure on experimental group status is conditional—that is, it depends on whether the patients are male or female.

TABLE 10.6 Coding of Interactions for Two Dummy Variables

Cell	group X_1	sex X_2	interact X_3
Intervention Group, Female	1	1	1
Intervention Group, Male	1	0	0
Control Group, Female	0	1	0
Control Group, Male	0	0	0

A Note on the Link Between Regression and ANOVA

Since categorical variables and interaction terms can be represented as independent variables in multiple regression, you may wonder if there is a connection between multiple regression and ANOVA. In fact, ANOVA and multiple regression are virtually identical. All the examples used in the chapter on ANOVA could have been analyzed through multiple regression analysis, and the conclusions would have been identical. Both ANOVA and regression require a continuous dependent variable, and both involve partitioning variance into a component associated with the independent variables and a component for unexplained or error variance. Both techniques involve the computation of an F ratio to test for significant effects. And both provide information about the total amount of variation explained by the independent variable: through R^2 for multiple regression and through eta^2 for ANOVA.

By convention, researchers whose research design is experimental (i.e., those who manipulate and control the independent variable) usually use ANOVA, while those whose research is nonexperimental are more likely to use regression. Yet, any data for which ANOVA is appropriate could, through the use of coded nominal variables and interaction terms, be analyzed through multiple regression. When one or more independent variable is continuous, however, ANOVA cannot be used; the data must be analyzed by multiple regression.

SPECIAL ISSUES IN MULTIPLE REGRESSION

Multiple regression analysis is a complex procedure to which entire textbooks have been devoted. Although this book provides primarily an overview of the major features of regression, a few additional topics merit brief discussion.

Precision and Multiple Regression

The main results of multiple regression analysis are most often communicated as the value of R^2, along with information about whether R^2 is statistically different from zero. Yet, this information is not necessarily very informative: With multiple predictors, it is unusual to find an R^2 that is *not* significantly different from .00. Moreover, R^2 could be highly significant, yet very imprecise, especially if the sample size is small. Even when sample size adjustments are made to R^2, readers cannot grasp how reliable the estimate of the population R^2 is without confidence intervals.

As an example, suppose we did a regression analysis using five predictor variables for a sample of 50 people. Assume we obtained an R^2 of .40 (adjusted $R^2 = .33$), which is significant at $p < .001$—and so, we can be confident that the population multiple correlation between is not zero. Yet the 95% *CI* around the R^2 of .40 ranges from .22 to .58—a very substantial range of values despite the highly significant value of the coefficient.

It is extremely rare, however, for researchers to report *CI*s around R^2. This likely reflects the fact that most major software programs do not calculate such *CI*s. It is, however, possible to use Internet resources to calculate *CI*s, and we urge you to do so. One Internet resource, which requires you to input the value of R^2, the number of predictors, sample size, and the desired confidence interval, is the following: http://www.danielsoper.com/statcalc/calc28.aspx. It is simpler to state that "the R^2 of .40 was significant at the .001 level" than to state that "the confidence is 95% that the population R^2 lies between .22 and .58," but the latter statement communicates very meaningful information.

TIP: *Although SPSS and other major software do not currently calculate CIs around the value of* R^2, *they do provide options for calculating confidence intervals around regression coefficients.*

Sample Size and Power

One of the practical matters that needs to be considered in using multiple regression is whether the sample size is sufficiently large to support the analysis. Inadequate sample size can increases the risk of Type II errors. It also can yield unstable and meaningless regression coefficients. There are two ways of approaching the sample size issue, as discussed next.

RATIO OF PREDICTORS TO CASES   If the number of participants for the regression analysis is too small, the regression equation may yield a good solution for the sample data, yet be of little predictive value for a new sample. This is particularly likely to occur if there are many independent variables, and if a stepwise solution to variable selection has been used. Researchers usually collect data for numerous variables and, because multiple regression can readily be performed on a computer, it is sometimes tempting to put many independent variables into the analysis. Potential predictor variables should be chosen with care, however, because having too many predictors can reduce the utility of the regression equation and can raise the risk of Type I and Type II errors.

Various experts have offered sample size guidelines concerning the appropriate ratio of cases to predictors. Tabachnick and Fidell (2007) offer a simple guideline: $N \geq 50 + 8k$, where k is the number of predictors. So, if there were three predictors, there should be at least 74 participants for the regression analysis. They recommend, however, a ratio of 40 cases per predictor for stepwise regression. More cases are required for stepwise regression because it tends to capitalize on idiosyncracies of the specific data set. Also, by having a larger sample, cross-validation by splitting the sample in two halves may be a viable option.

These general guidelines may result in too small a sample under certain conditions. One of these conditions is a small effect size, an issue we discuss in the next section. Other situations that require a larger case-to-predictor ratio include having a dependent variable that is skewed rather than normally distributed and having variables with substantial measurement error.

POWER ANALYSIS   A more precise and reliable way to determine sample size requirements for multiple regression is to perform a power analysis. As we have seen, power analysis takes effect size—the estimated magnitude of the relationship between independent and dependent variables—into account in estimating the sample size needed to limit the risk of a Type II error.

The number of subjects needed to reject the null hypothesis that R^2 is zero is a function of effect size, number of predictors, desired power, and the significance criterion to be used. In multiple regression, the estimated effect size is often referred to as f^2 and is a function of the value of R^2. We do not show direct computations of f^2 here. Instead, we present a table for which the calculations have already been performed.

Table 10.7 presents the estimated sample size needed for a test of the basic multiple regression null hypothesis that $R^2 = .00$. This table shows sample size estimates to achieve a power of .80 with a significance criterion of .05 for 2 to 10 predictor variables, and for various values of R^2. (For other statistical criteria, more predictors,

TABLE 10.7 Sample Size Estimates for Test of Null Hypothesis That $R^2 = .00$, for Selected Values of R^2 and Various Number of Predictors, for Power = .80 and $\alpha = .05$

Number of Predictors	Estimated Population R^2													
	.02	.03	.04	.05	.06	.08	.10	.13	.15	.20	.25	.30	.40	.50
2	478	320	230	183	152	113	89	67	58	42	32	26	18	14
3	543	364	261	208	173	128	102	77	66	48	37	30	21	16
4	597	400	287	229	190	141	112	85	73	53	41	33	24	18
5	643	430	309	246	205	153	121	92	79	57	45	36	26	20
6	684	458	329	262	218	163	129	98	84	61	48	39	28	21
7	721	483	347	277	231	172	136	104	89	65	51	41	30	23
8	755	506	375	290	242	180	143	109	94	69	54	44	32	24
9	788	528	380	303	252	188	150	114	98	72	56	46	33	26
10	818	549	395	315	262	196	156	119	102	75	59	48	35	27

or different values of R^2, consult an online power calculator, such as this one: http://www.danielsoper.com/statcalc/calc01.aspx.)

As an example, suppose we were planning a study to predict patients' degree of preoperative anxiety on the basis of five predictor variables and had reason to believe—for example, based on pilot study evidence—that R^2 would be approximately .10. Table 10.7 indicates that a sample of at least 121 patients would be needed to detect a population R^2 of .10 using five predictors, with a 20% risk of a Type II error and a 5% risk of a Type I error.

In the absence of specific predictions about the size of R^2, researchers can, as a last resort, use Cohen's (1988) conventions. These guidelines suggest that effect size is *small* when $R^2 = .02$, *moderate* when $R^2 = .13$, and *large* when $R^2 = .30$.

Note that power analysis can also be used to determine the sample size requirements to test null hypotheses about individual regression coefficients, which is often a major research purpose. The procedures are described in Cohen, Cohen, West, and Aiken (2003), and can be performed online in certain power calculators, or with power software.

Relative Importance of Predictors

If the main purpose of a regression analysis is for prediction—as in our example of a nursing school predicting graduate GPA for admissions purposes—the goal is to achieve the most accurate prediction possible by maximizing R^2. However, multiple regression analysis is also used to help researchers better *understand* phenomena of interest, and for this reason they often seek to determine which independent variables in the regression are most important in explaining the dependent variable.

When predictor variables in a regression analysis are correlated—which is almost always the case—the assessment of the relative importance of the predictors is difficult. There is no totally satisfactory way of untangling the effects of correlated independent variables. It should be clear that the solution is *not* to compare the *b*-weights in the regression equation. Regression coefficients are in the original units of measurement, and so their values cannot be compared. In the regression equation for predicting graduate GPA, the *b* for undergraduate GPA was .672, while that for GRE Verbal scores was .003. Undergraduate GPA is not 224 times more important than verbal GRE scores, but the weight is 224 times larger because of differences in the units of measurement.

Perhaps, then, the solution is to compare standardized regression coefficients, which are all in the same unit of measurement. In the standardized regression equation for predicting graduate GPA, the β weight for undergraduate GPA (.460) was under 1% larger than that for verbal GRE scores (.457). Does that mean that undergraduate GPA has only about 1% more explanatory power than verbal GRE scores? Unfortunately, although some researchers compare beta weights in this fashion, it is not usually judicious to do so. Beta weights tend to be unstable, fluctuating in value from sample to sample. Moreover, beta weights change as variables are added to or subtracted from the regression equation. For example, if we were to omit GRE Verbal scores (X_2) from the regression analysis, the standardized regression equation would be as follows:

$$z_Y = .63z_{x1} + .14z_{x3} + .28z_{x4}$$

In this new equation, the beta weights for all three remaining variables are higher than before. The biggest change is the beta weight for GRE Quantitative, which was previously negative and is now positive. Because beta weights are not fixed relative to other beta weights in the analysis, it is difficult to attach much theoretical importance to them.

Another approach is to consider the proportion of Y's variability that is explained by different predictors, but this is problematic, too. In our graduate GPA example, the most highly correlated predictor was undergraduate GPA, which accounts for .76 of Y's variance ($r^2 = .87^2 = .76$). When GRE Verbal is added to the equation, R^2 increases to .83, a .07 increase. Should we conclude, then, that undergraduate grades are about 11 times as important as GRE Verbal scores (.76 ÷ .07 = 10.85) in explaining graduate school grades? This would not be appropriate, because the relative contribution of the two variables is determined by which one is entered into the regression first. If GRE Verbal were the first variable used to predict graduate GPA, the proportion of variance it would account for would be $r^2 = .76^2 = .58$. If undergraduate GPA were *then* added, the R^2 for the two predictors would stay the same at .83, so that the apparent contribution of undergraduate GPA is only .25 (.83 − .58 = .25); this is more than 200% *less than* the proportion for verbal GRE scores, rather than 11 times greater. This situation results from the fact that overlapping variability in the predictors (area *b* in Figure 10.1) is attributed to the first variable in the equation.

One of the better solutions is to compare the squared semipartial correlations of the predictors. This would mean comparing the area labeled *a* with that labeled *c* in Figure 10.1. The semipartial correlations are useful because they indicate a predictor's unique contribution to Y, i.e., the contribution after the effect of other predictors is taken into account. Semipartial correlations can be produced by major software packages. In the present example, the semipartial correlation of graduate GPA and undergraduate GPA while partialling GRE Verbal scores is .50, while that of graduate GPA and verbal GRE with undergraduate grades partialled is .29. Thus, when these two independent variables are used to predict graduate grades, the unique contribution of undergraduate grades is about 60% greater than that for GRE Verbal scores.

Example of evaluating relative importance:

Corless and colleagues (2008) studied factors that predicted fatigue in HIV/AIDS patients, using hierarchical multiple regression. Their regression tables presented information about both the betas and the squared semipartial correlation coeffcieints for each predictor.

Suppression in Multiple Regression

There are instances in which a predictor variable has an effect on the regression equation that appears inconsistent with that variable's relationship with the dependent variable. This can occur through a phenomenon called **suppression**.

For example, it is sometimes possible for an independent variable to contribute significantly to R^2 even though it is totally uncorrelated with the dependent variable. This situation, which is sometimes called **classical suppression**, is illustrated in Figure 10.4(A). Here, X_1 is correlated with Y, but X_2 is not. Yet, because of the correlation between the two predictors, the inclusion of X_2 in the regression equation increases the variance accounted for in the dependent variable by suppressing some of the variability in X_1 that is irrelevant to Y.

An illustration may clarify how this works. Suppose we wanted to predict new nurses' clinical performance as rated by their supervisors (Y) on the basis of the nurses' score on a nursing achievement test (X_1). Test scores are influenced not only by actual nursing knowledge, but also by test anxiety (X_2). Test anxiety does not affect the nurse's day-to-day performance in clinical settings, and so these two variables are uncorrelated. However, part of the reason that test scores and clinical performance do not correlate more highly than they do is because the test scores of some nurses are lowered by their anxiety—their real nursing knowledge is artificially masked. By removing the portion of test score variability that reflects the influence of test anxiety, the prediction of clinical performance based on test scores improves.

There are other types of suppression, one of which is illustrated in Figure 10.4(B). In **net suppression**, there are correlations among all the variables. That is, $r^2_{y1} > .00$, $r^2_{y2} > .00$, and $r^2_{12} > .00$. However, the correlation between Y and X_2 is relatively small, and yet the contribution of X_2 in the regression equation is not insubstantial. This results from the fact that the contribution of X_2 occurs mainly through suppressing a portion of the variance of X_1 that is uncorrelated with Y.

The presence of suppressors can be detected by comparing the bivariate correlations of Y and each X with the corresponding beta weights for each X. If the regression coefficients are significant, suppression is present when the bivariate correlation and the beta weight have opposite signs, or when the value of the correlation coefficient is substantially smaller than the value of the beta weight. There is some suppression in our graduate GPA example, as evidenced by the fact that the bivariate correlation

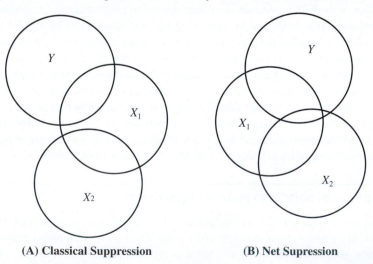

(A) Classical Suppression   (B) Net Supression

FIGURE 10.4   Venn diagram illustrating suppression in multiple regression.

between graduate grades and GRE Quantitative scores is positive, and the regression coefficient is negative. This coefficient is not statistically significant, however, so that a suppression effect in the population cannot be inferred.

Assumptions and Problems in Multiple Regression

Multiple regression is a powerful procedure, but researchers need to pay attention to potential problems in using it—many of which relate to underlying assumptions. This section discusses some issues of concern.

MULTICOLLINEARITY   A problem known as **multicollinearity** can occur in multiple regression analysis when the independent variables are too highly intercorrelated. Multicollinearity should be avoided for several reasons. First, if the independent variables are highly correlated, they add little new information to the regression when used in combination—and, a degree of freedom is used up for each redundant predictor, making it more difficult to reject the null hypothesis. Second, regression results when multicollinearity is present tend to be unstable. And third, as a result of the second problem, the regression coefficients can be misleading and render interpretation of the results problematic.

The easiest way to prevent multicollinearity is to avoid including highly intercorrelated independent variables in the regression equation. In general, researchers should avoid the use of a set of independent variables when there are intercorrelations that are .85 or higher. However, it is not always possible to detect multicollinearity by simply inspecting bivariate correlation coefficients, because *combinations* of variables sometimes create multicollinearity.

Computer programs that perform regression can be instructed to avoid multicollinearity by establishing a tolerance. **Tolerance** is computed by treating each predictor as the dependent variable in a multiple regression analysis, and determining the R^2 when the other independent variables are used as predictors; tolerance is 1 minus this R^2 value. Thus, if a predictor variable were totally uncorrelated with other independent variables, tolerance would be 1.00. Tolerance would be .00 if the predictor variables were perfectly intercorrelated. Tolerance is usually between .00 and 1.00, with higher values being more desirable. The computer can be instructed to automatically exclude any predictor whose tolerance falls below a specified level (e.g., .10). However, it might be preferable to make your own choice about variables to exclude, rather than letting the computer mechanically rule out predictors. This can be accomplished by inspecting the tolerances for all variables and then re-running the analysis after deciding which, if any, should be omitted.

TIP: *A problem called* singularity *occurs if independent variables are* perfectly *correlated. The calculation of regression coefficients is done through* matrix algebra, *and singularity prohibits some of the necessary operations. Singularity would occur if, for example, four rather than three dummy variables were included in a regression analysis to represent a four-category nominal variable.*

VIOLATION OF ASSUMPTIONS   Like all inferential statistics, the use of multiple regression as an inferential tool is based on certain assumptions. First, **multivariate normality** is the assumption that each variable and all linear combinations of the variables are normally distributed. Second, linearity is assumed—i.e., it is assumed that there is a straight line relationship between all pairs of variables. Third, there is

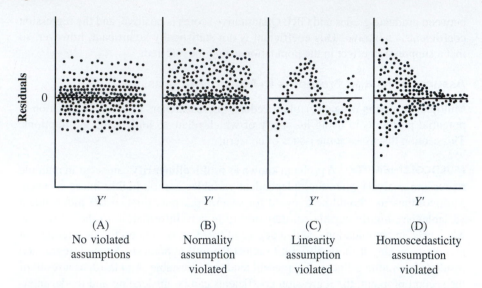

FIGURE 10.5 Residual scatterplots illustrating violations of assumptions.

an assumption of homoscedasticity, i.e., that the variability in scores for one variable is approximately the same at all values of another variable.

In bivariate statistics, frequency distributions of individual variables and scatterplots of the two variables in the analysis are used to assess the violation of underlying assumptions. In multiple regression, researchers examine **residual scatterplots** that plot errors of prediction on one axis and predicted values of the dependent variable on the other. Residual scatterplots can be produced by major software packages.

When the assumptions for multiple regression are met, the residuals are distributed approximately in a rectangular form, with a concentration of values along a straight line in the center. Figure 10.5(A) presents an example of a residual scatterplot in which all assumptions are met. When multivariate normality is achieved, the errors of prediction are normally distributed around each value of Y', and so there should be a clustering of residuals along the center line, with residuals trailing off on either side. Figure 10.5(B) illustrates a residual scatterplot in which the distribution of residuals is skewed (i.e., there are more values above the center line than below it). If nonlinearity is present, the overall shape of the scatterplot would be curved rather than rectangular, as illustrated in Figure 10.5(C). Finally, Figure 10.5(D) illustrates a violation of the assumption of homoscedasticity, showing that the errors of prediction are not comparably distributed for all predicted values of Y.

If there is evidence that assumptions have been violated, it may be possible to address the problem through transformations of the original data. Transformations such as computing the square root, taking logs, or computing the reciprocal of variables can help to stabilize the variance and achieve linearity and normality (see Table 2.4 in Chapter 2). A fuller discussion of transformations and their effects may be found in Tabachnick and Fidell (2007) or Cohen et al. (2003).

TIP: *Another assumption in multiple regression is that errors of prediction are independent of one another. This might not be the case if, for example, systematic changes occurred over the course of collecting data (e.g., systematic improvements over time when implementing an intervention). If there is a reason to suspect nonindependence of errors that is related to the order of cases, there are tests (e.g., the Durbin-Watson statistic) to detect this problem.*

OUTLIERS   Extreme cases that are legitimate outliers can have a strong impact on the regression solution and therefore need to be diagnosed and addressed. Outliers for individual variables can be detected by examining frequency distributions for variables in the analysis and using methods described in Chapters 2 and 3. Even when there are no univariate outliers, however, there can be multivariate outliers that represent extreme combinations of independent variables in the context of the dependent variable.

Multivariate outliers can also be detected through an analysis of the residuals. Standardized residual values that are greater than 3 or less than -3 are considered multivariate outliers. In our example of predicting graduate GPA, the standardized residuals ranged from $-.35$ to .22, indicating the absence of outliers. Computer programs for multiple regression provide other residual analyses that help the researcher evaluate extreme cases. When extreme cases are found, they should be eliminated from the analysis or rescored.

COMPUTER ANALYSIS AND MULTIPLE REGRESSION

Multiple regression analyses are almost always performed by computer, and therefore it is important to know how to read output from a regression analysis. This section discusses printouts for the analysis of the graduate GPA data presented in Table 10.1.

Computer Example of Simultaneous Regression

Figure 10.6 presents portions of the SPSS printout for the standard (simultaneous) regression of graduate GPA regressed on the four predictor variables, which were produced through the Analyze ➜ Regression ➜ Linear commands. Panel A shows that all four predictors were entered as a block (Method = Enter) for the dependent variable Graduate GPA. Panel B summarizes features of the overall regression model. The value of the multiple R (.940) and R^2 (.883) are presented, followed by the value of the adjusted R^2 (.852) and the standard error of estimate (.170). The standard error could be used to build confidence intervals around predicted values of graduate grades.

The overall test for the significance of the regression is presented in Panel C, labeled ANOVA. The printout shows the sums of squares, degrees of freedom, and mean squares due to two sources: regression and residuals. The overall F ratio for this analysis is 28.427, similar to the value we computed manually. The significance (probability) is .000, i.e., less than 1 in 1,000 that an F this large occurred by chance alone. Thus, the independent variables as a group were significantly correlated with the dependent variable.

The next two panels (Coefficients) provide information about individual predictors. In Panel D, the first column lists all predictor variables, and the column headed by B shows the regression coefficients (b-weights) associated with each. These values and the value of the intercept constant (Constant) are the ones we presented earlier as the regression equation. The next column indicates the standard errors for each b-weight. Coefficients with large standard errors are unreliable, and their values may vary from sample to sample. Next, the standardized regression coefficients (β-weights) are shown in the column headed Beta. The next two columns of panel D provide information on statistical tests for individual regression coefficients. The t statistic is computed by dividing the b-weight by its standard error, and the value is shown in the column titled t. The next column (Sig.) indicates the probability that the regression coefficients reflect sampling fluctuation. In this example, the coefficients for undergrad GPA, GRE Verbal, and Motivation are significant beyond the .05 level. GRE Quant, however, is not statistically significant. Its inclusion in the

Regression

A
Variables Entered/Removed[b]

Model	Variables Entered	Variables Removed	Method
1	Motivation Score, GRE Quant, Undergrad GPA, GRE Verbal[a]	.	Enter

a. All requested variables entered.
b. Dependent variable: Graduate GPA

B
Model Summary

Model	R	R Square	Adjusted R Square	Std. Error of the Estimate
1	.940[a]	.883	.852	.1700

a. Predictors: (Constant), Motivation Score, GRE Quant, Undergrad GPA, GRE Verbal

C
ANOVA[b]

Model	Sum of Squares	df	Mean Square	F	Sig.
1 Regression	3.285	4	.821	28.427	.000[a]
Residual	.433	15	.029		
Total	3.718	19			

a. Predictors: (Constant), Motivation score, GRE Quant, Undergrad GPA, GRE Verbal
b. Dependent variable: Graduate GPA

D
Coefficients[a]

Model	Unstandardized Coefficients B	Unstandardized Coefficients Std. Error	Standardized Coefficients Beta	t	Sig.	95% CI for B Lower Bound	95% CI for B Upper Bound
1 (Constant)	-1.215	.446		-2.727	.016	-2.165	-.266
Undergrad GPA	.672	.200	.460	3.364	.004	.246	1.097
GRE Verbal	.003	.001	.457	3.189	.006	.001	.005
GRE Quant	.000	.001	-.113	-.898	.383	-.002	.001
Motivation Score	.012	.005	.268	2.307	.036	.001	.022

a. Dependent variable: Graduate GPA

FIGURE 10.6 SPSS printout of simultaneous regression.

E   **Coefficients**

Model	Correlations			Collinearity Statistics	
	Zero-order	Partial	Part	Tolerance	VIF
1 (Constant)					
Undergrad GPA	.866	.656	.296	.415	2.409
GRE Verbal	.761	.636	.281	.379	2.640
GRE Quant	.466	-.226	-.079	.493	2.029
Motivation Score	.710	.512	.203	.577	1.733

a. Dependent variable: Graduate GPA.

FIGURE 10.6 Continued

regression analysis does not significantly improve the prediction of graduate grades, over that which is achieved through the other three predictors. Finally, the last two columns present confidence intervals around the b-weights. For example, the 95% CI for the first b coefficient of .672—the one for undergraduate GPA—is from .246 to 1.097. This interval does not include 0.00, consistent with the t-statistic results indicating that the coefficient is significantly different from zero.

Panel E, a continuation of the previous Coefficient panel, presents various statistics for each predictor. Three columns under the heading Correlations show the zero-order, partial, and semipartial (Part) coefficients, respectively, for each independent variable with graduate GPA. Note that the semipartial correlation coefficients for the full equation indicate that the unique contribution of undergrad GPA and GRE Verbal is about equal when the other two predictors are in the equation (i.e., just under .30). The next two columns show statistics on possible multicollinearity. In the Tolerance column, we see that all values are well above the default for excluding a multicollinear variable, which is .0001 in SPSS. The lowest tolerance is .379 (GRE Verbal), indicating no multicollinearity in this example. The final column shows the **variance inflation factor** (**VIF**), which is the reciprocal of tolerance (i.e., $1 \div$ tolerance).

Computer Example of Stepwise Regression

Figure 10.7 shows SPSS output for a stepwise regression of the same data set, i.e., the data in Table 10.1. Panel A summarizes what happens in the three steps. In Model 1, we see that undergrad GPA was entered first. The variable stepped in first is the predictor with the highest correlation, which in this case is undergrad GPA. We also see in the right column that stepwise was the method, that the criterion for the probability of F-to-enter was .050, and that for F-to-remove was .100. In stepwise regression, statistical criteria must be indicated for variables to enter and exit the equation. Probability to enter is the level that must be achieved by a regression coefficient for a variable to go *into* the equation. Probability to remove is used to determine variables going *out*. The two values shown (.050 and .100) are default values that could be modified by the analyst. Next, we see that in Model 2, the variable GRE Verbal was stepped into the equation. This is the variable that, when added to the equation with Undergrad GPA, results in the biggest increment to graduate GPA and adds significant predictive power. Finally, in Model 3, Motivation score is stepped into the equation along with the previous two. The fourth predictor, GRE Quant, was not entered into the equation because it failed to meet the criterion for the probability of F to enter.

Regression

A
Variables Entered/Removed[a]

Model	Variables Entered	Variables Removed	Method
1	Undergrad GPA	.	Stepwise (Criteria: Probability-of-F-to-enter <= .050, Probability-of-F-to-remove >= .100).
2	GRE Verbal	.	Stepwise (Criteria: Probability-of-F-to-enter <= .050, Probability-of-F-to-remove >= .100).
3	Motivation Score	.	Stepwise (Criteria: Probability-of-F-to-enter <= .050, Probability-of-F-to-remove >= .100).

a. Dependent variable: Graduate GPA

B
Model Summary

Model	R	R Square	Adjusted R Square	Std. Error of the Estimate	R Square Change	F Change	df 1	df 2	Sig. F Change
					Change Statistics				
1	.866[a]	.751	.737	.2270	.751	54.157	1	18	.000
2	.912[b]	.832	.812	.1917	.081	8.239	1	17	.011
3	.937[c]	.877	.854	.1689	.045	5.890	1	16	.027

a. Predictors: (Constant), Undergrad GPA
b. Predictors: (Constant), Undergrad GPA, GRE Verbal
c. Predictors: (Constant), Undergrad GPA, GRE Verbal, Motivation Score

C
ANOVA[d]

Model		Sum of Squares	df	Mean Square	F	Sig.
1	Regression	2.791	1	2.791	54.157	.000[a]
	Residual	.927	18	.052		
	Total	3.718	19			
2	Regression	3.093	2	1.547	42.089	.000[b]
	Residual	.625	17	.037		
	Total	3.718	19			
3	Regression	3.261	3	1.087	38.094	.000[c]
	Residual	.457	16	.029		
	Total	3.718	19			

a. Predictors: (Constant), Undergrad GPA
b. Predictors: (Constant), Undergrad GPA, GRE Verbal
c. Predictors: (Constant), Undergrad GPA, GRE Verbal, Motivation Score
d. Dependent variable: Graduate GPA

FIGURE 10.7 SPSS printout of stepwise regression.

D **Coefficients**[a]

Model	Unstandardized Coefficients B	Std. Error	Standardized Coefficients Beta	t	Sig.
1 (Constant)	-.981	.572		-1.716	.103
Undergrad GPA	1.264	.172	.866	7.359	.000
2 (Constant)	-1.299	.495		-2.622	.018
Undergrad GPA	.936	.185	.641	5.064	.000
GRE Verbal	.002	.001	.363	2.870	.011
3 (Constant)	-1.282	.437		-2.936	.010
Undergrad GPA	.662	.198	.454	3.340	.004
GRE Verbal	.003	.001	.377	3.374	.004
Motivation Score	.012	.005	.278	2.427	.027

a. Dependent variable: Graduate GPA

E **Excluded Variables**[d]

Model	Beta In	t	Sig.	Partial Correlation	Collinearity Statistics Tolerance
1 GRE Verbal	.363[a]	2.870	.011	.571	.616
GRE Quant	.109[a]	.827	.420	.197	.810
Motivation Score	.259[a]	1.782	.093	.397	.585
2 GRE Quant	-.143[b]	-1.013	.326	-.245	.498
Motivation Score	.278[b]	2.427	.027	-.519	.583
3 GRE Quant	-.113[c]	-.898	.383	-.226	.493

a. Predictors in the model: (Constant), Undergrad GPA
b. Predictors in the model: (Constant), Undergrad GPA, GRE Verbal
c. Predictors in the model: (Constant), Undergrad GPA, GRE Verbal, Motivation Score
d. Dependent variable: Graduate GPA

FIGURE 10.7 Continued

Panel B summarizes the regression analysis for the three models. For each of the three models, the output shows the value of R, R^2, adjusted R^2, the standard error of estimate, and then statistics associated with change. In model 1, the value of R is simply the bivariate correlation between the predictor entered first (undergrad GPA) and the dependent variable, graduate GPA. The R^2 change is the difference between .00 and .751, i.e., .751. The next row shows statistics for the second model, in which both undergrad GPA and GRE Verbal scores are in the equation, as indicated in footnote b. We see that R^2 has increased from .751 to .832, and that the amount of R^2 change is .081. The F for testing the significance of adding this predictor is 8.239 which, with 1 and 17 degrees of freedom, is significant at $p = .011$. The bottom row shows comparable information for the model in which three predictors are in the equation. The R^2 change of .045 is significant at $p = .027$.

Panel C shows three sets of ANOVA results in which the sum of squares due to regression for each of the three models is contrasted with sum of squares residual. In all three models, the total sum of squares (total variability) is 3.718, but each successive model has a larger value for $SS_{\text{Regression}}$, because each new predictor "explains" more variability in graduate school grades. Note, however, that although $SS_{\text{Regression}}$ gets larger in each model, the F statistic gets smaller because the degrees of freedom in the numerator increases—a good lesson in why it may be unwise to include too many predictors when sample size is small. The overall regression equation is, in each model, significant at $p < .001$.

Panel D shows information about individual predictors in each of the three models. These coefficients indicate what the regression equation for predicting new values of graduate GPA would be with the model's predictors in the equation. For example, in Model 2, which predicts graduate GPA on the basis of undergrad GPA (X_1) and GRE Verbal scores (X_2), the regression equation would be $Y' = -1.299 + .936\,(X_1) + .002\,(X_2)$. For the variables in the equation in each model, the printout lists the regression coefficient (B), standard error of B, Beta weight, t statistic for the regression coefficient, and significance of t. In all three models, all variables are significant beyond the .05 level.

Finally, Panel E shows information about variables not yet entered in the regression. In Model 1, there are three variables not yet entered—GRE Verbal, GRE Quantitative, and motivation scores. The statistical information indicates *what would happen if each variable were entered in the next step*. The value under Beta In is the standardized regression coefficient for each predictor *if* the variable were to enter the regression equation in step 2, and the next two columns shows the t value for this coefficient, if entered next, and its significance. The partial correlation for the predictor, holding undergrad GPA constant, is shown in the next column, followed by information on the minimum tolerance. This represents the smallest tolerance any variable *already in* the equation would have if the specified predictor were included. In this example, all of the Tolerance values for the three predictors exceed .01, indicating no problem with multicollinearity for any variables that might enter. In Model 1, we see that the variable with the highest partial correlation with graduate GPA, holding undergrad GPA constant, is GRE Verbal (.571), which is the variable chosen to enter in the next step of the analysis, Model 2. When we look at the information for Model 3, we see that the t for GRE Quantitative is $-.898$, which does not meet the criterion to enter the equation: The significance of .383 for this fourth variable exceeds the criterion of .05. Thus, the stepwise regression stopped at this point.

RESEARCH APPLICATIONS OF MULTIPLE REGRESSION

Multiple regression is a widely used statistical procedure in nursing research. This section describes the major research applications of multiple regression and discusses the presentation of multiple regression results in research reports.

The Uses of Multiple Regression

Nurse researchers use multiple regression to address a variety of research questions regarding the relationships among variables. Multiple regression is also used for prediction and for other purposes as well.

1. *Answering research questions* Multiple regression can help to answer a number of different types of questions, including the following:

   • How well does a particular group of independent variables explain or predict a dependent variable? (For example, how well do undergraduate grades, GRE scores, and achievement motivation explain graduate grades?)

- How much does any single independent variable add to the prediction of a dependent variable, over what is accomplished by other independent variables? (For example, how much do motivation scores add to the prediction of graduate GPA, over what undergraduate GPA and GRE scores contribute?)
- What is the relationship between any given independent variable and the dependent variable, once other predictors are taken into account? (For example, what is the relationship between undergraduate GPA and graduate GPA, once the relationship between graduate GPA and the other three predictors is controlled?)
- What is the relative importance of one predictor in explaining a dependent variable in comparison with other predictors? (For example, what is the relative importance of verbal versus quantitative GRE scores in predicting graduate GPA?)

As discussed earlier, the fourth question is difficult to answer unequivocally when predictors are correlated. Multiple regression, however, is the basis for a sophisticated technique known as path analysis, which is an approach to **causal modeling**. Although correlations cannot be used to establish causality, path analytic procedures can provide some evidence about the nature and direction of causal influence among variables. Path analysis and other methods of causal modeling are described in advanced textbooks such as those by Tabachnick and Fidell (2007), Cohen et al. (2003), and Olobatuyi (2006).

2. *Prediction*   Multiple regression provides an excellent vehicle for making predictions about a dependent variable when only information on the independent variables are available. Such predictions are typically undertaken for utilitarian purposes. As an example, Ellett, Beckstrand, Flueckiger, Perkins, and Johnson (2005) used multiple regression analysis to predict the insertion distance for placing gastric tubes in adults, on the basis of numerous clinical and demographic variables. The best model used three predictors: sex, weight, and the measurement from nose to the umbilicus, with the adult's head flat on the bed.

3. *Missing values imputation*   As noted in earlier chapters, researchers often face the problem of missing data for some participants on one or more variable. There are several different solutions to the missing values problem, as we discuss in Chapter 14. Here we note only that one approach is to use multiple regression to "predict" what the missing value would have been, had it not been missing, and to substitute that predicted value for the missing data.

The Presentation of Multiple Regression in Research Reports

Multiple regression analyses are typically so complex that they cannot adequately be summarized in the text of a report without tables. The exception is when the main focus of the analysis is to determine the value of R^2, information that can readily be reported in one or two sentences. However, this is rarely the only information sought in a multiple regression analysis, so tables are almost always needed.

Unfortunately, there is no standard format for the tabular presentation of regression results. This stems in part from the fact that regression is used to address many different questions, but it also is due to the absence of widely accepted guidelines. Often, multiple tables are needed—one to show the means and *SD*s of variables in the regression and correlations among them, and another presenting regression results. In this section we discuss elements that we believe should be included in regression tables, along with some options. The overall guiding principle in laying out a regression table is to be parsimonious while conveying critical pieces of information about the analysis.

TABLE 10.8 Example of a Table for Simultaneous Regression

Predictor Variable	b	SE	β	t	p
Constant	−1.215	.45		−2.73	.016
Undergraduate GPA	.672	.20	.46	3.36	.004
GRE Verbal scores	.003	.001	.46	3.19	.006
GRE Quantitative scores	.0007	.001	−.11	−.90	.383
Achievement Motivation scores	.012	.005	.27	2.31	.036

Overall R^2 = .88, Adjusted R^2 = .85, $F(4, 15)$ = 28.43, $p < .001$

Graduate Grade Point Average Regressed on Four Predictors (N = 20)

TABLES FOR SIMULTANEOUS REGRESSION RESULTS   Regression tables are most straightforward when simultaneous regression has been used. Table 10.8 summarizes the standard regression of the graduate GPA data (i.e., for the computer printout shown in Figure 10.6). At a bare minimum, a table for standard regression should include the following: sample size; name of the dependent variable; names of all predictor variables; regression coefficients (either b or β, or both) for the predictors; the value of R^2; significance of the overall regression; and the significance of individual predictors. Table 10.8 has all of these elements.

Sample size is sometimes specified in the title of the table, as it is in this example, or sometimes in a table footnote. The name of the dependent variable should appear in the title. In tables reporting more than one regression analysis with the same set of predictors, the dependent variables should be named in column headings, which could also indicate Ns if they differ from one analysis to another.

Predictor variables are typically reported in the first column of the table, in sufficient detail that a person can understand the nature of the variable without having to refer to the text. In standard regression, the order of the variables in the list is not important. Many researchers present standardized regression coefficients (βs) for each predictor and omit unstandardized b-weights and their standard errors. If an aim of the report is to communicate a regression equation for prediction purposes, however, unstandardized b-weights (and the intercept constant) should be used instead of, or in addition to, beta weights.

Statistical tests for individual predictors can be presented in various ways. In this example, we showed the values of the t statistics associated with each regression coefficient, and the associated p values. Information on t statistics is often omitted, however, if the table presents regression results for two or three outcomes. In such a case, researchers usually use the system of asterisks next to the beta weights to indicate p thresholds, rather than giving actual p values.

The value of R^2 for each analysis must be reported and, unless the sample size is large, it is also wise to report the adjusted R^2, as in this example. Some researchers report the value of R in addition to R^2, but it is unnecessary to do so because it is redundant. We also suggest reporting the F for the overall test of the regression equation, degrees of freedom, and probability level, as we did at the bottom of this table.

Other elements are sometimes included in addition to, or instead of, some of the statistics reported in Table 10.8. For example, if a separate correlation matrix has not been presented, the regression table could show the value of r between each predictor and the dependent variable. Another option is to include a column for squared semipartial correlations, showing the unique proportion of variance associated with each predictor.

TABLES FOR HIERARCHICAL REGRESSION   All the basic elements for a standard regression should also be included in a hierarchical regression table—i.e., sample size, names of dependent and predictor variables, regression coefficients, the value of R^2, and results of significance tests. In addition, information on the changes to R^2 at each step of the analysis and the significance of the changes should be presented.

Table 10.9 presents results for three hierarchical regression analyses using data from a large sample of teenage mothers. Depression scale scores, Parenting Stress scale scores, and scores on a measure of alcohol abuse were regressed on three blocks of predictors. Block 1 consists of variables about household composition—whether the young mother's own mother (the maternal grandmother) lives in the household, whether her partner lives in the household, and number of her own children. Block 2 involves variables on the young woman's economic situation—whether she receives cash welfare assistance, whether she is employed, and whether she has a high school diploma. The third block includes psychosocial variables—scores on a Difficult Life Circumstances scale (items include whether someone close to the teen is in jail, whether she was mugged in the past year, etc.); scores on a Self-Esteem scale, and scores on a Social Support scale. These predictors are shown in the left column, grouped in blocks in the order of entry into the regression.

Standardized regression coefficients (βs) for each independent variable are shown in the column labeled "Beta," for each dependent variable. Asterisks next to the beta weights indicate whether t tests for the predictors were statistically significant. For the Depression outcome variable, for example, all three psychosocial predictors, plus educational attainment, were statistically significant. For each dependent variable

TABLE 10.9 Example of a Table for Hierarchical Regression

Step	Predictor	Depression Beta[a]	Depression R^2 Change	Parenting Stress Beta[a]	Parenting Stress R^2 Change	Alcohol Abuse Beta[a]	Alcohol Abuse R^2 Change
1	*Household Composition*		.01**		.01***		.02***
	Mother present	−.03		−.01		−.08***	
	Partner present	−.03		−.07**		−.09***	
	No. of children	.00		.07*		−.09***	
2	*Economic Variables*		.02**		.01**		.00
	Receiving welfare	.00		.07**		.00	
	Employed	−.03		.01		.00	
	Has HS diploma	−.11***		−.04*		.06**	
3	*Psychosocial Variables*		.24***		.07*		.04***
	Diff. Life Circs.	.39***		.18***		.19***	
	Self-Esteem scale	−.24***		−.18***		.02	
	Social Support scale	−.07***		.04		−.02	
	Cumulative R^2		.27***		.09***		.06***

[a]Betas shown are for the last step.

*$p < .05$ **$p < .01$ ***$p < .001$

Hierarchical Multiple Regression of Depression, Parenting Stress, and Alcohol Abuse in Low-Income Teenage Mothers (N = 1892)

there is also a column labeled "R^2 Change" that shows the increment to R^2 as each of the three blocks enters the equation. The asterisks next to this value indicate whether the F test for the increment to R^2 is statistically significant. In this example, even though the increments to R^2 are often small, each change is significant because of the large sample ($N = 1,892$). The final row of the table shows the cumulative R^2—the amount of variance explained when all predictors are in the equation—which equals all of the R^2 changes added together. Asterisks are used again here to indicate the probability level for the overall equation. In this example, the cumulative R^2s range from .06 (Alcohol abuse) to .27 (Depression), and all are statistically significant. Adjusted R^2s are not included in this table because original and adjusted R^2 values were virtually identical with this large sample.

> **TIP:** *To economize on space, some researchers label the column for changes to* R^2 *as* R^2 *Δ (delta); Δ is the standard scientific symbol for change.*

A dilemma in creating tables for hierarchical regression is how to present the regression coefficients. The betas change at each step, and yet the format shown in Table 10.9 presents only one beta per predictor. It is probably best to present betas for the final step (i.e., for the final equation), as we did in this table—which we mention in the footnote. An alternative would have been to use the heading "Beta for Last Step." Regrettably, most tables for hierarchical regression in research reports fail to specify whether the betas shown are the values when the predictor first entered the equation or at the final step.

If it is theoretically important to show how the betas change as successive blocks of predictors are stepped into the equation—or if the addition of blocks dramatically changes the betas and these changes are of interest—all beta values should be shown in the table. Usually, however, changes to betas can only be presented for one or two dependent variables in one table, especially if there are more than three blocks of predictors. An example of this type of table, for the regression of the Depression and Parenting Stress scores from the previous analysis, is shown in Table 10.10. Beta weights are shown for each block of variables entered in successive steps. The R^2 changes and cumulative R^2 values are shown in the bottom two rows of the table, corresponding to values at each of the three steps. In this example, the changes to beta for predictors entered in the equation early tended to be relatively small (e.g., for mother present in the household, the betas were $-.01$, $-.01$, and $-.03$ at steps 1 through 3, respectively), and so in this example the expanded format is not especially informative. Variants of the format used in Table 10.9 are more common in research journals than that used in Table 10.10.

These tables illustrate how dummy-coded predictor variables can be handled in tables. When effect coding or orthogonal coding is used, coding *must* be explicitly specified, either as part of the label for the predictor or in a footnote. This is not usually necessary, however, for dummy variables. Five of the variables in Tables 10.9 and 10.10 are dummy coded: mother present, partner present, receiving welfare, employed, and has high school diploma. The labels for these variables indicate the condition that is coded 1. For example, the variable "employed" is, by convention, understood to represent the employed condition, which is coded 1, while the unemployed condition is coded 0. The coding scheme *can*, of course, be explicitly indicated. For example, the employment variable could have had the following label: Employment status (1 = employed, 0 = not employed).

TABLE 10.10 Example of a Table for Hierarchical Regression

		Depression			Parenting Stress		
		Step 1	Step 2 Beta Weights	Step 3	Step 1	Step 2 Beta Weights	Step 3
Step	Predictor						
1	*Household Composition*						
	Mother present	−.01	−.01	−.03	−.01	−.01	−.01
	Partner present	−.04	−.03	−.03	−.09***	−.07**	−.07**
	No. of children	.04	.02	.00	.09***	.08***	.07*
2	*Economic Variables*						
	Receiving welfare		.01	.00		.08**	.07**
	Employed		−.04	−.03		.00	.01
	Has HS diploma		−.14***	−.11***		−.06**	−.04*
3	*Psychosocial Variables*						
	Diff. Life Circs.			.39***			.18***
	Self-Esteem scale			−.24***			−.18***
	Social Support scale			−.07***			.04
	R^2 Change	.01**	.02*	.24***	.01***	.01**	.07*
	Cumulative R^2	.01**	.03***	.27***	.01***	.02***	.09***

$*p < .05 **p < .01 ***p < .001$

**Hierarchical Multiple Regression of Depression and Parenting Stress
in Low-Income Teenage Mothers (N = 1892)**

TIP: *Regression tables in journals are often flawed in their omission of
information on how to read dummy variables. For example, if a predictor
is listed as "Sex" or "Gender," readers cannot interpret the direction of sex
differences on the dependent variable unless there is explicit information
on how males and females were coded.*

TABLES FOR STEPWISE REGRESSION   Basic information for stepwise regression is
similar to that for standard regression. In stepwise regression, however, the listing of
independent variables is critical, because it indicates the order of entry of predictors. It
is usually not necessary to show the amount of change and significance of R^2 changes.
Thus, for each dependent variable included in the table there might simply be two
columns showing values for beta weights and cumulative R^2. (The reader can compute
the R^2 change at each step simply by subtracting the value of R^2 in one row from the
value of R^2 in the preceding row.) The names of predictors that did *not* get stepped into
the equation at statistically significant levels should be specified in a footnote.

NARRATIVE PRESENTATION OF REGRESSION RESULTS   The features of a regression table that a researcher chooses to highlight in the text depend on the nature of the
research questions posed. We present one example of the narrative that might be used
to describe Table 10.9, and urge you to consult journal articles for other examples.

> In this large sample of adolescent mothers, maternal household characteris-
> tics, economic circumstances, and psychosocial state did a modest job of explaining
> variation in the three dependent variables, as shown in Table 10.9. The overall R^2 for

predicting alcohol abuse was especially low ($R^2 = .06$), and was only slightly better for Parenting Stress scores ($R^2 = .09$). The regression was substantially more successful in predicting Depression scores ($R^2 = .27$). In all three cases, the overall regression was statistically significant beyond the .001 level.

Variables in the Household Composition block, entered in the first step, accounted for a very small (albeit significant) proportion of explained variance in all three analyses. None of the three household variables were, taken individually, significantly related to Depression scores, once other factors were taken into consideration. However, the presence of a husband or boyfriend in the teen mothers' household was associated with significantly less parenting stress and lower abuse of alcohol. Their own mothers' presence in the household was also associated with less alcohol abuse. The larger the number of children in the household, the greater is the amount of parenting stress, but the lower is the amount of alcohol abuse.

The block of Economic Variables also made only modest contributions to explained variance for all three outcome variables, with R^2 increments ranging from .00 to .02. The young mothers' employment status was unrelated to any of the three outcomes. Receipt of cash welfare assistance was associated with increased parenting stress but was unrelated to depression and alcohol abuse, once other predictors were controlled. Educational attainment was significantly related to all three dependent variables: Women who had a high school diploma were less depressed, had less parenting stress, but were *more* likely to abuse alcohol.

The inclusion of the three Psychosocial Variables greatly improved the predictive power of all three regressions. The increments to R^2 ranged from .04 for alcohol abuse to .25 for depression scores; all increments were statistically significant. The single most powerful predictor was scores on the Difficult Life Circumstances scale, a measure of ongoing, daily stress. Young women with a lot of daily stress were significantly more likely to be depressed, to feel stressed as parents, and to abuse alcohol. High self-esteem was associated with a lower risk of depression and parenting stress, but was unrelated to alcohol abuse. Women with greater amounts of social support tended to be less depressed, but social support was not related to parenting stress or alcohol abuse.

Research Example

The following study illustrates the use of multiple regression to test relationships predicted on the basis of a theory.

Study: "Effects of caregiving demand, mutuality, and preparedness on family caregiver outcomes during cancer treatment" (Schumacher et al., 2008)

Study Purpose: The purpose of this study was to explore the degree to which three caregiver constructs based on role theory would predict caregiving-specific outcomes among caregivers caring for family members during their cancer treatment.

Methods: A cross-sectional correlational design was used to explore relationships among theoretically relevant variables. Data were obtained from a sample of 87 caregivers, who were recruited from outpatient units of three cancer centers in the mid-Atlantic region of the United States.

Caregivers were asked to complete a series of questionnaires, which included nine outcome measures relating to the strain and burden of the caregiving role, as well as scales for three variables posited to contribute to strain: the time demands associated with caregiving tasks (Demand), the extent of mutually positive relationships between caregiver and patient (Mutuality), and degree of preparedness for caregiving (Preparedness).

Analysis: Simultaneous multiple regression was used to explore the degree to which the various caregiving outcomes could be predicted on the basis of the three caregiving role variables. Two control variables, the caregiver's age and sex, were included as predictors in the analyses.

Results: The five predictor outcomes, as a set, explained a significant proportion of variance in all nine caregiver burden outcomes, with the value of adjusted

TABLE 10.11 Simultaneous Regression Predicting Outcomes for Family Caregivers of Cancer Patients During Cancer Treatment ($N = 87$)

Predictor	Caregiver Outcomes					
	Global Strain		Fatigue		Anger	
	Beta	p	Beta	p	Beta	p
Caregiver sex (1 = female)	.14		−.03		−.15	
Caregiver age	.00		−.07		−.01	
Caregiving time demand	.44	< .01	.25	< .05	.15	
Mutuality/positive relationship	−.24	< .05	−.16		−.49	< .01
Preparedness for caregiving	−.18	< .05	−.25	< .05	−.13	
R^2	.40		.21		.33	
Adjusted R^2	.36		.16		.29	
Overall Significance	< .01		< .01		< .01	

Adapted from Table 4, Schumacher et al., 2008

R^2 ranging from .09 for scores on a Vigor scale, to .36 for scores on a scale measuring Caregiving Difficulty. Neither age nor sex was significantly associated with any outcomes, when other predictors were in the analysis. The three role variables were persistently significant predictors of the burdens of caregiving. Table 10.11 presents beta weights and the overall value of R^2 for three illustrative outcomes. For Global Strain scores, 36% of the variance was explained, and all three role variables were significant independent predictors; time demand seemed to play an especially important role in explaining overall strain. With regard to Fatigue scores, the value of R^2 was much lower (.16), but both Demand and Preparedness were significant predictors. Finally, the only significant predictor of scores on the Anger scale was Mutuality: Caregivers who had a less favorable relationship with their family member expressed a higher degree of anger regarding their role. Each 1 standard deviation (SD) decrease in Mutuality was associated with nearly one-half (.49) SD increase in Anger. The researchers concluded that the three role variables, derived from a theoretical model of caregiving, were predictive of negative caregiving outcomes and suggest avenues for tailoring interventions.

Summary Points

- **Multiple regression** is a statistical procedure for understanding and predicting a dependent variable on the basis of two or more independent variables. The basic multiple regression equation for predicting Y (Y') involves an intercept constant, plus the values of the predictor variables weighted by corresponding regression coefficients (b weights).
- When the equation is specified in standardized form, the regression coefficients are called **beta weights** (β).
- The **multiple correlation coefficient** (R) represents the magnitude (but not direction) of the relationship between the dependent variable and the predictor variables, taken together.
- The square of R (R^2) indicates the proportion of variance in Y accounted for by the predictors.

- R^2 is sometimes presented after a sample size adjustment is made. The new value is called **adjusted R^2**.
- Multiple regression offers the potential for **statistical control**: The regression coefficients indicate the number of units Y' is expected to change for each unit change in a given predictor, when the effects of the other predictors are held constant.
- Control is achieved through partialling overlapping variability in the predictors. The **partial correlation** between X_1 and Y ($r_{y1.2}$) is the degree to which X_1 and Y are correlated after the influence of a third variable, X_2, is removed.
- **Semipartial correlation** ($r_{y(1.2)}$) is the correlation between all of Y and X_1, from which X_2 has been partialled out. Squared semipartial correlation

coefficients are sometimes used to compare the relative importance that predictors uniquely make to the prediction of Y.

- An F-ratio statistic that contrasts the sum of squares due to regression against the sum of squares due to residuals is used to test the overall significance of the regression.
- An F statistic can also be used to test the significance of variables added to the regression equation—i.e., the significance of the increment to R^2.
- The significance of individual regression coefficients is determined through t statistics.
- Predictor variables are entered into the regression equation either through a **simultaneous regression model** (all predictors entered at the same time); a **hierarchical regression model** (variables entered in a sequence determined by the researcher); or a **stepwise regression model** (variables entered in the order that contributes most to the increment of R^2). An important difference between these methods concerns what happens to overlapping variability among intercorrelated independent variables.
- In multiple regression, the dependent variable should be a continuous variable measured on an interval or ratio scale.

- Independent variables can be continuous, but they can also be coded nominal-level variables. Alternative coding schemes for nominal-level variables include **dummy coding**, **effect coding**, and **orthogonal coding**.
- Interaction terms can also be included in the analysis, and thus data that are amenable to ANOVA can also be analyzed through multiple regression.
- Researchers using multiple regression need to attend to potential problems, such as **multicollinearity**—the inclusion of independent variables that are too highly correlated. Multicollinearity can be detected by examining the **tolerance** of predictors.
- Researchers should also check to determine that the assumptions for multiple regression have not been violated, and this is usually done through inspection of **residual scatterplots**.
- In interpreting regression results, researchers should also be alert to the possibility of **suppression**, a phenomenon that makes a predictor with little or no correlation with the dependent variable look important, because it suppresses irrelevant variability in other predictors.
- Care should be taken to ensure an adequate sample size for multiple regression, preferably through a power analysis.

Exercises

The following exercises cover concepts presented in this chapter. Appendix C provides answers to Part A exercises that are indicated with a dagger (†). Exercises in Part B involve computer analyses using the datasets provided with this textbook, and answers and comments are offered on this book's Web site.

PART A EXERCISES

† **A1.** Using the regression equation for predicting graduate GPA presented in this chapter, compute the following for the last two students in Table 10.1: (a) the predicted value of Y; and (b) the squared error term.

† **A2.** Using the following information for R^2, k, and N, calculate the value of the F statistic for testing the overall regression equation and determine whether the F is statistically significant at the .05 level:
  (a) $R^2 = .53, k = 5, N = 120$
  (b) $R^2 = .53, k = 5, N = 30$
  (c) $R^2 = .28, k = 4, N = 64$
  (d) $R^2 = .14, k = 4, N = 64$

† **A3.** Which, if any, of the tests described in Exercise A2 would be statistically significant with $\alpha = .001$?

† **A4.** Following is a correlation matrix:

	VARA	VARB	VARC	DVAR
VARA	1.00			
VARB	.62	1.00		
VARC	.77	.68	1.00	
DVAR	.54	.36	.48	1.00

  (a) If DVAR were regressed on VARA, VARB, and VARC, what is the *lowest* possible value of R^2?
  (b) In a stepwise regression, what would be the first predictor variable into the equation?
  (c) In a stepwise regression, what would be the second predictor variable into the equation?

† **A5.** Suppose that, using dummy codes, smokers were coded 1 and nonsmokers were coded 0 on SMOKSTAT, and that males were coded 1 and females were coded 0 on GENDER. What would be the 4 codes for the interaction term?

† **A6.** Using the Internet resource recommended in this chapter (or another similar online calculator), find the 95% confidence limits of R^2 for the following situations:

(a) $R^2 = .22$, $k = 6$, $N = 100$

(b) $R^2 = .22$, $k = 6$, $N = 200$

(c) $R^2 = .22$, $k = 10$, $N = 100$

† **A7.** For the following situations, estimate how large a sample would be needed for a multiple regression analysis to achieve standard statistical criteria, using Table 10.7.

(a) Estimated $R^2 = .20$, $k = 6$

(b) Estimated $R^2 = .13$, $k = 8$

(c) Estimated $R^2 = .08$, $k = 4$

PART B EXERCISES

† **B1.** For these exercises, you will be using the SPSS dataset Polit2SetC to do multiple regression analyses to predict level of depression in the sample of low-income urban women. You will need to begin by dummy coding the variable race/ethnicity. First, create a frequency distribution for *racethn* (Analyze → Descriptive Statistics → Frequencies), then answer these questions: (a) What percentage of women in this sample was African American, Hispanic, and White or other? (b) Are there any women whose information for *racethn* is missing? (c) How many new variables need to be created so that race/ethnicity can be used in regression analyses? (d) Which category do you think should be omitted?

† **B2.** Now you can create the new dummy-coded variables. Select Transform → Recode → Into Different Variables. Find *racethn* in the variable list and move it into the slot for "Numeric Variable > Output Variable." On the right, under Output Variable, type in a name for your first new variable (e.g., *black, afamer)*. In the slot for Label, you can type in a longer label, such as "African American" if you so choose. Then click Change, which will confirm the new variable as the output variable. Next, click the "Old and New Values" button, which will bring up a new dialog box. Under "Old Value," enter 1, which is the code for African Americans in the original ("old") variable *racethn*. Then, on the right under New Value, click "Copy old value," and then click the Add button. Women who were coded 1 on *racethn* will also be coded 1 on the new African-American variable. Next, under Old Value, click Range and enter 2 and then "through" 3 (the two codes for Hispanic and White/other women on *racethn*). On the right under New Value, enter 0, then click Add, which will code all non–African-American women as 0. Finally, under Old Value, click "System- or user-missing," and then under New Value click "System missing," then click Add. Women who have missing data for *racethn* will now have a missing values code for the new variable. Click Continue to go back to the original dialog box, then click OK to run the command. If you look at the last variable in your file in Data View, you should see the new variable with values of .00 and 1.00 (which can be changed to 0 and 1 by going into Variable View and changing the number of decimals to 0). Do the analogous procedure for the next new race/ethnic group—

except remember to change the values coded 1 and 0. Now, run frequencies on your new variables, and compare the results to those from Exercise B1, making sure that your new variables accurately reflect the original racial/ethnic distribution.

† **B3.** In this exercise, you will run a simultaneous multiple regression analysis to predict the women's level of depression (scores on the CESD depression scale, *cesd*) based on several demographic characteristics, socioeconomic characteristics, health status, and self-reported incidence of abuse in the prior year. The list of predictors is as follows: the two race/ethnicity dummy variables you created in exercise B2; *age; educatn* (educational attainment); *worknow* (a dummy variable for currently employed); *nabuse* (number of different types of abuse experienced in the past year, including verbal abuse, efforts to control, threats of harm, and physical abuse); and *poorhlth* (a dummy coded variable indicating self-reported poor health at the time of the interview. Bring up the regression dialog box by selecting Analyze → Regression → Linear. Insert the variable *cesd* in the box labeled Dependent. Insert the 7 predictor variables that we just mentioned into the box for Independent(s). Make sure that Method is set to "Enter," the command for entering all predictors simultaneously. Click the Statistics pushbutton and then select the following options: Estimates (under "Regression Coefficients"); Model Fit; Descriptives; and Collinearity Diagnostics. Then click Continue, and OK to run the analysis. Answer the following questions: (a) How large is the sample on which the regression analysis was run? (b) Interpret the mean value for poor health self-rating. (c) Which predictor has the highest zero-order correlation with *cesd*? (d) What were the values of R^2 and adjusted R^2? (e) Which predictors in the analysis were significantly predictive of the women's depression scores, once other predictors were included? Which were *not* significantly predictive? (f) For this sample of women, which predictor variable appeared to be the most powerful in predicting depression? (g) Did any of the tolerance levels suggest a problem with multicollinearity?

† **B4.** In this exercise, run a stepwise multiple regression to predict depression scores, using the same predictors as in Exercise B3. In the first SPSS Linear Regression dialog box, enter *cesd* as the Dependent variable and the list of predictors in the Independent slot, as in the previous exercise. For Method, select "Stepwise." For the Statistics options, you can omit Descriptives and Collinearity Diagnostics because you have already examined these, but this time you should select R squared change. Run the analysis and then answer the following questions: (a) How many predictors were entered before the regression stopped? (b) Which predictor variables made it into the regression—and which did not? Was the order of entry of predictors consistent with the values of the zero-order correlations? (c) Looking at the Model Summary panel, what was the progression of the value of R^2 from one step to the next—and were these changes significant? What happens to the standard error of the estimate with each progressive step? (d) Were all models statistically significant—that is, was the value of R^2 greater than zero at each step? (e) Looking at the

"Excluded Variables" panel—and focusing on Model 4, were any of the remaining predictors statistically significant?

B5. In this exercise, run a hierarchical multiple regression analysis to predict *cesd*, using the same predictors as in Exercises B3 and B4. Select the variables you would like to enter in each step, being sure to think of a reasonable rationale for the order of entry. In the first SPSS Linear Regression dialog box, enter *cesd* as the Dependent variable, and the predictor(s) you wish to enter in the first step in the Independent slot. Then, click the pushbutton Next in the area labeled "Block." Now you can select your second block of predictors. Keep clicking Next Block for each set of predictors, until all seven predictors are included. The Method box should say "Enter." Examine your output, and pay special attention to changes in R^2 for each successive block of variables.

† B6. It is tempting to think of the results obtained in the previous three analyses as suggesting a causal link between the women's abuse experiences and their level of depression—that is, inferring that being abused *caused* higher levels of depression. However, the opposite might be the case. For example, women who are depressed, lethargic, or absorbed with personal problems might incite others to yell at them, threaten them, or hit them. In the next analysis, we explore the issue of direction of influence, though we caution against firm causal conclusions. In this hierarchical regression, we will statistically control the women's level of depression 2 years earlier and then see if recent abuse experiences affected current depression, with earlier depression held constant. This is analogous to asking whether recent abuse was related to *changes* in depression. (Remember from Chapter 6 that we have Wave 1 CES-D scores for only a small subsample of women.) In the first SPSS Linear Regression dialog box, enter *cesd* as the Dependent variable, and *cesdwav1* as the predictor in the Independent slot. Then, click the pushbutton Next in the area labeled "Block." Now enter *nabuse* (number of types of abuse) as the predictor in the second block. The Method box should say "Enter." For statistical options select Estimates for the Regression Coefficients, Model Fit, and R squared change. Then run the analysis and answer these questions based on the output: (a) What was the correlation between the CES-D scores in the two waves of data collection? (b) Was R^2 statistically significant at both steps of the analysis? (c) What was the change to R^2 when abuse was added to the regression? Was this significant—and, if so, what does this suggest? (d) If you wanted to predict a woman's current CES-D score based on this analysis, what would the unstandardized regression equation be?

B7. Using output from one of the previous four exercises (B3 through B6), create a table to summarize key results of the analyses. Then write a paragraph summarizing the findings.

11

Analysis of Covariance, Multivariate ANOVA, and Related Multivariate Analyses

This chapter, which focuses on multivariate extensions of analysis of variance, continues to move us into new realms of analytic complexity. The extensions, while conceptually not difficult to grasp, are mathematically formidable, and so our discussion of computations and formulas is even briefer here than in previous chapters. We begin with a very simple overview of the general linear model.

THE GENERAL LINEAR MODEL

The **general linear model (GLM)** encompasses a broad class of statistical techniques, and underlies most analyses used in nursing research. The GLM is the foundation for such procedures as the *t* test, ANOVA, and regression analysis. The GLM is an important model because of its generality and applicability to numerous research situations, but a thorough understanding of the GLM requires advanced statistical training. Because this is an introductory textbook, we present a fairly superficial description of it, and we restrict our discussions of sophisticated multivariate procedures to overviews without detailed explanations.

As the name implies, the GLM encompasses analytic procedures that fit data to straight-line (linear) solutions. The basic GLM is an equation that looks similar to the regression equation we discussed in the previous chapter, except that it is more general. Each term in a basic GLM equation can represent a *set* of variables:

$$Y = b_0 + bx + e$$

where Y = a set of outcome variables
x = a set of independent and control variables
b = a set of coefficients, one for each x
b_0 = a set of intercepts (values for each y when each $x = 0$)
e = error

This model allows tremendous diversity, including multiple dependent variables, multiple independent variables that are nominal or continuous, between-group and within-group comparisons, and a host of other possibilities that are too complex to explain. For example, it allows analysts to include fixed effects versus random effects (which we do not explain here), to analyze data from balanced and unbalanced designs (designs in which groups being compared are of different sizes), and to use different mathematic options for calculating sums of squares. We mention these features primarily because software for running the types of analyses discussed in this chapter require analysts to specify which options are to be used. In this chapter, we focus on fixed effects models and **Type III sum of squares.**

A fundamental principle of the least squares estimation approach is that variation on a dependent variable can be partitioned into different sources of variation. The statistical procedures discussed in previous chapters use a *whole model* approach in partitioning variance. In complex designs, however, different models are often advantageous. The models differ in how variance is partitioned—i.e., in the calculation of the sums of squares—although this topic is too complex for elaboration. There are four commonly used types of sums of squares, all of which are options within SPSS and other statistical software. In SPSS, Type III is the default. The Type III sum of squares is calculated by comparing the full model to the full model without the variable of interest. Although computations are different, all models involve the same overall hypothesis-testing strategy: Variation attributable to an independent variable is tested against an appropriate error term.

TIP: *SPSS and other software offer a wealth of options within their GLM programs. The GLM procedure is not, however, available in the Student Version of SPSS. Moreover, not all SPSS systems carry GLM Multivariate and Repeated Measures options that are described in this chapter.*

ANALYSIS OF COVARIANCE

Researchers use **analysis of covariance (ANCOVA)** to make comparisons between two or more group means, after statistically removing the effect of one or more variables on the dependent variable. The central question for ANCOVA is the same as for ANOVA: Are mean differences between groups likely to be true population differences, or are observed mean differences in a sample likely to have occurred by chance?

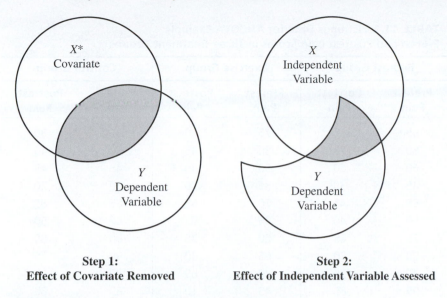

Step 1:
Effect of Covariate Removed

Step 2:
Effect of Independent Variable Assessed

FIGURE 11.1   Venn diagram depicting analysis of covariance.

Basic Concepts for ANCOVA

Conceptually, it is useful to think of ANCOVA as a combination of multiple regression and ANOVA. In the first stage of the analysis, the effects of confounding variables (called **covariates** in the context of ANCOVA) are removed from further consideration, similar to the first step in a hierarchical regression. In the next stage, variability in the dependent variable *that remains to be explained* is analyzed as in ANOVA. That is, the group means are compared after they have been statistically adjusted for the effect of the covariates. Because error variance is reduced, ANCOVA permits a more sensitive test of group differences than is achieved with ANOVA.

Figure 11.1, which shows a visual representation of ANCOVA, is similar to the depiction of hierarchical regression in Figure 10.3. The shaded area of the circle in Step 1 shows the extent to which the dependent variable Y is correlated with the covariate X^*. The dependent variable is regressed on X^*, and the portion of Y's variability that is accounted for by X^* is removed from further consideration. In Step 2, the analysis focuses on the ability of the independent variable X to explain any *remaining* variability in Y. The independent variable in ANCOVA is always a nominal-level variable, such as experimental versus control, male versus female, and so on.

As an example, suppose we wanted to test the effectiveness of an intervention to improve motor function in nursing home residents. The dependent variable is a measure of motor performance administered after the intervention, and the independent variable is group status (i.e., membership in the group that received the intervention or in a control group that did not). The covariate is motor performance scores prior to the intervention. Preintervention motor performance scores would likely be highly correlated with postintervention scores: Regardless of the intervention, some people would have better motor performance than others. In this example, we have controlled individual differences in motor function by using preintervention motor performance scores as the covariate. ANCOVA would be used to examine the effect of the intervention on what remains of the variability in postintervention motor performance scores after individual differences in motor function are statistically controlled.

TABLE 11.1 Fictitious Data for ANCOVA Example: Pretest and Posttest Pain Scores in Three Treatment Groups

Bedrest Group		Exercise Group		Control Group	
Pretest Pain	Posttest Pain	Pretest Pain	Posttest Pain	Pretest Pain	Posttest Pain
95	85	75	60	35	30
80	70	80	45	50	40
60	50	50	30	45	45
45	30	85	70	30	20
55	45	70	55	85	85
50	40	85	65	60	50
75	65	60	35	90	85
80	70	65	40	90	75
40	35	80	60	80	65
95	85	45	10	60	60
Means:					
67.50	57.50	69.50	47.00	62.50	55.50

ANOVA AND ANCOVA   It may be recalled from Chapter 7 on ANOVA that the total sum of squares for the dependent variable (SS_T) can be partitioned into variance attributable to the independent variable (sum of squares between groups or SS_B) and to variance associated with other factors such as individual differences (sum of squares within or SS_W). The F ratio contrasts these two sources of variation. In ANCOVA, the F ratio contrasts sums of squares that have been adjusted for the covariate's relationship with the dependent variable—although variance partitioning is complex because ANCOVA is not a whole model test within the GLM procedures of most software packages.

As an example, suppose that we randomly assigned 30 people with lower back pain to three treatment groups: a bedrest group, an exercise group, and a control group. Pain is measured both before the treatment (the covariate) and after the treatment (the dependent variable) on a visual analog scale that can range from 0 to 100. Hypothetical data for this example are shown in Table 11.1. As the means at the bottom of this table show, the pretest pain scores (the covariates) for the bedrest, exercise, and control groups were 67.5, 69.5, and 62.5, respectively. An ANOVA on these pretest means indicates that the groups were not significantly different at the outset of the study ($F = 0.35$ [2, 27], $p = .71$) and so we can conclude that initial group differences in pain reflect chance sampling fluctuations.

The posttest means are more variable, ranging from a low of 47.0 for the exercise group to a high of 57.5 for the bedrest group. The null hypothesis is that these means are equal, and the research hypothesis is that the three group means differ. An ANOVA on these data yields an F of 0.74, which has an associated p of .49. On the basis of ANOVA, we would not be able to infer that either a bedrest or an exercise intervention had an effect on lower back pain. Yet, ANCOVA could alter these conclusions.

The correlation between pretest and posttest pain is high: $r = .90$ ($p < .001$), indicating that 81% of the variation in posttest pain is accounted for by variation in pretest pain. This strong correlation reflects the fact that people who started out in especially severe pain tended to end up with high levels of pain, regardless of which group they were in, while people with less pain initially also tended to have less pain later.

Analysis of covariance involves examining the effect of the intervention on what remains in Y's variability after removing the effect of the covariate (preintervention pain). In this example, the F for the effect of the intervention on posttest pain scores, after controlling pretest pain, is 20.08. With 2 and 26 df, this F is significant at $p < .001$. The conclusion now is that, after controlling for initial pain levels, there is a statistically significant difference in mean posttest pain levels resulting from exposure to different treatments.

This example was deliberately contrived to have the ANCOVA results differ from the ANOVA results—the results typically are less dramatic. Nevertheless, if you can select good covariates, then ANCOVA usually will result in a more sensitive test than ordinary ANOVA. The increased sensitivity results from the fact that the error term, against which treatment effects are compared, is almost always smaller in ANCOVA.

TIP: *ANCOVA can be used with a single independent variable, as in this example, and can also be used in multifactor designs (e.g., a two-way ANCOVA).*

ADJUSTED MEANS The posttest pain scores for the three groups in our example reflect not only treatment effects, but also individual differences in pain. It is possible, and often desirable when reporting the results of ANCOVA, to adjust the group means. **Adjusted means** allow researchers to portray **net effects**—i.e., group differences on the dependent variable *net* of the effect of the covariate.

Adjusted means are produced in many statistical packages, including SPSS. In our example, the original means for posttest pain scores were 57.5, 47.0, and 55.5 for the bedrest, exercise, and control groups, respectively. After adjusting for pretest pain scores, the respective posttest means were 56.5, 43.9, and 59.6.

ANCOVA tests the null hypothesis that the *adjusted* means for the groups being compared are equal. In this example, an inspection of the adjusted means clarifies why the ANCOVA resulted in statistically significant group differences, while the ANOVA did not. The original unadjusted group means ranged from 47.0 to 57.5, a spread of 10.5 points. The range for the adjusted means is from 43.9 to 59.6, a spread of 15.7 points. In essence, the ANCOVA takes into consideration how much the groups *changed* from pretest to posttest. Table 11.1 indicates that the mean pretest–posttest changes in pain scores ranged from a low of 7.0 points for the control group, to a high of 22.5 points for the exercise group.

Reporting adjusted means in reports can communicate important information to readers, but adjusted means should be interpreted with caution because they rarely correspond to an actual situation in the real world. Adjusted means are the means that would have occurred *if all participants had the same scores on the covariate.* This would not occur in reality—yet, adjusted means are often a good way to highlight treatment effects.

MULTIPLE COMPARISONS AMONG ADJUSTED MEANS When ANCOVA results in a significant F test, as in this example, the researcher can reject the null hypothesis that the adjusted group means are equal. However, as in ANOVA, further analysis is needed to determine which pairs of adjusted group means are significantly different from one another if there are three or more groups.

Post hoc tests, you may recall from Chapter 7, protect against the heightened risk of a Type I error that can occur when multiple pairwise comparisons are run. In ANOVA, several alternative post hoc tests can be used. Fewer post hoc tests for *adjusted* group means are typically available, however. In fact, within SPSS, when covariates are named, the "pushbutton" for post hoc tests within the GLM program cannot be selected. Yet it is still possible to pinpoint group differences. We will show the relevant output in a subsequent section. Suffice it to say here that, in our example, the post hoc comparisons revealed that adjusted mean posttest pain scores for the exercise group were significantly different from those in the other two groups, but that other group comparisons were nonsignificant.

TIP: *As in ANOVA, group comparisons can be planned in advance, in which case the omnibus* F *test could be avoided. With planned comparisons, researchers establish explicit contrasts in which they are interested; protection against an inflated risk of a Type I error is achieved by running a small set of orthogonal contrasts.*

SELECTION OF COVARIATES   Covariates are usually continuous interval- or ratio-level variables. Sometimes, however, researchers want to statistically control nominal-level variables. This can be achieved by using dichotomous variables (e.g., married versus not married) as separate independent variables. (If a nominal dummy-coded value has a mean close to .50—i.e., close to a 50–50 split, which might occur with the variable *sex*—then it can be treated as a continuous variable and included in the model directly as a covariate.)

ANCOVA can be used to make adjustments for multiple covariates simultaneously. It is not usually wise to use more than three or four covariates, however. With small samples even fewer are recommended. When many covariates are included, it is inevitable that they will be intercorrelated, which could result in multicollinearity. Moreover, if covariates are highly correlated, they are redundant in reducing error variance, and they actually *lower* the power of the analysis. This is because degrees of freedom are subtracted from the denominator of the error term, even though error variance is not subtracted from the numerator.

TIP: *When multiple covariates are used, all covariates enter the first step simultaneously and are treated as a set, as in simultaneous regression. Within that set, the significance of each covariate is assessed as if it were the last to enter the equation. Thus, an individual covariate is significant in the ANCOVA only if its unique contribution to explaining variance in the dependent variable is significant.*

A pretest (baseline) measure of the dependent variable is almost always a powerful covariate. Important demographic characteristics such as age or sex are correlated with a broad array of human attributes and may therefore be attractive as covariates. The stronger the correlation between a covariate and the dependent variable, the better is the covariate. It is usually prudent to consult the research literature for factors that have been found to influence the dependent variable, and to use these as covariates.

Care should be taken to choose covariates that can be measured reliably. Measurement errors can lead to either overadjustments or underadjustments of the mean, and can contribute to either Type I or Type II errors. For many clinical and demographic variables (length of stay in hospital, age), measurement error is not typically a problem, but the same cannot be said for psychosocial variables. Tabachnick and Fidell (2007) recommend limiting covariates to those whose reliability is .80 or greater.

Assumptions for ANCOVA

As with all other inferential statistics, ANCOVA is based on a number of assumptions, including all of those we discussed with regard to ANOVA in Chapter 7—random selection of subjects, a normally distributed dependent variable, and homogeneity of variance among the groups. With a reasonably large sample size—and if the number of people in the groups is approximately equal—ANCOVA, like ANOVA, is robust to the violation of the latter two assumptions.

ANCOVA also assumes that the relationship between the dependent variable and covariates is linear, and relationships between all pairs of covariates are linear. When this assumption is not true, the power of the test is reduced, and the risk of a Type II error increases. Scatterplots can be used to evaluate for possible curvilinearity. When a covariate is found to have a curvilinear relationship with the dependent variable, it is probably best to eliminate it from the analysis, although transformations of the covariate may be an alternative.

Another assumption is **homogeneity of regression across groups**: The covariate should have the same relationship with the dependent variable in every group. Homogeneity of regression is illustrated in Figure 11.2 (A). Here we see that the slopes of the three groups are equal—that is, the regression lines are parallel. When there is heterogeneity of regression—illustrated in Figure 11.2 (B)—there is an interaction between the covariate and the independent (group) variable. Regression lines are no longer parallel. We illustrate how to test the null hypothesis that the slopes for the covariate are equal in a subsequent section. If the slopes are significantly different, ANCOVA typically should not be used. If you use ANCOVA when this assumption is violated, there is a heightened risk of a Type II error.

Applications of ANCOVA

Strictly speaking, ANCOVA is appropriate primarily in clinical trials in which participants have been randomly assigned to groups. In a randomized design, groups are in theory already equivalent across an infinite number of traits. In reality, however, groups are never perfectly equal, and so ANCOVA can enhance their comparability. Moreover, ANCOVA increases the sensitivity of the F test for the effect

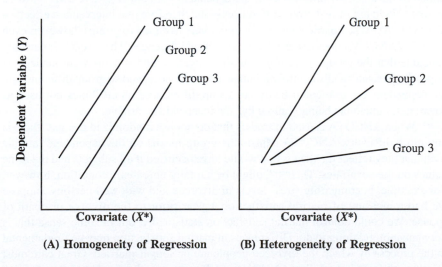

(A) Homogeneity of Regression   (B) Heterogeneity of Regression

FIGURE 11.2   Homogeneity and heterogeneity of regression.

of the independent variable by removing the variability attributable to the covariates from the error term (the sum of squares within groups). Unless covariates are uncorrelated with the dependent variable, ANCOVA increases the power of the analysis and can reduce the risk of a Type II error.

Although the use of ANCOVA in nonexperimental and quasiexperimental studies has been controversial, it is precisely in these situations where ANCOVA has been used most extensively. When participants are not randomly assigned to groups, researchers face the possibility that groups being compared are not equivalent, thereby potentially threatening the study's internal validity via the threat of bias called *selection*.

As an example, suppose we implemented a pain management strategy for patients in clinic A and compared them to patients in clinic B, who did not receive the intervention (a nonequivalent control group design). If we compared mean posttreatment pain scores for the two groups, we could not be sure that any differences were the result of the intervention, rather than due to preexisting differences in pain levels, because patients were not randomized to treatments. By using preintervention pain scores as a covariate, however, the two groups would essentially be equated on initial levels of pain. Differences between the two groups on the covariate (initial pain level) are removed so that, presumably, remaining differences can be attributed to the effect of the intervention. ANCOVA can thus be viewed as a form of "what if" analysis—*what* would postintervention pain differences be *if* all participants had equal (statistically equivalent) scores on the covariate?

ANCOVA is also used by some as a statistical matching procedure to enhance the comparability of groups being compared in observational (nonexperimental) studies, especially case-control studies. For example, if the stress levels of recently widowed and recently divorced persons were being compared, we would want to take steps to make the two groups comparable with respect to characteristics that might influence stress (e.g., age, length of marriage, and so on). These characteristics could be statistically controlled through ANCOVA.

The use of ANCOVA in nonrandomized studies is sometimes criticized because of misinterpretations of the results—particularly with regard to causal inferences. When people are randomly assigned to treatment groups, statistically significant group differences usually justify an inference of causality: The treatment variable (X) is presumed to have *caused* differences in the dependent variable (Y). ANCOVA allows a more sensitive test of real group differences—and therefore real intervention effects—than ANOVA. When participants are not randomly assigned to groups, however, even the use of ANCOVA does not usually justify causal inferences. The researcher can only conclude that the groups were *different* after covariate adjustments were made. It is impossible to statistically control *all* human characteristics, and so group differences in the dependent variable could be due to group differences on attributes not used as covariates, rather than being "caused by" the independent variable.

When ANCOVA is used in studies that do not use randomized designs, there is one more difficulty. ANCOVA adjusts the group means on the dependent variable such that they reflect the means that would have occurred *if* all subjects had the same values on the covariates. This "if" might be a totally unrealistic condition, however. For example, in comparing stress levels in divorced and widowed persons, suppose we had a measure of marital satisfaction 1 year prior to the divorce or death of spouse. We could control marital satisfaction statistically, but in some sense this is not a meaningful thing to do: Differences in marital satisfaction may be fundamental to the process by which the divorced people are no longer married. Great care must be taken, then, in interpreting ANCOVA results in nonrandomized studies.

Special Issues in ANCOVA

This section briefly covers a few additional issues relating to ANCOVA that deserve mention.

THE MAGNITUDE OF THE RELATIONSHIP Researchers and consumers of researchers are increasingly interested in learning the magnitude of effects of an independent variable on a dependent variables, and effect size can also be estimated in an ANCOVA context. Eta-squared, discussed as an effect size index for ANOVA, can be adjusted for the covariate, in which cases the index is a **partial eta-squared.** Essentially this *adjusted eta^2* contrasts the sum of squares due to the independent variable after removing the effect of the covariate against the sum of squares for the independent variable plus error—both with covariate adjustments.

Although we do not show full computations (computer output will be presented later), the adjusted value of eta^2 in our example of posttest pain scores is 1343.6 ÷ 2213.5 = .61. In this contrived example, 61% of the variance in the adjusted posttest pain scores is associated with the independent (treatment) variable. Said another way, 61% of the variance *remaining* in posttest pain scores, after removing variance accounted for by pretest pain scores, is attributable to the treatment variable. In a real study, the value of adjusted eta^2 would typically be lower.

POWER AND ANCOVA In general, when ANCOVA is used appropriately with carefully selected covariates, the analysis of group differences is more powerful than with ANOVA because error variance is reduced. The degree of increased power is a function of *how much* error variance is removed—i.e., how correlated the covariates are with the dependent variable. In our example, we calculated the adjusted eta^2 to be .61, but the value of *un*adjusted eta^2 is only .05.

Power analysis for ANCOVA can be used to estimate required sample size before the study begins, using adjusted eta^2 as the estimated effect size. The procedures and table described in the power analysis section of Chapter 7 for ANOVA are appropriate for ANCOVA, substituting the adjusted eta^2 for eta^2.

In the example used in this chapter, the value of adjusted eta^2 was .61. If the data for our contrived example were from a pilot study, we could use this effect size to estimate sample size needs for a full-blown test of the two treatments, using the power analysis information in Table 7.5. Because our adjusted eta^2 in this example is so large, we would estimate that we needed only three participants per group, using standard criteria for power and α. In most studies, the value of eta^2 is less than .14, the value designated as a "large" effect in Cohen's guidelines.

TIP: *It is also possible to compute a partial eta^2 for contrasts between groups—for example, to compute the effect size contrasting, say, the bedrest group against the other two groups. SPSS has an option for such computations.*

PRECISION AND CONFIDENCE INTERVALS Similar to ANOVA, confidence intervals (*CI*s) can be built around individual adjusted means, as we will see when we look at SPSS output. *CI*s, showing the precision of the statistics as estimates of population parameters, can also be constructed around differences in adjusted group means.

MULTICOLLINEARITY As with multiple regression, researchers must be careful not to include in the ANCOVA analyses independent variables and covariates that are too highly intercorrelated. The possibility of multicollinearity is most likely to occur when there are multiple covariates. Some software packages automatically protect against multicollinearity by computing the tolerance, as we described for multiple regression. Other packages (such as SPSS) do not. If there is a potential risk of multicollinearity, one option is to use a multiple regression program to examine tolerance levels prior to running the ANCOVA.

Alternatives to ANCOVA

Researchers sometimes consider alternatives to ANCOVA for analyzing their data. Alternatives are most readily available if the covariate and the dependent variable are measures of the same attribute, as in the example we have used in this chapter. When this is the case, one option is to use a repeated measures ANOVA with both a within-subjects factor (time of measurement) and a between-subjects factor (treatment group)—an approach we discuss later in this chapter. This option may be less attractive than ANCOVA, however, because the effect of the independent variable is evaluated as the interaction between the independent variable and the pretest versus posttest scores, rather than as a main effect.

Another alternative is to compute difference scores between the pretest and posttest measures, and to then treat these differences—called **change scores**—as the dependent variable in ANOVA. For example, using the data in Table 11.1, the change score for the first person in group A would be 10 (95 − 85). One of the main problems with change scores (as well as with RM-ANOVA) is that there are often **ceiling effects** or **floor effects** than constrain the magnitude of change. That is, the amount of change may be artificially small simply because pretest scores are at the upper or lower end of the scale, leaving little room for changes resulting from the treatment. To illustrate with our previous example, the pretest pain score of the first person in group A (95) could not have increased by more than 5 points, no matter how much more pain was felt at posttest. Another problem with change scores is that unreliability is compounded: Change scores tend to be less reliable that either the pretest or the posttest scores. ANCOVA is generally preferable to ANOVA with change scores.

TIP: *The alternative analyses ask slightly different questions. In ANCOVA, the question (using this chapter's example) is: Do treatment groups differ in levels of pain, after adjusting for pretreatment differences in pain? With change-score analysis and RM-ANOVA, the question is: Are* **changes** *in pain levels associated with participation or nonparticipation in a bedrest or exercise intervention?*

An option that does not require the covariate to be measured on the same scale as the dependent variable is **blocking.** This essentially involves using the covariate as another independent variable in a multifactor design, with ANOVA used to perform the statistical tests. If the covariate is a continuous variable, it must first be converted to a categorical variable (e.g., continuous pretest pain scores could be categorized as low, medium, and high based on some cutoff points). An advantage of this approach is that it can be used when the covariate's relationship with the dependent variable is curvilinear. Moreover, if there would have been heterogeneity of regression between the original covariate and the dependent variable in ANCOVA, this can be detected in multifactor ANOVA as an interaction between the blocked covariate and the independent variable. When ANCOVA's assumptions are met, however, ANCOVA is usually preferable to blocking because converting the covariate to a categorical blocking variable results in lost information and a smaller reduction of the error term.

Example of ANCOVA:

Peterson, Bergstrom, Samuelsson, Asberg, and Nygren (2008) analyzed data from a randomized controlled trial that tested an intervention to reduce stress and burnout among healthcare workers. Group differences on outcomes measured 12 months after the intervention were compared for the intervention and control group using ANCOVA. Baseline scores on the outcome variables were used as covariates. Statistically significant intervention effects were found for several outcomes (e.g., general health, perceived demands at work).

The Computer and ANCOVA

In this section we describe some SPSS printouts for analysis of covariance, using the data on pain scores presented in Table 11.1. The output is complex, and so we summarize only key features that are important to interpreting ANCOVA results.

We begin by testing the assumption of homogeneity of regression across groups, which is accomplished by including an interaction term in the analysis. That is, we instruct the computer to include a variable that represents the multiplicative interaction between the covariate (*Prepain*, pretest pain scores) and the treatment group variable (*Group*) as a "predictor" of posttest pain scores. If the interaction term is statistically significant, the null hypothesis of homogeneity of regression is rejected, and ANCOVA should not be used.

Figure 11.3 shows the relevant output for this test. (This figure was created in SPSS using Analyze ➜ General Linear Model ➜ Univariate with a custom model.) The focus here is on the row that is labeled *Group * Prepain* in the first column under the heading "Source," i.e., source of variation. In this row, which we have shaded, we see that the F statistic for the interaction terms is 1.361. With 2 and 29 *df*, this F is not significant, $p = .275$. We can therefore proceed with our analysis.

Figure 11.4 presents several panels of the SPSS printout for the ANCOVA, using the GLM univariate program and a full factorial model. Panel A shows the unadjusted

Tests of Between-Subjects Effects

Dependent Variable: Posttest Pain Score

Source	Type III Sum of Squares	df	Mean Square	F	Sig.
Corrected Model	11135.400[a]	5	2227.080	68.414	.000
Intercept	518.096	1	518.096	15.916	.001
Prepain	9629.884	1	9629.884	295.824	.000
Group	299.311	2	149.655	4.597	.020
Group * Prepain	88.618	2	44.309	1.361	.275
Error	781.267	24	32.553		
Total	97250.000	30			
Corrected Total	11916.667	29			

a. R Squared = .934 (Adjusted R Squared = .921)

FIGURE 11.3 SPSS printout for test of homogeneity of regression in ANCOVA.

A **Descriptive Statistics**

Dependent Variable: Posttest Pain Score

Experimental Group	Mean	Std. Deviation	N
Bedrest Group	57.50	20.173	10
Exercise Group	47.00	18.589	10
Control Group	55.50	22.417	10
Total	53.33	20.271	30

B Levene's Test of Equality of Error Variances[a]

Dependent Variable: Posttest Pain Score

F	df1	df2	Sig.
6.527	2	27	.005

Tests the null hypothesis that the error variance of the dependent variable is equal across groups.

a. Design: Intercept + prepain + group

C **Tests of Between-Subjects Effects**

Dependent Variable: Posttest Pain Score

Source	Type III Sum of Squares	df	Mean Square	F	Sig.	Partial Eta-Squared
Corrected Model	11046.782[a]	3	3682.261	110.059	.000	.927
Intercept	430.072	1	430.072	12.854	.001	.331
Prepain	10425.115	1	10425.115	311.596	.000	.923
Group	1343.608	2	671.804	20.080	.000	.607
Error	869.885	26	33.457			
Total	97250.000	30				
Corrected Total	11916.667	29				

a. R Squared = .927 (Adjusted R Squared = .919)

D **Parameter Estimates**

Dependent Variable: Posttest Pain Score

Parameter	B	Std. Error	t	Sig.	95% Confidence Interval Lower Bound	95% Confidence Interval Upper Bound	Partial Eta-Squared
Intercept	−8.006	4.036	−1.984	.058	−16.302	.290	.131
Prepain	1.016	.058	17.652	.000	.898	1.134	.923
[Group = 1]	−3.080	2.603	−1.184	.247	−8.430	2.270	.051
[Group = 2]	−15.613	2.618	−5.964	.000	−20.994	−10.231	.578
[Group = 3]	0[a]	.	.	.	.	.	.

a. This parameter is set to zero because it is redundant.

FIGURE 11.4 SPSS printout for ANCOVA.

Estimated Marginal Means
Experimental Group

E **Estimates**

Dependent Variable: Posttest Pain Score

Experimental Group	Mean	Std. Error	95% CI	
			Lower Bound	Upper Bound
Bedrest Group	56.484[a]	1.830	52.722	60.246
Exercise Group	43.952[a]	1.837	40.175	47.728
Control Group	59.564[a]	1.844	55.775	63.354

a. Covariates appearing in the model are evaluated at the following values: Pretest pain score = 66.50.

F **Pairwise Comparisons**

Dependent Variable: Posttest Pain Score

(I) Experimental Group	(J) Experimental Group	Mean Difference (I − J)	Std. Error	Sig.[a]	95% CI for Difference[a]	
					Lower Bound	Upper Bound
Bedrest Group	Exercise Group	12.532*	2.589	.000	5.906	19.158
	Control Group	−3.080	2.603	.247	−9.741	3.580
Exercise Group	Bedrest Group	−12.532*	2.589	.000	−19.158	−5.906
	Control Group	−15.613*	2.618	.000	−22.312	−8.913
Control Group	Bedrest Group	3.080	2.603	.247	−3.580	9.741
	Exercise Group	15.613*	2.618	.000	8.913	22.312

Based on estimated marginal means

*. The mean difference is significant at the .05 level.

[a] Adjustment for multiple comparisons: Bonferroni.

FIGURE 11.4   Continued

means (and *SD*s) for the three treatment groups—the same means shown at the bottom of Table 11.1. Panel B presents the results of the test of the assumption of homogeneity of variance using the Levene test (See Chapter 7). In this example, the probability for this test was $p = .005$, indicating significant group differences in the variances. However, an alternative test, described in the "Tip" below, suggests homogeneity is acceptable.

> **TIP:** *It has been argued (e.g., Field, 2005) that Levene's test is not necessarily the best way to evaluate whether variances are unequal enough to be problematic for ANOVA and ANCOVA. An alternative test is the* **variance ratio,** *which is the ratio of the largest group variance (the* SD *squared) divided by the smallest group variance. If the ratio is less than 2, heterogeneity of variance is not considered to be problematic. In our example, the variance for the control group (502.66) divided by the variance for the Exercise group (345.60) is only 1.45, and so we can proceed.*

Panel C summarizes the results of the ANCOVA analysis. The sources of interest—the shaded rows in this panel—are *Prepain*, the covariate, and *Group*, the independent variable. This output indicates that the F for the covariate is 311.596 ($df = 1, 26$), which is significant at $p < .001$. This F was computed by dividing the mean square for *Prepain* (10425.115) by the mean square for error (33.457). This result indicates that pretest pain scores were strongly related to posttest pain scores. With pretest pain scores statistically controlled, the F for the treatment group variable is 20.080, which reflects the mean square for *Group* (671.804) divided by the mean square for error (33.457). With 2 and 26 df, this F is highly significant, $p < .001$. We can reject the null hypothesis that the adjusted group means on posttest pain scores were equal. The far-right column of this panel indicates that the value of eta-squared, controlling for the covariate, is .607. At the bottom of this panel we see that the overall R^2 for all components in this model was .929, with an adjusted value of .919.

Panel D, Parameter Estimates, shows output similar to that for multiple regression—b weights, standard errors, t statistics, and significant levels for each component in the model. For this part of the analysis, SPSS created contrasts among the groups, and used Group 3 (the control group) as the reference group. (In SPSS, the default is to use the last group as the reference group.) The output indicates that Group 1 (bedrest) is not significantly different from the other two groups ($t = -1.84, p = .247$), but Group 2 (exercise) *is* significantly different from the other two ($t = -5.964, p < .001$). *CIs* around the b weight are also shown. In the case of group 1, the 95% *CI* around b includes the value of 0.00 (-8.43 to $+2.27$), showing that it is not significant. The final column shows that the partial eta-squared summarizing the net effect size for the exercise condition (Group 2), when contrasted to the other two and controlling pretest pain scores, was .578.

TIP: *Note that parameters in GLM cannot be interpreted as in ordinary least squares. That is to say, a unit change in an independent variable* X *does not correspond to a* b_X *change in the dependent variable.*

Panel E presents adjusted means—mean posttest pain statistically adjusted for pretest pain scores for the three groups—and the 95% *CI* around them. For example, the 95% *CI* around the adjusted mean posttest pain score for the bedrest group (56.484) is 52.722 to 60.246. This panel also indicates that the exercise group is significantly different than the other two: The upper bound of the 95% *CI* around the exercise group's adjusted mean (47.728) is lower than the lower bound for either of the other groups (52.722, bedrest and 55.775, controls). In other words, we can be 95% confident that the means are different.

Panel F shows Pairwise Comparisons using the Bonferroni multiple comparison procedure, which adjusts for the inflated risk of a Type I error with multiple comparisons. This panel confirms that adjusted mean for the exercise group was significantly different from those in the other groups, at $p < .001$ (shaded rows). Adjusted means for the bedrest and control groups did not differ significantly from each other.

TIP: *There are only two options in SPSS for post hoc comparisons of adjusted means—the Bonferroni test or the Sidak test. The Sidak procedure is less conservative than the Bonferroni, which means it is somewhat more susceptible to Type I errors, but less susceptible to Type II errors.*

MULTIVARIATE ANALYSIS OF VARIANCE AND COVARIANCE

Multivariate analysis of variance (MANOVA) is an extension of ANOVA that is used to test differences between two or more groups on two or more dependent variables simultaneously. For example, suppose an intervention with cancer patients is designed to both reduce stress and increase hopefulness. Or suppose a treatment for insomniacs is evaluated for its effect on several sleep measures (e.g., minutes of sleep, intrasleep awakenings, etc.). In such situations, MANOVA is likely to be appropriate. It is beyond the scope of this book to explain MANOVA in detail because of its extreme complexity, but major features are described.

Basic Concepts for MANOVA

The *F* statistic in ANOVA tests whether any group differences on the mean of one dependent variable are likely to have occurred by chance. In MANOVA, statistical tests evaluate whether mean group differences on *multiple* dependent variables are likely to have resulted by chance. MANOVA involves the creation of a new dependent variable that is a linear combination of the original dependent variables. Analysis of variance is performed on the composite dependent variable.

Like ANOVA, MANOVA involves partitioning variance into various components. For the most basic MANOVA situation—a one-way MANOVA—variance in the composite dependent variable is partitioned into variance attributable to differences between groups, and error variance, i.e., differences *within* groups. In ANOVA, the partitioned components are computed by summing the squared differences between individual scores and various means. By contrast, MANOVA involves a matrix of scores on the dependent variables, and complex matrix operations are required to partition variance in the composite dependent variable. These matrix operations are described in such texts as Tabachnick and Fidell (2007).

Typically, MANOVA is used in the context of experimental designs in which the investigator has randomly assigned participants to different treatment groups. Although MANOVA *can* also be used to analyze nonexperimental data, the interpretations of results are necessarily different. In practice, researchers analyzing nonexperimental data are more likely to use multiple regression than MANOVA.

TIP: *The dependent variables for MANOVA and MANCOVA should be measured on a scale that is ratio-level or interval-level. Covariates for MANCOVA are typically continuous variables, but dummy-coded dichotomous variables can also be included as described in the section on ANCOVA.*

THE USES OF MANOVA   When comparing group means on several dependent variables, most researchers perform multiple ANOVAs rather than MANOVA—yet, it is usually inappropriate to perform a series of ANOVAs with the same people. The problem with multiple ANOVAs is that the risk of a Type I error is inflated when the dependent variables are correlated, as they almost always are. This is a similar problem to using multiple *t* tests rather than ANOVA when there are more than two groups. MANOVA takes correlations among dependent variables into account when it creates the composite dependent variable, and therefore the risk of a Type I error is maintained at the desired level (i.e., at .05 or lower).

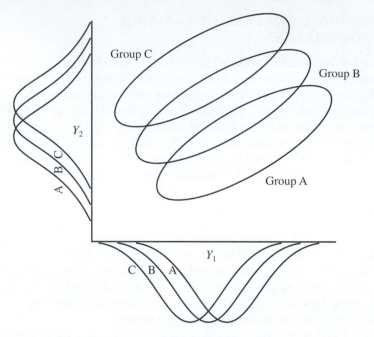

FIGURE 11.5 Composite of two dependent variables for three groups.

Another reason for using MANOVA is that it may reveal group differences that were nonsignificant with individual ANOVAs. Figure 11.5 illustrates how this might occur. In this figure, the axes of the coordinates represent two dependent variables, Y_1 and Y_2. Frequency distributions for three groups being compared (A, B, and C) are portrayed directly on the axes. These distributions indicate considerable overlap among the three groups on the two dependent variables when they are considered separately; the three group means on Y_1 and Y_2 are fairly close in value. Yet the ellipses in this figure, which represent the composite of the two dependent variables, make group differences stand out more clearly. Sometimes, then, MANOVA can be more powerful than a series of ANOVAs.

MANOVA may, however, be *less* powerful than ANOVA. Given the same effect size, significance criterion, and desired power, it usually requires a larger sample to reject the null hypothesis for MANOVA than for ANOVA. Moreover, MANOVA involves even more assumptions than ANOVA and may lead to ambiguities when interpreting the effects of the independent variable on any individual dependent variable. Nevertheless, if the research involves more than one dependent variable, MANOVA is often appropriate.

Tabachnick and Fidell (2007) note that MANOVA works best (from a statistical point of view) when the dependent variables are highly negatively correlated or moderately positively correlated. If the dependent variables are uncorrelated, or very highly positively correlated, MANOVA can be viewed as "wasteful" (Tabachnick & Fidell, 2007, p. 268). Researchers who opt to use multiple ANOVAs rather than a MANOVA should consider an adjustment to their alpha level to protect against the inflated risk of a Type I error, as discussed in the next section.

TIP: *Theoretically, there is no limit to the number of dependent variables that can be used in MANOVA. As the number increases, however, interpretation becomes more difficult, the likelihood of error based on complex interactions increases, and typically there is a loss of power.*

TABLE 11.2 Fictitious Data for MANOVA Example: Scores on Two Posttest Dependent Variables in Three Treatment Groups

Bedrest Group		Exercise Group		Control Group	
Pain	Medications	Pain	Medications	Pain	Medications
85	12	60	9	30	2
70	7	45	4	40	5
50	4	30	0	45	4
30	2	70	6	20	1
45	8	55	4	85	10
40	5	65	8	50	6
65	7	35	5	85	14
70	9	40	3	75	8
35	2	60	8	65	6
85	11	10	1	60	4
Means:					
57.50	6.7	47.00	4.8	55.50	6.0

STATISTICAL TESTS FOR MANOVA   To illustrate MANOVA, suppose that in our fictitious experiment to evaluate the effectiveness of bedrest versus exercise versus no intervention in reducing lower back pain, we had two dependent variables: post-treatment pain scores and number of pain medications taken in the 5 days following treatment. For the moment, we omit from the analysis the pretreatment pain scores. Data for this example are presented in Table 11.2.

The most basic research question in MANOVA is whether the mean group differences on the dependent variables are true population differences or whether sample mean differences likely occurred by chance. In ANOVA, an F statistic is computed, but in MANOVA there are four alternative statistics: **Pillai's trace criterion, Wilks' lambda (λ), Hotelling's trace criterion,** and **Roy's largest root criterion** (sometimes called *Roy's greatest characteristic* root or *gcr*). An F test in ANOVA is the ratio of the mean squares for the treatment to the mean squares for error. In MANOVA, there is no longer a single number to represent the two sums of squares, but rather there are several matrices with sums of squares and cross products. The matrices must be combined into a test statistic, and the four statistics just described use different criteria for creating the test statistic. When only two groups are being compared in a one-way MANOVA, the four statistics are identical. When there are three or more groups, the values of these statistics may differ, but the conclusions (i.e., whether to reject or accept the null hypothesis) are usually—although not always—the same.

For the data shown in Table 11.2, the MANOVA statistics for testing group differences are as follows: Pillai's trace criterion = .06; Wilks' lambda = .94; Hotelling's trace criterion = .07; and Roy's largest root = .06. Perhaps the most widely-reported of these test statistics is Wilks' lambda, especially when there are three or more groups. This statistic represents the pooled ratio of error variance in the composite dependent variable to error variance plus treatment variance. This may sound similar to the R^2 statistic—in fact, Wilks' lambda may be defined as follows:

$$\lambda = 1 - R^2$$

In other words, Wilks' lambda is a measure of the proportion of variance in the composite dependent variable that is *not* accounted for by the independent variable. Thus, one reason for the popularity of Wilks' lambda as the test statistic in MANOVA is that it provides a direct measure of the strength of the relationship between the independent variable and the dependent variables, taken together. In our example, the proportion of variance accounted for by the treatment variable is .06, i.e., $(1 - .94)$.

Pillai's criterion, however, is the most robust of the four statistics, meaning that it yields results that are most likely to be correct even when MANOVA assumptions are violated. When the sample is small, when there are unequal ns in the groups, or when basic assumptions (described below) are known to be violated, Pillai's criterion is the preferred test statistic.

Tables of the exact distributions for the four MANOVA test statistics can be found in advanced textbooks, but the more usual procedure is to transform the statistics to an approximate F distribution. For the Wilks' lambda statistic in our example, the F statistic is 0.44 (4, 52), $p = .78$. Based on this MANOVA analysis, we would conclude that the three groups do not differ significantly in terms of posttreatment pain scores or number of pain medications. We would have reached the same conclusion regardless of which of the four test statistics had been used.

If we *had* found statistically different group means for the overall MANOVA test, we would naturally want to identify which dependent variables had significant group differences. This is not a straightforward task if the dependent variables are correlated. One approach is to examine univariate ANOVA results for each dependent variable. Dependent variables can be rank ordered, in terms of their contribution to a significant MANOVA statistic, by the magnitude of *significant* univariate F statistics. When this approach is used, however, more stringent alpha levels should be used in determining which dependent variables are significant, using a Bonferroni-type adjustment described in Chapter 8. The formula for estimating the risk of a Type I error when evaluating multiple dependent variables via ANOVA is as follows:

$$\alpha = 1 - (1 - \alpha_1)(1 - \alpha_2) \ldots (1 - \alpha_j)$$

where α = overall risk of Type I error
$\alpha_1 \ldots \alpha_j$ = risk of Type I error for Y_1 to Y_j
j = number of dependent variables

Thus, if our significance criterion for the univariate F tests were .05, the overall risk of committing a Type I error in our example of two separate univariate ANOVAs would be as follows:

$$\alpha = 1 - (1 - .05)(1 - .05) = .098$$

With two dependent variables, there would be about a one in ten chance of committing a Type I error if we used .05 as the significance criterion for individual ANOVA tests. If we wanted our overall risk of a Type I error to be kept to the 5% level, we would have to conclude that a dependent variable was nonsignificant if the p value for the univariate ANOVA F test exceeded .025 (.05 $\times$ .05).

Another alternative for evaluating dependent variables in the context of significant overall MANOVA results is a **stepdown analysis.** This procedure is comparable to using hierarchical multiple regression to test the importance of independent variables. In the first step, the highest-priority dependent variable (as specified by the researcher) is tested via ordinary ANOVA. Remaining dependent variables are "stepped in" in a series of ANCOVAs that use previously entered dependent variables as covariates to see whether the new dependent variable adds anything to the combination of dependent variables already tested.

MANCOVA and Other Related Procedures

Like ANOVA, MANOVA can be extended in various ways to accommodate different research designs. For example, **multifactor MANOVAs** can also be performed. A two-way MANOVA would be used to test hypotheses about multiple dependent variables when there are two independent variables (e.g., the effect of three treatment conditions on posttreatment pain scores and pain medication usage, separately for those who have or have not had back surgery). In this case, the analysis provides tests of two main effects (treatment and surgical history) and an interaction effect on the composite dependent variable.

Another important extension of MANOVA is **multivariate analysis of covariance (MANCOVA).** MANCOVA involves adjustments to the composite dependent variable prior to assessing the effects of the independent variable. Just as ANCOVA generally adds power to the statistical test in comparison with ANOVA, so too does MANCOVA generally make it less likely that a Type II error will be committed in comparison with MANOVA. The power increases as the correlation between the covariates and the dependent variables increases.

In the example we used to illustrate MANOVA, we could use MANCOVA to first statistically remove the effect of pretreatment pain scores, and then examine the effect of the treatment variable on both posttreatment pain scores and medications. In fact, when we do this, the conclusions are different than when MANOVA is used. It may be recalled that without pretreatment pain scores controlled, the value of Wilks' lambda for the effect of the treatment variable on the composite dependent variable was .94—only 6% of the variance explained. After removing the effect of initial pain scores, the treatment group variable accounts for a full 62% of the variance in the composite dependent variable (i.e., $\lambda = .38$). This effect is significant beyond the .001 level. We examine SPSS output for this analysis in a subsequent section.

Assumptions for MANOVA and MANCOVA

Significance tests for MANOVA and MANCOVA assume random sampling from the population and a multivariate normal distribution. MANOVA is fairly robust to the normality assumption when there are at least 20 cases in each cell of the design, but if any dependent variable is known to be severely skewed, a transformation should be used.

The multivariate analog of the assumption of homogeneous variances for individual dependent variables is **homogeneity of the variance–covariance matrices**[1]. If sample sizes are equal in the groups being compared, MANOVA is robust to violations of this assumption. With unequal sample sizes, the **Box *M* test** should be used to assess homogeneity. This test tends to be overly sensitive, and so Tabachnick and Fidell (2007) recommend that an alpha of .001 be used as the criterion for concluding that the MANOVA may not be adequately robust. They also recommend using Pillai's criterion as the statistical test when the significance of the Box *M* test exceeds .001.

---

[1] A **variance–covariance matrix** is a square matrix with the variances of the variables on the diagonal and the covariances of pairs of variables off the diagonal. The **covariance** of two variables is the sum of the cross products of each variable's deviation scores, divided by degrees of freedom. The covariance can be thought of as an unstandardized correlation coefficient. When each covariance is divided by the standard deviations of the two variables, the result is the correlation between the two.

Linearity is also assumed—linearity between all pairs of dependent variables, all pairs of covariates in MANCOVA, and all covariate-dependent variable combinations. If there is reason to assume a curvilinear relationship, scatterplots of pairs of variables should be examined. Departures from linearity can reduce the power of the statistical tests.

In both stepdown analysis and MANCOVA, homogeneity of regression is assumed. If an interaction between a covariate and an independent variable exists, MANCOVA is not appropriate. An interaction implies that a different covariate adjustment on the dependent variable is needed in different groups.

Power and Sample Size in MANOVA

When using MANOVA or MANCOVA, there should always be more cases than dependent variables in every cell of the design. If a cell has more dependent variables than participants, the cell becomes singular and the homogeneity assumption becomes untestable. Sample sizes in each cell should, in any event, be reasonably large to ensure adequate power.

It is possible to do a power analysis for MANOVA and MANCOVA, but this typically requires specialized software. Some approximate projections of sample size needs can be made if you can estimate the lowest partial eta^2 for your various dependent variables. In other words, you can base your power analysis on the estimated effect of your independent variable on the dependent variable with the *smallest* expected group difference, using power analysis procedures discussed previously.

Power in MANOVA also depends on the relationships among the dependent variables. Power is lowered when correlations among the dependent variables are positive or moderately negative. If you anticipate such a situation, your sample size estimates should be increased accordingly to minimize the risk of a Type II error.

> **TIP:** *In SPSS, researchers can select an option for all GLM analyses, such as MANOVA and ANCOVA, that will indicate "observed power" (i.e., post hoc power) for each component of the model. This option yields an estimate of the power of the analysis to detect the obtained effect, given the sample size and a significance criterion, the default for which is .05.*

Computer Example of MANCOVA

Computer programs for MANOVA and MANCOVA typically offer dozens of options for statistical information and displays. Figure 11.6 presents selected minimal SPSS output for a MANCOVA, involving the analysis of data presented in Table 11.2, with the pretreatment pain scores from Table 11.1 as the covariate. In this analysis, which was run in SPSS using Analyze ➔ General Linear Model ➔ Multivariate, *Prepain* is the covariate and *Group* is the independent variable. We comment on major features of this printout in this section.

> **TIP:** *In SPSS, the term "multivariate" is used only when there are multiple dependent variables. Thus, ANCOVA is run within the GLM Univariate program, while MANOVA and MANCOVA are run with the Multivariate program.*

Panel A presents results of the test of the assumption regarding the homogeneity of the variance–covariance matrices. The Box M statistic is 1.010, which is transformed to an F value (.150) that is nonsignificant ($p = .989$). We can conclude that the assumption of homogeneity has not been violated.

Panel B (Multivariate tests) presents a particularly important table for our analysis. This panel shows the four MANOVA statistics for the intercept, the covariate *Prepain*, and the independent treatment group variable *Group*. All effects are statistically significant at $p = .001$ or lower, regardless of which of the four statistical tests for multivariate effects is used. Of particular importance are the rows for *Group*. With pretest pain scores controlled, group differences on the composite dependent variable are statistically significant. For example, we see that the value of the Wilks' lambda statistic is .379 (i.e., about 62% of the variance explained). Using this test, the partial eta^2 for the independent variable, shown in the last column, is .384. Although we do not show the MANOVA results (the same analysis without the

A Box's Test of Equality of Covariance Matrices[a]

Box's M	1.010
F	.150
df1	6
df2	18168.923
Sig.	.989

Tests the null hypothesis that the observed covariance matrices of the dependent variables are equal across groups.

[a] Design: Intercept + prepain + group

B   **Multivariate Tests[c]**

Effect		Value	F	Hypothesis df	Error df	Sig.	Partial Eta-Squared
Intercept	Pillai's Trace	.437	9.690[a]	2.000	25.000	.001	.437
	Wilks' Lambda	.563	9.690[a]	2.000	25.000	.001	.437
	Hotelling's Trace	.775	9.690[a]	2.000	25.000	.001	.437
	Roy's Largest Root	.775	9.690[a]	2.000	25.000	.001	.437
Prepain	Pillai's Trace	.926	155.291[a]	2.000	25.000	.000	.926
	Wilks' Lambda	.074	155.291[a]	2.000	25.000	.000	.926
	Hotelling's Trace	12.423	155.291[a]	2.000	25.000	.000	.926
	Roy's Largest Root	12.423	155.291[a]	2.000	25.000	.000	.926
Group	Pillai's Trace	.627	5.941	4.000	52.000	.001	.314
	Wilks' Lambda	.379	7.794[a]	4.000	50.000	.000	.384
	Hotelling's Trace	1.618	9.709	4.000	48.000	.000	.447
	Roy's Largest Root	1.607	20.893[b]	2.000	26.000	.000	.616

[a] Exact statistic
[b] The statistic is an upper bound on F that yields a lower bound on the significance level
[c] Design: Intercept + prepain + group

FIGURE 11.6 SPSS printout of MANCOVA.

C

Tests of Between-Subjects Effects

Source	Dependent Variable	Type III Sum of Squares	df	Mean Square	F	Sig.	Partial Eta-Squared
Corrected Model	Posttest pain score	11046.782[a]	3	3682.261	110.059	.000	.927
	Number of medications	261.489[b]	3	87.163	28.090	.000	.764
Intercept	Posttest pain score	430.072	1	430.072	12.854	.001	.331
	Number of medications	42.649	1	42.649	13.745	.001	.346
Prepain	Posttest pain score	10425.115	1	10425.115	311.596	.000	.923
	Number of medications	243.023	1	243.023	78.319	.000	.751
Group	Posttest pain score	1343.608	2	671.804	20.080	.000	.607
	Number of medications	33.258	2	16.629	5.359	.011	.292
Error	Posttest pain score	869.885	26	33.457			
	Number of medications	80.677	26	3.103			
Total	Posttest pain score	97250.000	30				
	Number of medications	1363.000	30				
Corrected Total	Posttest pain score	11916.667	29				
	Number of medications	342.167	29				

[a] R Squared = .927 (Adjusted R Squared = .919)
[b] R Squared = .764 (Adjusted R Squared = .737)

FIGURE 11.6   Continued

covariate), suffice it to say that all four multivariate tests were nonsignificant for the *Group* variable when pretest pain scores were not controlled.

The next panel of SPSS printout presented results of Levene's test for homogeneity of variances, which we do not show in Figure 11.6 in order to conserve space. Levene's test for the dependent variable posttest pain was statistically significant, as discussed previously, but the test for medications was not significant ($p = .761$), indicating that the assumption of homogeneous variances was not violated.

Panel C of Figure 11.6 (Between Subjects Effects) presents univariate results—i.e., statistics for each dependent variable separately. This panel essentially summarizes the results of analyses in which each dependent variable is regressed on *Prepain* and *Group*. For example, the footnotes at the bottom shows that R^2 for posttest pain scores regressed on the covariate and independent variable is .927 (adjusted value = .919), while that for the regression of number of medications on these two variables is .764 (adjusted value = .737). The first row of the table indicates that, for both dependent variables, the overall models are significant beyond the .001 level.

Panel C also shows individual ANCOVAs for the two dependent variables, for the independent variable *Group* (the shaded rows). Results for the first dependent variable, posttest pain scores, are identical to the ANCOVA results presented in Figure 11.4. For example, the F of 20.080 is the same in both analyses. The ANCOVA for the second dependent variable, number of medications, has an $F = 5.359$, which is significant at $p = .011$. Thus, these separate univariate tests indicate that *Group* had a significant effect on *both* dependent variables, considered separately, with pretest pain scores controlled. Remember, however, that with a desired overall α of .05, each univariate F test must have a p value equal to or less than .025, as previously noted. Both dependent variables meet this criterion, and thus we can conclude that, after controlling for initial levels of pain, the three treatments had different effects on both posttreatment pain and the use of pain medications. In this example, the stepdown analysis also resulted in significant *F* values for both dependent variables (not shown).

The MANCOVA output included several panels that we did not include in Figure 11.6. One is an optional table for Marginal Means, i.e., the adjusted group means on the dependent variables after removing the effect of the covariate (analogous to panel D of Figure 11.4). Figure 11.6 also does not show the panel for Pairwise Comparisons (analogous to panel E of Figure 11.4). The pairwise comparisons for number of medications were similar to those for posttest pain scores: The exercise group was significantly different from the bedrest and control groups, but the two latter groups were not significantly different from each other.

> **TIP:** *In a MANOVA performed within SPSS, a full range of post hoc tests is available to pinpoint differences between the means of paired groups while adjusting for the inflated risk of a Type I error. Several such tests were discussed in Chapter 7 on ANOVA. When there are covariates in the model, however, only the Bonferroni and Sidak procedures are available for comparing adjusted means in MANCOVA.*

Example of MANCOVA:

Good and Ahn (2008) used MANCOVA to test the effect of a music intervention on pain among Korean women who had had gynecologic surgery. Women in the treatment group chose between several types of music, while those in the control group had no music. Pain levels were assessed using two pain measures, a sensory component and an affective (distress) component. The two groups were compared on the two postintervention pain measures using a multivariate model with baseline pain levels controlled.

REPEATED MEASURES ANOVA FOR MIXED DESIGNS

In Chapter 7, we discussed one-way repeated-measures ANOVA (RM-ANOVA), which is appropriate for within-subject designs in which one group of people is measured at multiple points. In such situations, the null hypothesis is that the means have not changed over time, or under different conditions in a crossover design.

Many clinical trials involve randomly assigning participants to different treatment groups such as an experimental and control group, and then collecting data at multiple points. When there are only two data collection points (e.g., a pretest and a posttest), ANCOVA is often used to test the null hypothesis that group means are equal, after removing the effect of pretest scores. When data are collected at three or more time points, the appropriate analysis usually is a **repeated measures ANOVA for mixed designs.** The design is called *mixed* because there is a within-subjects time factor, as well as a between-subjects treatment factor. That is, the analysis compares means for the *same* people over time, as well as means for *different* people in the treatment groups. Because there are two factors (time and treatment), there is an interaction term, and in fact, it is the interaction term that is of primary interest in clinical trials. When people are randomized to treatment groups, we would expect their mean values at baseline to be equal—but if the treatment is beneficial, group means would be different at subsequent points of data collection, thus resulting in a time $\times$ treatment interaction. The general linear model can be used to analyze data from such mixed-design studies.

TIP: *Because RM-ANOVA is undertaken within the GLM, there is considerable flexibility. For example, there can be two or more between-subjects independent variables, covariates, and many different points of data collection.*

Basic Concepts for Mixed-Design RM-ANOVA

To make our discussion more concrete, consider the data in Table 11.3, which extends our example of experimental interventions for lower back pain. Suppose we collected preintervention data on pain levels at T1, randomly assigned participants to three groups, administered the interventions to the two treatment groups, and then measured pain 1 month (T2) and 2 months (T3) later. A mixed-design RM-ANOVA would be appropriate for analyzing these data. In this situation, the RM-ANOVA addresses the questions of whether (1) mean pain scores changed significantly over time, regardless of treatment group; (2) group means were different, regardless of when data were collected; and (3) mean pain scores for the groups are different conditional upon the timing of the data collection. With regard to the first question, the mean pain scores at T1, T2, and T3 for the three groups combined were 66.50, 53.33, and 55.50, respectively—but are these differences significant? The second question, in the context of this RCT, is of limited interest. But with regard to the third question, there were declines in pain scores over time in all three groups, but were declines significantly greater in some groups—that is, did an intervention lead to significantly greater improvements in pain? These are questions addressed in the RM-ANOVA.

Many of the assumptions for a mixed-design RM-ANOVA are similar to others we have noted in this chapter, because they reflect basic assumptions of the

TABLE 11.3 Fictitious Data for RM-ANOVA Example: Pain Scores at Three Time Points (T1–T3) for Three Treatment Groups

Bedrest Group			Exercise Group			Control Group		
T1	**T2**	**T3**	**T1**	**T2**	**T3**	**T1**	**T2**	**T3**
95	85	80	75	60	65	35	30	35
80	70	75	80	45	55	50	40	45
60	50	55	50	30	35	45	45	45
45	30	45	85	70	65	30	20	25
55	45	40	70	55	55	85	85	80
50	40	45	85	65	60	60	50	50
75	65	60	60	35	40	90	85	85
80	70	70	65	40	50	90	75	80
40	35	30	80	60	60	80	65	70
95	85	85	45	10	20	60	60	60
Means:								
67.50	57.50	58.50	69.50	47.00	50.50	62.50	55.50	57.50
Overall Bedrest Mean = 61.17			Overall Exercise Mean = 55.67			Overall Control Mean = 58.50		
Overall time means: T1 = 66.50; T2 = 53.33; T3 = 55.50 Grand mean = 58.44								

general linear model. These include the assumptions of multivariate normality, homogeneity of variances, and homogeneity of the variance–covariance matrix, as in MANOVA. However, as discussed in Chapter 7, RM-ANOVA has some unique assumptions—the assumption of *sphericity* (the variance of the difference between the estimated means for any pair of time points is the same as for any other pair) and the related assumption of *compound symmetry* (homogeneity of within-treatment variances and homogeneity of covariance between pairs of treatment levels).

Although ANOVA and its variants are fairly robust to violations of such assumptions as the normality and homogeneity of variances, the same cannot be said about violations of sphericity and compound symmetry. There are differences of opinion about what to do if these assumptions are violated, as well as differences in how to assess violations. The most widely used test, as noted in Chapter 7, is **Mauchly's test,** which tests the null hypothesis that sphericity holds true. If this test is statistically significant, it suggests that the assumption has been violated. The test has been criticized, however, on several grounds. First, the test is not robust to violations of the normality assumption, and it has low statistical power. When samples are small, Mauchly's test is often unable to detect violations that actually exist, even when such violations are extreme. Yet with a very large sample, Mauchly's test can be statistically significant even if there are minor violations of sphericity. An alternative approach to assessing sphericity is discussed subsequently.

CORRECTIONS TO SIGNIFICANCE TESTS FOR SPHERICITY VIOLATIONS   If sphericity is violated, two alternative strategies are most often proposed. One approach is to make an adjustment when testing the *F* statistic, to correct for the inflated risk of a Type I error that can occur when sphericity does not hold. To make this adjustment, it is necessary to compute a statistic called **epsilon,** which is a measure of the degree to which sphericity has been violated. When sphericity is met perfectly, epsilon is 1.0. The lower the value of epsilon, the worse is the violation of sphericity. The *lower bound* of epsilon depends of the number of measurements on the repeated measures factor. When there are three measurements (as in our example), the lower bound of epsilon is 0.50. In general, the larger the number of measurements, the greater is the potential for violating the sphericity assumption. Because epsilon is an index of magnitude of violation of sphericity, some have suggested inspecting values of epsilon rather than relying exclusively on Mauchly's test. If epsilon is close to 1.0, then violations to sphericity are likely to be minor. If epsilon is close to the lower bound, then it is more important to use the correction, or to use the alternative approach discussed in the next section.

TIP: *The lower bound of epsilon can be calculated through a simple formula: $1 \div (k - 1)$, where k is the number of measurements in the within-subjects factor. For example, if k = 4, the lower bound for epsilon = .33 and if k = 4, the lower bound = .25. Thus, when k = 2 (only two time periods), epsilon always equals one and sphericity necessarily holds.*

Epsilon, which is used as a correction factor in evaluating the *F* statistic, can be estimated using different methods. The two most widely used formulas are called the Greenhouse-Geisser correction and the Huynh-Feldt correction. The **Greenhouse-Geisser correction** is a conservative correction that tends to underestimate epsilon. The **Huynh-Feldt correction,** by contrast, tends to overestimate epsilon, which has led some statisticians to suggest averaging the two when their values are very different. The more conservative correction is especially appropriate when departures from sphericity are severe—for example, when epsilon is less than .75.

Whichever estimate of epsilon is used, the correction works the same way: Degrees of freedom for the F test are multiplied by epsilon. When epsilon is 1.0, df are unchanged. But when epsilon is low, df are lowered as well, which makes it more difficult to obtain a significant result. For example, if epsilon were .50, the correction would turn an F test with 2 and 60 df into an F test with 1 and 30 df ($2 \times .50 = 1$ and $60 \times .50 = 30$). The value of F would need to be 3.15 to be statistically significant at the .05 level for the first test, but would need to be 4.17 for the second one. In SPSS, the values of epsilon using both correction formulas are calculated, and then the results of the F tests with both corrections (and also without the correction) are shown.

THE MANOVA ALTERNATIVE   An alternative to correcting for violations to sphericity is to use a test that does not assume sphericity, which usually means switching to MANOVA. In a mixed-design RM-ANOVA, the various measurements of the dependent variable (Time 1 to Time 3 in our example) are considered a within-subjects independent variable representing time. If the same data were analyzed by MANOVA, each measurement would be used as a separate dependent variable. In our example, there would be three dependent variables, one for each pain score.

The reason for preferring univariate mixed-method RM-ANOVA with epsilon corrections over the MANOVA solution is that the former tends to be more powerful, meaning fewer Type II errors. SPSS routinely produces the results both ways when an RM-ANOVA is requested within the GLM routine. This leads to a confusing array of output, but the advantage is that the results can be compared immediately.

The Computer and Mixed-Design RM-ANOVA

Figure 11.7 presents selected panels of output from a mixed-design RM-ANOVA. In this analysis, the data presented in Table 11.3 were analyzed using SPSS (Analyze → General Linear Model → Repeated Measures). We have omitted from this figure the output for Descriptive Statistics (which shows means and SDs for each cell of this 3×3 design), and for the Box M test. In this example, the Box M test had a p value of .015, which is greater than the recommended criterion of $p < 001$. Thus, we can conclude that the assumption of the homogeneity of the variance–covariance matrix has not been markedly violated.

Panel A in Figure 11.7 (Multivariate Tests) shows the MANOVA results for the *Time* (within subjects) factor and the *Time * Group* interaction. For each effect, SPSS computed the four multivariate tests described earlier—Pillai's trace, Wilks' lambda, Hotelling's trace, and Roy's largest root. Regardless of which test is used, both time and the interaction effect are significant. The three sets of pain measures are significantly different at $p < .001$. The treatment factor, conditional upon time of measurement, is also significant at $p < .001$. Values for partial eta^2 are shown in the far-right column.

Panel B presents results for Mauchly's test of sphericity for the within-subjects factor *Time*. As shown in the shaded area, the test is not significant, $p = .628$ and so we can retain the null hypothesis of sphericity. This panel also shows values for epsilon. The first, Greenhouse-Geisser epsilon, is .966, which is only a minor departure from a "perfect" epsilon of 1.0. The less conservative Huynh-Feldt epsilon is 1.00. Thus, there appears to be sufficient evidence that the sphericity assumption has not been violated, which means we can use the tests of within-subjects effects in the next panel, rather than using MANOVA results.

As it turns out, results for both univariate and multivariate tests lead to the same conclusions. Panel C (Within Subjects Effects) shows that the F test for *Time*, with sphericity assumed and also with corrections, is significant at $p < .001$. Note that degrees of freedom were adjusted when correction factors were applied. For

General Linear Model

A   **Multivariate Tests**[c]

Effect		Value	F	Hypothesis df	Error df	Sig.	Partial Eta-Squared
Time	Pillai's Trace	.888	103.537[a]	2.000	26.000	.000	.888
	Wilks' Lambda	.112	103.537[a]	2.000	26.000	.000	.888
	Hotelling's Trace	7.964	103.537[a]	2.000	26.000	.000	.888
	Roy's Largest Root	7.964	103.537[a]	2.000	26.000	.000	.888
Time * group	Pillai's Trace	.699	7.248	4.000	54.000	.000	.349
	Wilks' Lambda	.311	10.310[a]	4.000	52.000	.000	.442
	Hotelling's Trace	2.184	13.650	4.000	50.000	.000	.522
	Roy's Largest Root	2.170	29.290[b]	2.000	27.000	.000	.685

[a]Exact statistic
[b]The statistic is an upper bound on F that yields a lower bound on the significance level
[c]Design: Intercept + group   Within-Subjects Design: Time

B   **Mauchly's Test of Sphericity**[b]

Measure: Pain

Within Subjects Effect	Mauchly's W	Approx. Chi-Square	df	Sig.	Epsilon[a]		
					Greenhouse-Geisser	Huynh-Feldt	Lower-bound
Time	.965	.931	2	.628	.966	1.000	.500

Tests the null hypothesis that the error covariance matrix of the orthonormalized transformed dependent variables is proportional to an identity matrix.

[a]May be used to adjust the degrees of freedom for the averaged tests of significance. Corrected tests are displayed in the Tests of Within-Subjects Effects table.
[b]Design: Intercept + group   Within-Subjects Design: Time

C   **Tests of Within-Subjects Effects**

Measure: Pain

Source		Type III Sum of Squares	df	Mean Square	F	Sig.	Partial Eta-Squared
Time	Sphericity assumed	2990.556	2	1495.278	105.091	.000	.796
	Greenhouse-Geisser	2990.556	1.932	1547.885	105.091	.000	.796
	Huynh-Feldt	2990.556	2.000	1495.278	105.091	.000	.796
	Lower-bound	2990.556	1.000	2990.556	105.091	.000	.796
Time * Group	Sphericity assumed	807.778	4	201.944	14.193	.000	.513
	Greenhouse-Geisser	807.778	3.864	209.049	14.193	.000	.513
	Huynh-Feldt	807.778	4.000	201.944	14.193	.000	.513
	Lower-bound	807.778	2.000	403.889	14.193	.000	.513
Error (Time)	Sphericity assumed	768.333	54	14.228			
	Greenhouse-Geisser	768.333	52.165	14.729			
	Huynh-Feldt	768.333	54.000	14.228			
	Lower-bound	768.333	27.000	28.457			

FIGURE 11.7   SPSS printout of mixed-design RM-ANOVA.

D   **Tests of Within-Subjects Contrasts**

Measure: Pain

Source	Time	Type III Sum of Squares	df	Mean Square	F	Sig.
Time	Level 2 vs. Level 1	5200.833	1	5200.833	160.943	.000
	Level 3 vs. Level 1	3630.000	1	3630.000	155.571	.000
Time * group	Level 2 vs. Level 1	1351.667	2	675.833	20.914	.000
	Level 3 vs. Level 1	1040.000	2	520.000	22.286	.000
Error (Time)	Level 2 vs. Level 1	872.500	27	32.315		
	Level 3 vs. Level 1	630.000	27	23.333		

E   **Tests of Between-Subjects Effects**

Measure: Pain

Transformed Variable: Average

Source	Type III Sum of Squares	df	Mean Square	F	Sig.	Partial Eta-Squared
Intercept	102472.593	1	102472.593	281.254	.000	.912
Group	151.296	2	75.648	.208	.814	.015
Error	9837.222	27	364.342			

F   **Estimated Marginal Means**

TIME

F1   **Estimates**

Measure: Pain

Time	Mean	Std. Error	95% CI Lower Bound	95% CI Upper Bound
1	66.500	3.531	59.256	73.744
2	53.333	3.734	45.671	60.995
3	55.500	3.312	48.703	62.297

F2   **Pairwise Comparisons**

Measure: Pain

(I) Time	(J) Time	Mean Difference (I − J)	Std. Error	Sig.[a]	95% CI for Difference[a] Lower Bound	95% CI for Difference[a] Upper Bound
1	2	13.167*	1.038	.000	10.518	15.816
	3	11.000*	.882	.000	8.749	13.251
2	1	−13.167*	1.038	.000	−15.816	−10.518
	3	−2.167	.995	.038	−4.707	.374
3	1	−11.000*	.882	.000	−13.251	−8.749
	2	2.167	.995	.038	−.374	4.707

Based on estimated marginal means

*The mean difference is significant at the .05 level.

[a]Adjustment for multiple comparisons: Bonferroni.

FIGURE 11.7   Continued

G   **Experimental Group * Time**

Measure: Pain

Experimental Group	Time	Mean	Std. Error	95% CI Lower Bound	95% CI Upper Bound
Bedrest Group	1	67.500	6.115	54.952	80.048
	2	57.500	6.468	44.229	70.771
	3	58.500	5.737	46.728	70.272
Exercise Group	1	69.500	6.115	56.952	82.048
	2	47.000	6.468	33.729	60.271
	3	50.500	5.737	38.728	62.272
Control Group	1	62.500	6.115	49.952	75.048
	2	55.500	6.468	42.229	68.771
	3	57.500	5.737	45.728	69.272

H   **Profile Plots**

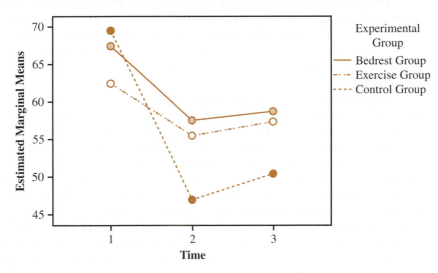

FIGURE 11.7   Continued

example, in the analysis for *Time*, the original *df* of 2, when multiplied by the Greenhouse-Geisser epsilon of .966, equals 1.932. In this univariate table, with or without corrections, both *Time* and *Time * Group* are statistically significant—the same result obtained earlier via MANOVA. Values for partial eta^2, however, are somewhat different from those shown in the multivariate table.

Panel D presents a series of within-subjects contrasts that are available through the "Contrasts" option within SPSS. Here, we requested that preintervention pain scores (referred to as Level 1 of the *Time* variable) be contrasted with the two post-treatment scores (Levels 2 and 3). For the main effect of *Time*, averaged across treatment groups, T1 pain scores are significantly different from both T2 and T3 pain scores at $p < .001$. The bottom of Panel D shows the contrast for the *Time * Group*

predictors that are weighted with *b* weights. The discriminant analysis solves for the values of *a* and *b* so as to maximize the separation of the groups, using the least-squares criterion. The discriminant equation can also be standardized, providing a better means for comparing the relative contribution of the predictors.

When the dependent variable involves three or more groups (categories), there is more than one discriminant function, and each has a separate equation for predicting discriminant scores. The number of discriminant functions is either the number of groups minus one or the number of predictor variables, whichever is smaller. For example, suppose that we wanted to use our four predictors (two GRE scores, motivation scores, and undergraduate GPA) to predict whether a graduate student would (1) obtain a graduate degree, (2) voluntarily drop out of the program, or (3) flunk out. In this case, there would be two discriminant functions (i.e., three outcome categories minus 1 = 2). When more than one discriminant function is derived, the first function extracts the maximum amount of variance possible. The second function has the second highest ratio of between-groups to within-groups sums of squares, but is subject to the constraint that it must be uncorrelated with the first function.

TIP: *In discriminant analysis, the dependent variable is a categorical variable measured on a nominal scale (or on an ordinal scale with a small number of values). Independent variables can be continuous interval- or ratio-level variables, or dummy-coded dichotomous variables. When predictors are all dichotomous, however, the discriminant function is not optimal.*

The relationship between discriminant (*D*) scores and individual predictors can be evaluated by computing correlations, which are called *structure coefficients* or *loadings,* as in canonical analysis. Such structure coefficients are useful for interpreting the results of a discriminant analysis when there are two or more functions. Different underlying dimensions may contribute to discrimination among multiple groups, and structure coefficients are used to interpret the pattern. For example, suppose we used the four predictors from our graduate program example to discriminate between completers, dropouts, and "flunkouts." A structure matrix for this example might have high loadings for motivation on the first function, and high loadings on the two GRE scores on the second function. The two separate dimensions captured in this analysis would be motivation on the one hand and cognitive ability on the other hand.

CLASSIFICATION IN DISCRIMINANT ANALYSIS   Based on discriminant scores, statistical criteria can be used to classify cases into groups. When the classification process is done for the original sample, the percent of correct classifications can be estimated by comparing actual group membership with projected group membership for each case. If classification is successful (i.e., a high percentage of correct classifications), the discriminant function equation can be used to classify new cases for which group membership is unknown—in our example, for predicting students who would complete graduate training.

Discriminant analysis develops a classification equation for each group. Then raw data for a case is inserted into each equation, and this yields that case's classification probability for each group. The case is assigned to the group for which it has the highest classification probability.

Discriminant analysis yields a summary classification table that indicates degree of success. Table 11.4 illustrates such a classification table for our fictitious example of predicting completion versus noncompletion of graduate school. This table shows that of 8 students who did not finish the program, 7 (87.5%) were correctly classified, and

TABLE 11.4 Summary Classification Table for Graduate School Completion Example

Actual Group Membership	Predicted Group Membership	
	0 = Did Not Graduate	1 = Graduated
0 Did not graduate ($N = 8$)	7 (87.5%)	1 (12.5%)
1 Graduated ($N = 12$)	1 (8.3%)	11 (91.7%)
Overall rate of successful classification = 90.0% (18 ÷ 20)		

1 (12.5%) was misclassified as finishing the program. Among the 12 students who *did* actually get a graduate degree, 1 (8.3%) was misclassified as a likely noncompleter but 11 (91.7%) were correctly classified. Thus, 18 of the 20 students (90.0% of the sample) were correctly classified on the basis of the discriminant analysis.

Classification rates are typically higher in the sample used to generate the discriminant function than in other samples from the same population, and so the percentage of correctly classified cases is usually an inflated estimate of actual performance in the population. Cross-validation of the discriminant function is highly recommended, and can be achieved within a single sample—by dividing it in half—if the sample is sufficiently large.

SIGNIFICANCE TESTS IN DISCRIMINANT ANALYSIS   The main significance test in discriminant analysis is the test of the null hypothesis that the discriminant functions reflect chance sampling fluctuations (i.e., that groups cannot be reliably distinguished on the basis of the predictors in the analysis). A test of the null hypothesis can be based on Wilks' lambda, and the significance level of the lambda statistic is based on a transformation that approximates a chi-square or F distribution. (Other statistics include the now-familiar Pillai's trace criterion and Hotelling's trace.)

When there is more than one discriminant function, the analysis typically evaluates whether each function contains reliable discriminatory power. Computer programs usually use a "peel-away" process to successively test discriminatory power as functions are removed, analogous to the process described for canonical correlation.

> **TIP:** *A significant Wilks' lambda does not necessarily imply successful classification. With a large sample, minor group differences can result in a significant Wilks' lambda without resulting in good discrimination among groups.*

Assumptions underlying the use of discriminant analysis are the same as for MANOVA. Multivariate normality is assumed, but this assumption is usually robust to violation when there are more than 20 cases in the smallest group. Discriminant analysis also assumes a linear relationship among all pairs of predictors within each group, as well as homogeneity of the variance–covariance matrix. When the sample size is large and groups are of approximately equal size, the homogeneity assumption is fairly robust.

STRATEGIES FOR ENTERING PREDICTORS IN DISCRIMINANT ANALYSIS   Standard discriminant analysis involves the direct entry of all predictors as a block, analogous to simultaneous multiple regression. Discriminant analysis can also be performed hierarchically—that is, researchers can specify the order of entry of the predictor variables, either for theoretical reasons or to control confounding variables.

Discriminant analysis can also be performed in an exploratory stepwise fashion, whereby variables are stepped into the discriminant function in the order in which they meet certain statistical criteria. Various statistical criteria can be used in entering predictors in a stepwise analysis. One criterion is the minimization of Wilks' lambda, whereby the variable that results in the smallest Wilks' lambda is selected for entry at each step. Another criterion is the **Mahalanobis distance (D^2),** a generalized measure of the distance between groups. The results are often the same regardless of which criterion is used.

Example of discriminant analysis:

Elliott, Horgas, and Marsiske (2008) used discriminant analysis to explore whether mild cognitive impairment (MCI), an indicator of early cognitive changes in the elderly, could be identified using fairly simple screening tools. A team of clinicians classified a sample of 130 elderly participants into one of three groups: cognitively intact, MCI, or probable dementia. Participants completed a series of cognitive tests, a demographic form, and a depression scale and scores were used to "predict" group membership. Overall, 95% of the participants were correctly classified. The first discriminant function differentiated those who were cognitively intact from those who were not (MCI and impaired), while the second one differentiated the MCI cases from all others. High loadings on the first function were found for tests of more generalized cognitive function. Loadings on the second function were high primarily on memory measures, indicating the disproportionate memory loss associated with MCI.

RESEARCH APPLICATIONS OF MULTIVARIATE GLM ANALYSES

The multivariate statistical procedures discussed in this chapter are used primarily to test research hypotheses and to address research questions—although discriminant analysis can be used in pragmatic applications when classification is desired. Many research questions lend themselves, in particular, to ANCOVA, MANOVA, and mixed-design RM-ANOVA. The remainder of this section discusses the presentation of results from these techniques.

The Presentation of ANCOVA in Research Reports

ANCOVA results are presented in much the same fashion as ANOVA results. When there is a single one-way ANCOVA to report, it may be efficient to simply describe the results in the text. As an example of a narrative presentation, here is how the ANCOVA results from Figure 11.4 might be reported:

> The posttreatment pain scores for the three treatment groups were analyzed using ANCOVA, with pretreatment pain scores as the covariate. After controlling for initial levels of pain, group differences in posttreatment pain scores were highly significant, $F(2, 26) = 20.08$, $p < .001$. The adjusted group means for the bed rest, exercise, and control groups were 56.5, 44.0, and 59.6, respectively. A multiple comparison procedure with a Bonferroni correction indicated that, net of pretreatment pain, patients in the exercise group experienced significantly less posttreatment pain than those in either the bedrest or the control group ($p < .05$). Posttreatment pain scores of the bedrest and control groups were not significantly different from each other.

TABLE 11.5 Example of an ANCOVA Results Table

Treatment Group	Adjusted Mean[a] (SE)	95% CI	Partial Eta^2
Bedrest Group (N = 10)	56.48 (1.83)	52.72, 60.25	.05[b]
Exercise Group (N = 10)	43.95 (1.84)	40.18, 47.73	.58[b]
Control Group (N = 10)	59.56 (1.84)	55.78, 63.35	—

[a]Means were adjusted for pre-intervention pain scores.

[b]Group effect, net of pre-treatment pain scores.

$F(2, 26)$ for groups = 20.08, $p < .001$.

Analysis of Covariance Results for Postintervention Pain Scores, Controlling for Preintervention Pain in Three Treatment Groups.

On the other hand, even with a single dependent variable, a table might be desirable if it is considered important to report other aspects of the analysis. For example, when the relationship between individual covariates and the dependent variable is of substantive interest, an ANCOVA summary table might be needed. A summary table would be similar to Panel B of Figure 11.4, showing mean squares for all sources of variation, together with all F tests.

In other cases, it might be important (or necessary, depending on the journal) to show 95% CIs or effect sizes. Table 11.5 illustrates another presentation that includes information about adjusted means, 95% CIs, partial eta-squared, and ANCOVA results. This table could be adapted for multiple ANCOVAs (i.e., multiple dependent variables) by including extra rows, and separate footnotes to show F and p value for each ANCOVA.

If it is important to show changes over two points in time, a table could be constructed to show pretest and posttest means, as in the example in Table 11.6. This table shows ANCOVAs for two different dependent variables (the second one was invented for illustrative purposes). In this table, the far-right columns show the ANCOVA F values and associated ps. If there were only one dependent variable, this information could be included as a footnote.

TABLE 11.6 Example of an ANCOVA Results Table with Unadjusted Pretest and Posttest Means

Outcome and Time of Measurement	Bedrest (n = 10) Mean (SD)	Exercise (n = 10) Mean (SD)	Control (n = 10) Mean (SD)	ANCOVA* F (2, 26)	p
Pain Scores					
Pretreatment	67.5 (20.2)	69.5 (14.2)	62.5 (22.6)		
Posttreatment	57.5 (20.2)	47.0 (18.6)	55.5 (22.4)	20.08	< .001
Anxiety Scores					
Pretreatment	15.3 (4.2)	15.8 (4.3)	15.6 (4.1)		
Posttreatment	16.7 (3.5)	14.8 (3.0)	16.0 (3.9)	3.30	.051

*ANCOVA results are for group differences on posttreatment scores, controlling pre-treatment scores on the same outcome.

Pretreatment/Posttreatment Means on Pain and Anxiety Scores for Three Treatment Groups, with ANCOVA Results.

TABLE 11.7 Example of a MANCOVA Results Table with Adjusted Means

Outcome Variable	Bedrest ($n = 10$) Mean[a] (SE)	Exercise ($n = 10$) Mean[a] (SE)	Control ($n = 10$) Mean[a] (SE)	Significance Tests	
				F (df)	p
Pain Scores	56.5 (1.8)	44.0 (1.8)	59.6 (1.8)	20.08 (2,26)[b]	<.001
Number of Medications	6.5 (0.6)	4.3 (0.6)	6.6 (0.6)	5.36 (2,26)[b]	.011
MANCOVA Test, Wilks' Lambda = .38				7.79 (4, 50)	<.001

[a]Means have been adjusted for pretreatment pain scores.

[b]Multiple comparison tests on adjusted means, with Bonferroni correction: Exercise group significantly different from Bedrest and Control groups (both $p < .05$)

Adjusted Posttreatment Means, by Treatment Group, with ANCOVA and MANCOVA Results.

In sum, there are alternative ways to summarize ANCOVA information because in different studies researchers may wish to highlight different information. A table such as our Table 11.6 would be especially attractive if, for example, improvements over time were notable and worthy of discussion. A figure showing mean changes over time for different groups might also be attractive. In other cases, pretest means might be of little interest, in which case adjusted means might be relevant. Also, if the covariate is not a pretest measure of the outcome, but is a control variable (e.g., participants' age), group means adjusted for the covariate would be appropriate.

The Presentation of MANOVA and MANCOVA in Research Reports

MANOVA and MANCOVA results are usually displayed in tables similar to those for ANCOVA. As with ANCOVA, the level of detail and the manner of presenting descriptive information such as means or adjusted means depends on the nature of the questions being asked, the pattern of results, and journal requirements.

Typically, results are shown for both univariate tests and for multivariate tests. Table 11.7 illustrates one such presentation, using data from our MANCOVA analysis of posttreatment pain scores and medications. This table shows the mean adjusted posttreatment scores on the two dependent variables, with associated univariate tests. These values were taken from the SPSS output shown in Panel C of Figure 11.6. MANCOVA test results (from Panel B of Figure 11.6) are then presented. We opted to report the value of Wilk's lambda, but another statistic such as Pillai's trace could also have been reported. We included the results of multiple comparisons tests in a footnote. The note indicates which multiple comparison procedure was used (Bonferroni), which adjusted group means were significantly different from others, and what the level of significance was.

Note that post hoc tests for analyses described in this chapter are typically reported either in the text or in a footnote to a table, as in this example. If a complex pattern of results for post hoc tests occurs, however—for example, the pattern of group differences varies from one outcome variable to another—then a separate table might be advantageous.

TABLE 11.8 Example of an RM-ANOVA Results Table[†]

Plasma Glucose/ Serum Lipid Levels (in mg/dL)	Means (*SD*)			F (*p*)		
	Baseline	3 Months	6 Months	Group	Time	G × T
Fasting Plasma Glucose				0.45 (.51)	0.48 (.62)	3.69 (.03)
Intervention Group*	156.2 (25.8)	145.5 (35.3)	151.6 (42.6)			
Control Group*	138.9 (25.0)	143.1 (34.1)	144.9 (35.7)			
2-hr Postmeal Glucose				1.58 (.23)	4.86 (.01)	12.49 (<.001)
Intervention Group	272.6 (86.2)	152.5 (64.3)	213.7 (52.8)			
Control Group	209.4 (75.3)	240.9 (78.7)	227.9 (67.1)			
Total Cholesterol				4.23 (.05)	0.64 (.51)	3.72 (.04)
Intervention Group	181.0 (27.2)	170.8 (28.7)	175.9 (22.3)			
Control Group	180.5 (21.7)	187.3 (28.9)	190.4 (28.6)			
HDL Cholesterol				0.09 (.77)	0.74 (.47)	2.59 (.09)
Intervention Group	44.4 (7.3)	47.3 (7.5)	47.3 (8.5)			
Control Group	43.3 (9.7)	43.7 (11.2)	43.3 (10.1)			

*Intervention Group $n = 18$; Control Group $n = 16$.
[†]Adapted from Tables 2 and 3 of Kim and Song (2008).

Repeated Measures ANOVA: Mean Plasma Glucose and Serum Lipid Levels Over Time, by Treatment Group.

The Presentation of Mixed-Design RM-ANOVA in Research Reports

As with other types of analyses described in this chapter, researchers have several options for summarizing their RM-ANOVA results in tables. Repeated measures analyses are particularly complex and can lead to cumbersome tables because there are two dimensions (time and a between-subjects factor), resulting in several statistical tests for each dependent variable. If there are more than three time periods, the sheer mass of numerical information can be daunting, so care must be taken to feature key patterns.

Table 11.8, which illustrates one type of presentation, will be more fully discussed in the research example in the next section. We see that this table shows the means and standard deviations for several plasma glucose and serum lipid level measures at three points in time (at baseline, 3 months, and 6 months), for both an experimental and control group of participants. The last three columns of the table show statistical test results contrasting means for groups, time periods, and group × time interactions. Thus, this table efficiently summarizes key results.

Graphs are especially suitable for displaying multiple group means for an outcome over multiple time periods. The graph shown in Panel H of Figure 11.7, for example, communicates quickly and directly the pattern of findings for mean pain scores at three points in time—although, of course, the figure does not tell the whole story because we cannot tell from this figure whether differences in means are statistically significant.

Research Example

This concluding section summarizes a study that used a mixed-design repeated measures analysis of variance.

Study: "Technological intervention for obese patients with type 2 diabetes" (Kim and Song, 2008).

Study Purpose: The purpose of this study was to test the effectiveness of a 6-month nursing intervention—a short message intervention via cell phones and the Internet—on levels of plasma glucose and serum lipids in obese Korean patients with type 2 diabetes.

Methods: A sample of 40 patients from the endocrinology department of a tertiary care hospital was recruited into the study and randomly assigned to an intervention or control group; 34 patients (18 in the intervention group and 16 in the control group) completed the study. Patients in the intervention group got weekly personalized messages via cell phone and Internet that reflected clinicians' recommendations based on the patients' daily self-checked blood glucose levels, which they transmitted to researchers on a project Web site. Researchers obtained measures of plasma glucose and serum lipids at baseline, 3 months, and 6 months.

Analysis: Repeated measures ANOVA was used to assess differences between the two groups over time on key indicators of plasma glucose (levels of HbA_{1c}, fasting plasma glucose, and 2-hour postmeal glucose) and serum lipids (total cholesterol, high density lipoprotein [HDL] cholesterol, and triglycerides). When a significant interaction was found, paired t tests with Bonferroni correction were used to pinpoint specific differences.

Results: Table 11.8 highlights selected results from the RM-ANOVA analyses. Although there were a few significant main effects for group (e.g., total cholesterol) and time (e.g., 2-hour postmeal glucose), the primary focus of the analyses were on the group × time interactions. These interactions tested whether plasma glucose and serum lipid levels had improved over time to a greater extent among those exposed to the intervention. As Table 11.8 shows, the interactions were significant for fasting plasma glucose, 2-hour postmeal glucose, and total cholesterol, but not for HDL cholesterol. Post hoc analyses indicated significant improvements over time for patients in the intervention group but not for those in the control group. In most cases, significant improvements were found at both the 3-month and the 6-month period.

Summary Points

- The **general linear model (GLM)** includes a broad class of statistical techniques often used in nursing research. The GLM allows tremendous diversity, including various options for calculating sums of squares. **Type III sums of squares** is typically the default in GLM analyses.
- **Analysis of covariance** (**ANCOVA**), a procedure within the GLM, tests differences in group means after statistically controlling for one or more **covariate.** ANCOVA is especially appropriate in randomized designs, but is often used to enhance internal validity in quasiexperimental or case-control studies.
- In ANCOVA, variability associated with confounding variables (or a pretest measures of the dependent variable) is removed in a first step, and then group differences in what remains of the variability in the dependent variable are analyzed.

F tests are used to test the significance of both covariates and independent variables.

- ANCOVA yields estimated **adjusted means** of the groups, i.e., the group means on the outcomes, net of the effect of the covariates.
- ANCOVA's assumptions are similar to other previously described procedures, but also include the assumption of **homogeneity of regression across groups** (parallel regression slopes for groups being compared).
- Effect size in ANCOVA can be estimated through **partial eta-squared.**
- **Multivariate analysis of variance** (**MANOVA**) is used to test differences in group means for two or more dependent variables simultaneously. In MANOVA, the dependent variables are linearly combined into a new composite variable whose variance is partitioned into different sources, much as in ANOVA.

- The two most widely used statistical tests for MANOVA are **Wilks' lambda (λ)** and **Pillai's trace** criterion, both of which can be transformed to an F distribution for significance testing. Wilks' lambda is a measure of the proportion of variance in the composite dependent variable that is *not* accounted for by the independent variables.
- A **stepdown analysis** is one method of evaluating the contribution of individual dependent variables to an overall significant MANOVA.
- When covariates are used in MANOVA, the analysis is called **multivariate analysis of covariance (MANCOVA)**.
- An important assumption for both MANOVA and MANCOVA is **homogeneity of the variance–covariance matrix.** The **Box M test** is used to evaluate violations of this assumption.
- **Mixed-design RM-ANOVA** is used to test mean differences between groups (the between-subjects factor) over time (the within-subjects factor).
- Assumptions for mixed-design RM-ANOVA include *compound symmetry* and the related assumption of *sphericity*, which are usually tested with **Mauchly's test for sphericity**.
- If the sphericity assumption is violated, a correction factor (**epsilon**) is usually applied to adjust the risk of a Type I error. Formulas for epsilon include the **Greenhouse-Geisser** and the **Huynh-Feldt** corrections, which are used to adjust degrees of freedom for the F test on the within-subjects factor. The alternative to a correction is to use MANOVA.
- **Canonical analysis** is used to study relationships between two sets of variables, each of which has at least two variables. In canonical analysis, linear composites (**canonical variates**) are formed, one for each of the two sets. Each pair of canonical variates yields a separate **canonical correlation (R_c)** that corresponds to a dimension of the relationship between the two sets. The dimension can be interpreted by examining the **structure coefficients** (or *loadings*) of the original variables on a canonical variate. Wilks' lambda is used to evaluate whether the R_cs are significantly different from zero.
- **Discriminant analysis** is used to predict a categorical dependent variable on the basis of several predictor variables. Discriminant analysis forms linear combinations of the predictors (**discriminant functions**) to predict group membership. **Discriminant (D) scores**, can be used to classify cases into groups. Predicted and actual classifications can be compared to evaluate the adequacy of the discriminant model. Structure coefficients indicate the correlation between the predictors and discriminant scores. The test of the null hypothesis that the discriminant functions reflect chance sampling fluctuations is usually based on Wilks' lambda.

Exercises

The following exercises cover concepts presented in this chapter. Appendix C provides answers to Part A exercises that are indicated with a dagger (†). Exercises in Part B involve computer analyses using the datasets provided with this textbook, and answers and comments are offered on this book's Web site.

PART A EXERCISES

† **A1.** Indicate which statistical procedure discussed in this chapter would most likely be used in the following circumstances:
   (a) Independent variables: age, length of time in nursing home, gender, marital status, number of kin living in 25-mile radius; dependent variables: functional ability, fatigue.
   (b) Independent variables: type of stimuli used with infants (visual, auditory, tactile), gender; dependent variables: postintervention heart rate, amount of crying; covariate: baseline heart rate.
   (c) Independent variable: presence versus absence of boomerang pillows; dependent variable: respiratory capacity before treatment and 1 and 2 days after treatment.
   (d) Independent variable: receipt versus nonreceipt of an intervention to facilitate coping with unexpected hospitalization; dependent variables: scores on a coping scale, an anxiety scale, and a fear of hospitals scale.
   (e) Independent variables: age, cognitive status, length of time in nursing home, sex; dependent variable: had a fall versus did not have a fall in the past 12 months.
   (f) Independent variable: Mediterranean diet versus regular (no special) diet; dependent variable: total cholesterol; covariate: body mass index at baseline.

A2. Suppose you were interested in studying the effect of a person's early retirement (at or below age 62 versus at age 65 or later) on indicators of physical and emotional health. What variables would you suggest using as covariates to enhance the comparability of the groups?

† **A3.** Use the following information to compute unadjusted and adjusted group means on patient satisfaction scale scores:

Grand Mean = 20.521

| | Unadjusted | |
Deviation	Deviation	Adjusted
No insurance	−2.56	−3.89
Private insurance	3.81	4.97
Public health insurance	−1.65	−2.47

† **A4.** Following are some means from a randomized controlled trial. Indicate at least two ways to analyze the data to test for treatment effects.

	Experimental Group	Control Group
Baseline score	53.88	52.99
Postintervention score	65.23	57.47

A5. Using data from Table 11.8, make a graph displaying group differences over time for one of the outcomes in the Kim and Song study.

PART B EXERCISES

† **B1.** You will be using the SPSS dataset Polit2SetC to do various analyses. For the first analysis (ANCOVA), you will be testing for racial/ethnic differences (*racethn*) in physical health scores (*sf12phys*), controlling for total household income (*income*). Begin by testing the assumption of homogeneity of regression across the three racial/ethnic groups (African American, Hispanic, and white/other). Select Analyze ➜ General Linear Model ➜ Univariate. In the opening dialog box, move the variable *sf12phys* into the slot for Dependent Variable; move *racethn* into the slot for Fixed Factors; and move *income* into the slot for Covariates. Click the Model pushbutton, which will have as the default the full factorial model. Click Custom and then on the left highlight both *racethn* and *income* in the Factors and Covariates box. Make sure that in the "Build Terms" section, the Type is set to Interaction, and then click the right arrow to move the interaction (*income* * *racethn*) into the Model box. Click Continue to return to the main dialog box and then click the Options pushbutton. Select Homogeneity tests as the option for Display. Then click Continue, and OK to run the analysis. Use the output to answer these questions: (a) What can you conclude from Levene's test about the homogeneity of error variance of physical health scores across the three groups? (b) Is the interaction between race/ethnicity and income significant? What does this suggest about the homogeneity of regression assumption?

† **B2.** Now we can proceed with the ANCOVA analysis described in Exercise B1. Open the GLM Univariate dialog box again, which should already have the necessary variable information (unless you run Exercise B1 and B2 on different days).

Click the Model pushbutton, select Full factorial model, then click Continue to return to the main dialog box. Click the Options pushbutton and in the top panel (Estimated marginal means), select *racethn* and use the right arrow to move it into the box labeled "Display means for:" Now click "Compare main effects" to generate multiple pairwise comparisons, and below that select the Bonferroni adjustment from the pull-down menu. At the bottom (under Display), select Descriptive statistics and Estimates of effect size. Then click Continue and OK to run the analysis. Use the output to answer these questions: (a) Before any adjustments for the covariate, what is the range of group means? (b) In the full factorial model, was the covariate significantly related to physical health scores? (c) With income controlled, were racial/ethnic differences in physical health significant? (d) Compare the adjusted group means with the unadjusted group means. What happened as a result of the adjustment? Why do you think this happened? (e) What do the pairwise comparisons indicate? Was this analysis necessary?

† **B3.** For this exercise, you will use MANOVA to test the hypothesis that there are racial/ethnic differences in scores on the SF-12, using scores from both the physical health component (*sf12phys*) and mental health component (*sf12ment*) as the dependent variables and *racethn* as the independent variable. Open the main dialog box through Analyze ➜ General Linear Model ➜ Multivariate. Move the two SF-12 variables into the box for Dependent Variables and *racethn* into the box for Fixed Factor. Click the Post Hoc pushbutton and make sure that *racethn* is in the box "Post hoc tests for:" Select Bonferroni, then click Continue. On the main dialog box click the Options pushbutton. From the list of Display options, select Descriptives, Estimates of effect size, Parameter estimates, and Homogeneity tests. Then click Continue and OK to run the analysis. Answer the following questions based on the output: (a) Is the assumption of homogeneous variance–covariance matrices violated? (b) Is the overall multivariate test for differences in racial/ethnic group means statistically significant? (c) Can we accept the assumption of homogeneous variances for this analysis? (d) In the panels for univariate results, were group differences statistically significant? (e) If overall group differences were significant, which groups were significantly different from other groups, and what was the nature of the differences?

B4. Re-run the analysis in exercise B3 as a MANCOVA by selecting a covariate from the data set. Was the covariate a significant predictor of the SF-12 scores? Did including the covariate in the analysis alter the relationship between *racethn* and SF-12 scores?

† **B5.** In this exercise, we will test racial/ethnic differences in depression over time, using CES-D scores from the two waves of interviews with a subsample of these women. You will need to begin by excluding women in the white/other group because there were too few of them in this small

subsample to permit their inclusion. Go to Data ➔ Select Cases and click Select "If condition is satisfied" in the opening dialog box. Click the If pushbutton, and then type the following into the box to exclude whites/others, who are coded 3: "racethn NE 3." Click Continue, then OK to restrict the analysis to African-American and Hispanic women. Now run the main analysis, using Analyze ➔ General Linear Model ➔ Repeated. You will first be asked to give the within-subjects factor a name. We used "Wave" to designate Wave 1 or Wave 2 measurement of depression. The number of levels to enter, in the next box, is 2 (i.e., two waves). Click Add then go to the bottom, where you can name the dependent variable in a slot labeled Measure Name. Enter Depression, then click Add. Now click the Define pushbutton, which brings up a dialog box for defining variables. Select *cesdwav1* and click the right arrow to move this variable into the list as the first Within-Subjects Variable. Then select *cesd* (Wave 2 scores) and move it into the list as the second Within-Subjects Variable. Next, move *racethn* into the slot for the Between-Subjects Factor. Now click the pushbutton Plots and in the dialog box that appears move *wave* into the Horizontal Axis box and *racethn* into the Separate Lines box. Click Add, then Continue. Back on the original dialog box, click Options and at the bottom of the next dialog box select the following Display options: Descriptives, Estimates of effect size, and Homogeneity tests. After clicking Continue and OK to run the analysis, answer the following questions: (a) What are the null hypotheses in this analysis? (b) How many women were in this analysis, by race? (c) Was the assumption of homogeneity of the variance–covariance matrix upheld? What are the implications for this analysis? (d) Was the assumption of sphericity upheld? What are the implications for this analysis? (e) Was the assumption of homogeneity of variances upheld? What are the implications for this analysis? (f) What are the results for the null hypotheses being tested in this RM-ANOVA, as identified in question a? (g) Should post hoc tests be run for this analysis? Why or why not? (h) What does the profile plot tell us about changes over time?

B6. Using output from one of the previous three exercises (B3 through B5), create a table to summarize key results of the analyses. Then write a paragraph summarizing the findings.

CHAPTER

12

Logistic Regression

Logistic regression (sometimes called *logit analysis*) is similar to multiple linear regression in that it analyzes the relationship between multiple independent variables and a single dependent variable, and yields a predictive equation. Logistic regression, however, is used when the dependent variable is categorical and so is similar to discriminant analysis (Chapter 11). Logistic regression, however, is based on an estimation procedure that has less restrictive assumptions than techniques based on the general linear model (GLM), and is usually preferred to discriminant analysis. Indeed, logistic regression is one of the more widely used types of statistical analysis among nurse researchers.

TIP: *Not all SPSS systems include a logistic regression program. The SPSS add-on Regression module, which includes logistic regression, must be separately purchased. Check in the Analyze ➔ Regression menu to see if there is an option called Binary Logistic Regression.*

BASIC CONCEPTS FOR LOGISTIC REGRESSION

This section provides an overview of some basic concepts that are important to understanding logistic regression. Computations are kept to a minimum, but a few are shown to communicate how logistic regression works. Later sections describe tests of statistical inference associated with logistic regression, as well as assumptions and requirements for this method of analysis.

Maximum Likelihood Estimation

Multiple regression (and most other statistical techniques we have discussed thus far) estimates parameters using a least-squares criterion. As discussed in Chapter 10, the unknown parameters, such as the intercept constant and regression coefficients, are estimated by minimizing the sum of the squared deviations between the data and the linear model.

In logistic regression, estimation of parameters is based on **maximum likelihood estimation (MLE),** a major alternative to least squares estimation. Maximum likelihood estimators are ones that estimate the parameters that are most likely to have generated the observed data. Maximum likelihood estimation can be used in several multivariate statistical techniques, including factor analysis, which is discussed in Chapter 13.

Least squares regression is a closed-form solution, which means that it is does not arrive at a solution in a series of iterations. Maximum likelihood estimation, by contrast, has to be solved by an iterative procedure that starts with an initial estimate of what the parameters are likely to be.

The MLE algorithm then determines the direction and size of the change in the logit coefficients that meet certain statistical criteria. The goal of MLE is to find the best combination of predictors to maximize the likelihood of obtaining the observed frequencies on the outcome variable. After the initial estimate, the residuals are tested and a re-estimate is made with an improved function. The process is repeated, typically about three to five times, until *convergence* is reached, that is, until the change in the statistical criterion is no longer significant.

> **TIP:** *An excellent primer on maximum likelihood estimation is available on the following Web site: http://statgen.iop.kcl.ac.uk/bgim/mle/sslike_1.html.*

Logistic Regression Models

Logistic regression develops models for estimating the probability that an event occurs. For example, we might be interested in modeling the factors that affect the probability of being HIV positive; or the probability of a woman practicing breast self-examination; or the probability of death occurring while in an intensive care unit. Logistic regression is most often used to predict dichotomous outcomes such as these, and in such situations is sometimes called **binary** (or *binomial*) **logistic regression.** Logistic regression can also be used to model dependent variables that have more than two categories, such as a prediction of whether a pregnancy would end in a miscarriage, stillbirth, preterm birth, or full-term birth. When there are multiple categories in the dependent variable, researchers use **multinomial logistic regression.** This chapter focuses on binary logistic regression.

In Chapter 10, we illustrated multiple regression with an example in which we predicted the grade point average (GPA) of nursing students in a graduate program, using undergraduate GPA, verbal and quantitative GRE scores, and scores on an achievement motivation scale as predictors. In the previous chapter, we modified this example to illustrate discriminant analysis, using the same predictor variables to predict a dichotomous outcome: completion versus noncompletion of graduate school. We will use the dichotomous graduate school outcome again as an example of logistic regression, but we will make a change to the motivation scores so that we can better illustrate some features of logistic regression. Instead of using the original motivation scores, we will substitute a dummy code to signify high motivation: Students with a

TABLE 12.1 Fictitious Data for Logistic Regression Analysis Predicting Graduate School Completion

	Independent (Predictor) Variables				Dependent Variable
Student	Undergrad GPA X_1	GRE Verbal X_2	GRE Quantitative X_3	High Motivation* X_4	Completion Status** Y
1	3.4	600	540	1	1
2	3.1	510	480	0	1
3	3.7	650	710	1	1
4	3.2	530	450	0	0
5	3.5	610	500	1	1
6	2.9	540	620	0	0
7	3.3	530	510	1	1
8	2.9	540	600	0	0
9	3.4	550	580	1	0
10	3.2	700	630	0	1
11	3.7	630	700	1	1
12	3.0	480	490	1	1
13	3.1	530	520	0	0
14	3.7	580	610	0	1
15	3.9	710	660	1	1
16	3.5	500	480	1	1
17	3.1	490	510	0	0
18	2.9	560	540	0	0
19	3.2	550	590	0	0
20	3.6	600	550	0	1

*High motivation is coded 1 for high motivation, and 0 for low motivation.

**Completion status is coded 1 for completion of graduate program, and 0 for noncompletion.

score over 70 are coded 1 (highly motivated) and students with a score of 70 and below are coded 0 (not highly motivated). Table 12.1 presents the data for the logistic regression example.

Logistic regression converts the probability that an outcome will occur (e.g., the probability of completing the graduate program) into its odds. You may recall from Chapter 4 that the *odds* of an event are defined as the ratio of two probabilities: The probability of an event occurring to the probability that it will not occur. For example, if 40% of all entering graduate students completed the program, the odds would be as follows:

$$\text{Odds}_{\text{Completing}} = \frac{\text{Prob (Completing)}}{\text{Prob (Not completing)}} = \frac{.40}{.60} = .667$$

In a logistic regression analysis, the dependent variable is transformed to be the natural log of the odds, which is called a **logit** (short for *log*istic probability un*it*). As a result of the transformation, the dependent variable ranges from minus to plus infinity. Maximum likelihood is then used to estimate the coefficients associated with the independent variables, with the logit as a continuous dependent variable.

The logistic regression model can be written as follows:

$$\log \left[\frac{\text{Prob (event)}}{\text{Prob (no event)}} \right] = b_0 + b_1 X_1 + \ldots b_k X_k$$

where b_0 = constant
k = number of independent (predictor) variables
b_1 to b_k = coefficients estimated from the data
X_1 to X_k = values of the k predictor variables

In other words, the logit (log of the odds) is predicted from a weighted combination of the independent variables, plus a constant. In our graduate school example, the logistic regression equation, which we obtained through SPSS, is as follows:

$$\log \left[\frac{\text{Prob (completing)}}{\text{Prob (not completing)}} \right] = -19.260 + 4.603 X_1 + .028 X_2 - .022 X_3 + 2.336 X_4$$

The right-hand side of the logistic regression equation essentially takes the same form as the equation for multiple regression. The dependent variable (logit) is predicted as a combination of a constant, plus unstandardized regression coefficients that are used to weight each predictor variable. The interpretation, however, is different than in multiple regression because we are no longer predicting actual values of the dependent variable. In logistic regression, a b coefficient can be interpreted as the change in the log odds associated with a one-unit change in the associated independent variable. For example, a b of 2.336 for X_4 (high motivation) means that when the variable changes from 0 to 1 (from not highly motivated to highly motivated), the log odds of completing graduate school increases by 2.336. A b of 4.603 for X_1 (undergraduate grades) means that when grade point average increases by one point (e.g., from 2.0 to 3.0), the log odds of completing the program increases by 4.603.

The Odds Ratio in Logistic Regression

It is difficult to comprehend what the logistic regression equation means because we are not accustomed to thinking in terms of log odds. However, we can transform the logistic equation so that the left-hand expression is the odds rather than the log odds, as follows:

$$\frac{\text{Prob (event)}}{\text{Prob (no event)}} = e^{b_0 + b_1 X_1 + \ldots + b_k X_k}$$

where e = the base of natural logarithms (approximately 2.7183)

Written to solve for the odds, the equation tells us that e raised to the power of, for example, b_4, is the factor by which the odds change when X_4 increases by one unit, after controlling for all other variables in the model. When the coefficient is positive, the odds increase, and when the coefficient is negative, the odds decrease. In our example, when X_4 (high motivation) changes from 0 to 1 and all other predictors are the same, the odds of completing the graduate program are increased by a factor of about 10.0 ($e^{2.336} = 10.337$).

The factor by which the odds change is the *odds ratio* (OR), a concept we introduced in Chapter 4. To fully convey what the OR represents in the context of logistic regression, we must present the logistic regression equation in yet another form, this time solving for the probability of an event, as follows:

$$\text{Prob (event)} = \frac{e^{b_0 + b_1 X_1 + \ldots + b_k X_k}}{1 + e^{b_0 + b_1 X_1 + \ldots + b_k X_k}}$$

Written in this fashion, we can use the logistic equation to estimate the probability that a particular student will complete the graduate program. To illustrate, suppose we had a highly motivated student ($X_4 = 1$) with an undergraduate grade point average of 3.0 and scores of 600 for both verbal GRE and quantitative GRE. Using the coefficients we presented earlier, the probability of this particular student completing the graduate program would be as follows:

$$\text{Prob (completing)} = \frac{e^{(-19.260) + (4.603)(3.0) + (.028)(600) - (.022)(600) + (2.336)(1)}}{1 + e^{(-19.260) + (4.603)(3.0) + (.028)(600) - (.022)(600) + (2.336)(1)}}$$

$$\text{Prob (completing)} = 0.6893$$

The estimated probability that this student will complete the program is, thus, .6893 and the estimated probability of *not* completing it is .3107 (i.e., $1 - .6893 = .3107$). The *odds* of completion for this student are then estimated as 2.2185 (i.e., $.6893 \div .3107 = 2.2185$).

Suppose now that this same student had been classified as *not* highly motivated ($X_4 = 0$), but that all other independent variables stayed the same. Inserting 0 instead of 1 for X_4 in the previous formula, we would now estimate that the student's probability of completing is .1767, and the probability of not completing is .8233. If the student were not highly motivated, the *odds* of completion are $.1767 \div .8233 = .2146$. We can now calculate the *odds ratio* for the motivation predictor as follows:

$$\text{Odds ratio}_{X_4} = \frac{\text{odds}_{\text{If Motivated}}}{\text{odds}_{\text{If Not Motivated}}} = \frac{2.2185}{.2146} = 10.337$$

By changing the value of motivation from 1 to 0 with all else constant, the odds change from 2.2185 to .2146, and the odds ratio changes by a factor of 10.337. This is the same value we obtained earlier by raising e to the power of 2.336, the value of the logistic coefficient for the motivation variable X_4. The OR provides an estimate of the risk of the event occurring given one condition, versus the risk of it occurring given a different condition. In our example, we would estimate that the odds of finishing graduate school are about 10 times greater if a student is highly motivated than if he or she is not, with other variables controlled. (Sometimes odds ratios from multiple logistic regression are called *adjusted odds ratios* because they represent the odds ratios after controlling other factors.)

TIP: *Logistic regression programs can be used to compute odds ratios when there is only one predictor, similar to simple regression as described in Chapter 9. (In SPSS, it may be recalled, the Crosstabs procedure can also be used to calculate ORs.) Results from simple least-squares regression are rarely reported in the literature, but ORs from simple logistic regression are often reported. When more than one predictor is used in binary logistic regression, the analysis is sometimes called* multiple *logistic regression, analogous to multiple regression using least-squares estimation.*

Classification in Logistic Regression

As in discriminant analysis, logistic regression can be used to classify cases within categories of the dependent variable, thereby providing a mechanism for evaluating the predictive success of the model. For the purposes of classification, each person's **predicted probability** is computed based on the logistic regression equation, as we illustrated in the previous section. By default, if Prob (event) is greater than .50, the case is classified as a positive case. In the example we just worked through, the motivated student with the specified GRE scores and undergraduate GPA would be classified as completing the graduate program (probability = .689) but the unmotivated student would be classified as a noncompleter (probability = .177).

Classification information for the 20 students whose data are shown in Table 12.1 is presented in Table 12.2. This table shows the students' *actual* completion status in the second column. For example, the first student, who completed the graduate school program, has a code of 1 (completed) for actual completion status. This student's predicted classification, shown next, is completed (1), which is correct. The predicted (estimated) probability based on the logistic regression is shown in the next column. The first student's predicted probability of completion is quite high—.98. The asterisks in the column for predicted completion status indicate that there were four misclassifications: Students 2 and 12 actually finished graduate school but were predicted to be noncompleters, while students 4 and 9 failed to complete the program but were predicted to be completers. Overall, 80.0% of the 20 cases were correctly classified.

TABLE 12.2 Predicting Graduate School Completion Through Logistic Regression

Student	Actual Completion Status 1 = Completed 0 = Did not complete	Predicted Status 1 = Completed 0 = Did not complete	Estimated Probability of Completing
1	1	1	.98
2	1	0*	.27
3	1	1	.95
4	0	1*	.66
5	1	1	.99
6	0	0	.02
7	1	1	.90
8	0	0	.02
9	0	1*	.84
10	1	1	.83
11	1	1	.94
12	1	0*	.45
13	0	0	.21
14	1	1	.71
15	1	1	.99
16	1	1	.95
17	0	0	.10
18	0	0	.14
19	0	0	.14
20	1	1	.91

*Misclassification

> **TIP:** *The estimated probabilities shown in the fourth column of Table 12.2 were obtained in SPSS through the Save feature within the logistic regression program. When you instruct the program to save predicted probabilities (or predicted group membership), the values are added as a new variable to the end of the data file for each participant.*

In some situations, particularly if you have a large sample, it is a good idea to develop the logistic regression model with a random subset of participants. The classification accuracy of the logistic regression equation can then be tested on both the original random subset used to generate the equation, and on the remaining unselected subset for cross-validation purposes. If the percent correctly classified is about the same in the two subsets and is reasonably high, greater confidence can be placed in classifying other people from the same population.

We illustrate this approach using data that will be used throughout this chapter. In this example, we will predict whether a woman has had a tubal ligation (coded 1 for *yes* and 0 for *no*). The four predictors include the woman's age, number of live births, educational attainment, and whether or not any of her children have any type of disability. In the full sample, there were 3,960 women. We selected a random subset of 2,500 women for building the logistic regression model. Classification of the remaining (unselected) subset was then tested.

Classification results are shown in Figure 12.1. With the original random subset of 2,363 cases with complete data (the selected cases), 255 women who actually had a tubal ligation (52.3%) were classified as having one, and 1,265 women who did not have a tubal ligation (67.5%) were classified as not having one. The overall rate of successful classification was 64.3%, which is not a particularly strong success rate. Yet, the logistic regression equation was equally successful in classifying the 1,401 unselected cases: 65.2% of unselected cases were correctly classified. We can conclude, at least, that the parameter estimates are stable.

Classification Table[d]

			Predicted					
			Selected Cases[a]			Unselected Cases[b,c]		
			Ever Had Tubal Ligation		Percentage Correct	Ever Had Tubal Ligation		Percentage Correct
Observed			No (0)	Yes (1)		No (0)	Yes (1)	
Step 1	Ever Had Tubal Ligation	No (0)	1265	233	84.4	759	126	85.8
		Yes (1)	610	255	29.5	362	154	29.8
		Overall Percentage			64.3			65.2

[a]Selected cases random subset EQ 1
[b]Unselected cases random subset NE 1
[c]Some of the unselected cases are not classified due to either missing values in the independent variables or categorical variables with values out of the range of the selected cases.
[d]The cut value is .500

FIGURE 12.1   SPSS printout of a classification table for selected and unselected cases in logistic regression: tubal ligation example.

In practical applications, researchers might want to establish a different rule for classifying probabilities if the consequences of making a mistake in one direction are more severe than misclassification in the other direction. For example, a graduate program administrator might be more willing to accept students with a risk of not completing than to reject students who would have successfully finished. In such a situation, a probability value other than .50 can be used for classification. Computer programs such as SPSS allow you to establish classification probabilities. In the example shown in Figure 12.1, footnote d indicates that the cut value on the predicted probabilities was .500, but different cut values can be established.

TIP: *In SPSS, you can request a classification plot that generates a histogram of estimated probabilities. Predicted probability of the dependent variable is plotted on the horizontal (X) axis, ranging from .00 to 1.00. Frequency of cases with the predicted probability is plotted on the vertical (Y) axis. The ideal plot is essentially U shaped, with high frequencies for the two categories of the dependent variable clustering at their respective ends of the plot. The histogram is sometimes useful for making decisions about whether a probability value other than .50 would be better in classifying cases.*

Example of classification in logistic regression:

Shishani (2008) used logistic regression to predict the need of chronically ill adults for education on self-medication. Need for education was predicted on the basis of patients' knowledge about the benefits and side effects of medications, and knowledge about how to manage side effects. The model was successful in classifying 82% of the patients.

PREDICTOR VARIABLES IN LOGISTIC REGRESSION

As previously indicated, the dependent variable in binary logistic regression is a dichotomous variable. Usually this variable is coded 1 to represent an event (e.g., had a tubal ligation) or the presence of a characteristic (e.g., is hypertensive), and is coded 0 to represent the absence of the event or characteristic (no tubal ligation, no hypertension). Binary logistic regression in SPSS by default predicts the higher of the two code categories of the dependent variable, using the lower one as the reference category.

In this section we focus on options for predictor variables. In brief, predictors can be continuous variables, categorical variables, interaction terms, and combinations of all of these. Although there are no strict limits to the number of predictors that can be included, in practice it is best to achieve a parsimonious model with strong predictive power using a small set of good predictors. A large number of predictors increases the risk of a Type I error and can result in problems with multicollinearity. The selection of predictors for a logistic regression model should be judicious, based on a theoretical framework or a solid foundation of existing evidence.

TIP: *In SPSS, the independent variables (predictors) are entered into a slot called "Covariates."*

Continuous Predictors

As in multiple regression, predictors in logistic regression can be continuous variables—that is, interval- or ratio-level variables or ordinal values that approach interval characteristics. In our example of predicting graduate school completion, GRE scores and undergraduate GPA are continuous variables.

In the tubal ligation example, the woman's age and number of live births are continuous variables. As we shall see in a subsequent section, the odds ratio for number of live births is 1.323. This means that for every additional birth, the odds of having a tubal ligation increased by about 32%, with everything else in the model held constant.

Categorical Predictors

We saw in Chapter 10 that nominal-level variables can be used as predictors in multiple regression, and this is also true in logistic regression. Dummy-coded variables, also called **indicator variables,** are a common method of representing a dichotomous predictor, such as male (1) versus female (0) or smokes cigarettes (1) versus does not smoke cigarettes (0). In our example of predicting whether a woman would opt for a tubal ligation, there is one such dummy variable—whether the woman has any children with a disability (1) or has no children with a disability (0).

In Chapter 10 we described procedures for creating a series of dummy variables for multicategory nominal-level variables such as race/ethnicity or marital status. For example, if there were three marital status groups (e.g., currently married, never married, and previously married), two new variables (the number of categories, minus 1) would have to be created to represent marital status as a predictor in the regression equation. One variable might be currently married or not, and the other might be never married or not. Previously married people in this case would be the reference category. In the SPSS logistic regression program, it is not necessary to create new variables prior to the analysis—the program can do this for you.

In our tubal ligation example, one of the predictors is the woman's educational attainment (*edstat*), which in this dataset is a three-category variable: no high school diploma (1), high school diploma (2), or college degree (3). In SPSS, there are numerous options for setting up contrasts with such multicategory variables. The default is *indicator coding* (dummy coding), using the last category as the reference category. If educational attainment is declared as a categorical variable, the logistic regression program would create two new variables: no diploma (1) versus all others (0), and diploma (1) versus all others (0). These would be named *edstat(1)* and *edstat(2)*, respectively, on some panels of the output. Those with a college degree, the reference group, would be zero on both these new variables. The SPSS output displays these codes and the group sizes, as shown in the first panel of Figure 12.2.

With indicator coding, the coefficients for the new variables represent the effect of each category compared to the reference category. For example, the logistic coefficient for *edstat(1)* represents the change in the log odds for not completing high school compared to having a college degree, and the coefficient for *edstat(2)* is the change in the log odds for having a high school diploma versus having a college degree.

The SPSS logistic regression program will automatically create a series of new variables for any original variable declared as categorical, and several contrast options are available. For example, if you want to compare the effect of each category to the average effect of all categories, you would select *deviation coding* rather than indicator coding. As shown in the second panel of Figure 12.2, deviation contrasts

A **Indicator Coding of Educational Status**

Categorical Variables Codings

			Parameter Coding	
		Frequency	(1)	(2)
Educational Status	No HS diploma	1725	1.000	.000
	HS diploma	1347	.000	1.000
	AA or BA degree	692	.000	.000

B **Deviation Coding of Educational Status**

Categorical Variables Codings

			Parameter Coding	
		Frequency	(1)	(2)
Educational Status	No HS diploma	1725	1.000	.000
	HS diploma	1347	.000	1.000
	AA or BA degree	692	−1.000	−1.000

FIGURE 12.2 SPSS printout of two alternative codings for categorical variables in logistic regression.

involve assigning the code of -1 to the last category for each newly created variable. When deviation coding is used, the logistic coefficients indicate how much better or worse each category is in comparison with average effects for all categories. SPSS offers seven different types of categorical contrast options, but indicator and deviation coding are the ones most often used.

TIP: *In SPSS, there is a separate dialog box for coding categorical variables, accessed through the Categorical pushbutton on the main dialog box. You first identify which variables are categorical, and then indicate whether you want the first or last category to be the reference group, and which type of contrast coding is desired. If you have an original variable in your dataset that is already dummy coded, do not declare it as a categorical variable.*

Interaction Terms

When a variable is entered into a logistic model, the assumption is that the effect of the variable on the outcome is the same for all values of other variables in the model. In our graduate school completion example, the model implies that being highly motivated has the same effect on program completion at all values of GRE scores and undergraduate grades. If this is not the case, there is an interaction. In logistic regression, as in least-squares regression, interaction terms can be added to the model.

For continuous predictors, an interaction term can be created as the product of two existing variables. (In SPSS, this can be achieved in the main dialog box.) For categorical variables, multiplication can be used directly to create an interaction term if the variables in the original dataset were dichotomous dummies. If you use the Define Categorical Variables option to create new variables within the logistic regression program, care is needed in setting up the interaction terms. We strongly recommend further reading on this topic if interaction terms are considered necessary (e.g., Norušis, 2008; Hosmer & Lemeshow, 2000; Tabachnick & Fidell, 2007).

Example of different predictor types in logistic regression:

McInerney and a team of coresearchers (2007) studied factors associated with antituberculosis medication adherence in South Africa. Their final model included continuous variables (e.g., number of days with no food, number of missed clinic appointments) and categorical variables (sex). The researchers also tested the interaction between days without food and missed appointments, and the interaction term was statistically significant: The effect of days without anything to eat on medication adherence was different for those with and without missed clinic appointments.

Entering Predictors in Logistic Regression

As with multiple regression and discriminant analysis, there are alternative methods of entering predictors into the logistic regression equation. In our graduate school example, we used simultaneous (standard) entry of all predictors in one block.

Hierarchical (also called sequential) logistic regression is another important option. In hierarchical logistic regression, researchers specify the order of entry of variables into the model, and can evaluate how much the prediction improves at each step.

Stepwise entry of predictors is also available in logistic regression. Stepwise regression is considered appropriate only for exploratory work because model building relies on statistical rather than theoretical criteria. There are several approaches to doing a stepwise logistic regression, using different statistical criteria to select predictors. Variables can either be entered *into* the model on a step-by-step basis (forward stepwise), or can be removed *from* the model in successive steps (backward stepwise). Forward selection is the usual option, which involves adding variables one at a time in an order that maximizes a statistical criterion. Backward selection starts with all variables and deletes one at a time, in the order they are least desirable according to a statistical criterion.

> **TIP:** *The stepwise variants available in SPSS include forward conditional, forward LR (which stands for likelihood ratio), forward Wald, and three corresponding backward options. The LR options are most often preferred.*

Confirmation of the parameter estimates achieved in stepwise regression is highly desirable, to rule out serendipitous results. Thus, when stepwise methods are used, it is advisable to divide the sample into subsets and run the logistic regression with both subsets to assess whether similar parameter estimates are achieved. If they are, greater confidence can be placed in the logistic regression model. Of course, such a cross-validation strategy requires a large sample.

Example of stepwise entry of predictors:

Mak and colleagues (2008) used logistic regression to predict the incidence of lymphedema among patients with breast cancer who were undergoing axillary lymph dissection. Predictors included clinical, demographic, and lifestyle risk factors. The researchers first identified significant predictors using stepwise logistic regression. Then they re-ran the model using forced entry of several demographic variables (e.g., age, body mass index) to ensure that these variables were statistically adjusted in the final model.

SIGNIFICANCE TESTS IN LOGISTIC REGRESSION

As with most analytic procedures described in this book, logistic regression is most often used to estimate population parameters, not merely to describe a sample. A variety of inferential statistics can be used to evaluate the reliability of different aspects of the logistic regression results.

Tests of the Overall Model and Model Improvements

Researchers want to know whether their overall model is reliable—whether the set of predictors, taken as a whole, are significantly better than chance in predicting the probability of the outcome event. The null hypothesis is that the predictors, as a set, are unrelated to the outcome variable. This is analogous to the null hypothesis in least-squares multiple regression that R^2 is zero.

Assessing the goodness of fit of a logistic regression model can be confusing because there are several different tests, and different authors use different names for the tests. Another potential source of confusion is that some tests indicate goodness of fit by a significant result, and others indicate goodness of fit by a *non*significant result. Two of the more widely used overall tests are discussed in this section.

LIKELIHOOD RATIO TESTS   One basic omnibus test in logistic regression involves comparing the model *with* a set of predictors to a model *without* any predictors. A two-step approach is used, and in the first step (called Block 0 in SPSS) parameters are estimated simply on the basis of how the outcome variable is distributed. Figure 12.3 presents three panels of SPSS output for the *null model* (sometimes called the *constant-only model*) in our example of predicting a woman's decision to have a tubal ligation. In the classification table in Panel B, we see that 1,381 women in this sample had had a tubal ligation and 2,383 had not had one, which means that 36.7% of the sample had had the procedure and 63.3% had not. In the null model, in the absence of any further information, the prediction is that everyone will have the outcome with the highest prevalence— in this case, *not* having a tubal ligation. Thus, this null model is correct 63.3% of the time, because 63.3% of the women had not had a tubal ligation.

Panel C of Figure 12.3 presents the logistic regression equation for the null model, which is of little inherent interest. We can see here, however, that the odds ratio for the null model is .580—the value shown in the cell labeled Exp(B) for exponentiation of the regression coefficient b. We can easily compute the odds ratio in the null model as the odds of having a tubal ligation (1,381 ÷ 3,764 = .3669) divided by the odds of not having a tubal ligation (2,383 ÷ 3,764 = .6331), which is .580, the value shown in the output as Exp(B).

An important index in logistic regression is called the **likelihood index,** which is the probability of the observed results, given the parameters estimated from the analysis. Like any probability, the likelihood index varies from 0 to 1. If the model

Logistic Regression
Block 0: Beginning Block

A   **Iteration History[a,b,c]**

Iteration	−2 Log Likelihood	Coefficients
		Constant
Step 0 1	4948.181	−.532
2	4948.030	−.546

[a]Constant is included in the model.
[b]Initial −2 Log Likelihood: 4948.030
[c]Estimation terminated at iteration number 2 because log-likelihood decreased by less than .010%.

B   **Classification Table[a,b]**

			Predicted		
			Ever Had Tubal Ligation		
	Observed		No (0)	Yes (1)	Percentage Correct
Step 0	Ever Had Tubal Ligation	No (0)	2383	0	100.0
		Yes (1)	1381	0	.0
		Overall Percentage			63.3

[a]Constant is included in the model.
[b]The cut value is .500

C   **Variables in the Equation**

	B	S.E.	Wald	df	Sig.	Exp(B)
Step 0 Constant	−.546	.034	260.200	1	.000	.580

FIGURE 12.3 SPSS printout for the null model (block 0) in logistic regression: tubal ligation example.

fits the data perfectly, the likelihood is 1.00. The likelihood index is almost always a small decimal number, and so it is customary to transform the index by multiplying −2 times the log of the likelihood. (The log likelihood varies from 0 to minus infinity and is negative because the log of any number less than 1 is negative.) The transformed index (**−2LL**) is a small number when the model fit is good; when the model is perfect, −2LL equals zero. Maximum likelihood estimation seeks to maximize likelihood (i.e., minimize −2LL), and iterations stop when likelihood does not change significantly. In our example, Panel A shows that −2LL was 4948.03 in the null model, and that two iterations were required (footnote c).

The overall model with predictors can be tested against the null model by computing the difference in their log likelihoods. This **likelihood ratio test** is sometimes called a *chi-square goodness-of-fit test* because −2LL has approximately a chi-square distribution. The likelihood ratio statistic can be defined as follows:

$$\chi^2 = (-2LL \text{ [reduced model]}) - (-2LL \text{ [larger model]})$$

Logistic Regression
Block 1: Method = Enter

A Omnibus Tests of Model Coefficients

		Chi-Square	df	Sig.
Step 1	Step	450.567	5	.000
	Block	450.567	5	.000
	Model	450.567	5	.000

B   Model Summary

Step	−2 Log Likelihood	Cox & Snell R Square	Nagelkerke R Square
1	4497.463[a]	.113	.154

[a]Estimation terminated at iteration number 5 because parameter estimates changed by less than .001.

C   Hosmer-Lemeshow Test

Step	Chi-Square	df	Sig.
1	151.747	8	.001

FIGURE 12.4   SPSS printout for tests of the overall model in logistic regression: tubal ligation example.

In the context of our discussion about an overall test, the "reduced model" is the null model and the "larger model" is the model predicting tubal ligation with the full set of predictors (the woman's age, number of births, educational status, and having a child with a disability). This likelihood ratio test would be used to test the null hypothesis that all the b_1 to b_k coefficients for the set of predictors are zero. In our tubal ligation example, the relevant values of $-2LL$, as shown in Panel A of Figure 12.3 and Panel B of Figure 12.4, are as follows:

$$-2LL, \text{ null model with only a constant} = 4948.030$$
$$-2LL, \text{ full model} \qquad\qquad\quad = 4497.463$$
$$\text{Model chi-square} \qquad\qquad\qquad = \overline{\quad 450.567}$$

Degrees of freedom for the likelihood ratio test are the difference between df for the larger and the reduced models. The null model has 1 df (for the constant) and the larger model has 6 df (one for each individual effect and the constant). In this example, the model chi-square is evaluated with $df = 5$. As shown in Panel A of Figure 12.4, the omnibus test of the full model for predicting the odds of having a tubal ligation is statistically significant at $p < .001$. We can reject the null hypothesis that all of the predictor effects are zero.

Panel A of Figure 12.4 shows three chi-square values (Step, Block, and Model), and in this case they are all the same, 450.567. This is because all the predictors were added in one block via simultaneous entry. (This is shown as Method = Enter near the top of the SPSS output.) When predictors are entered in blocks via hierarchical entry, or in steps via stepwise entry, the likelihood ratio test can be used to evaluate the significance of *improvement* to $-2LL$ with successive entry of

Logistic Regression
Block 1: Method = Enter

A   Omnibus Tests of Model Coefficients

		Chi-Square	df	Sig.
Step 1	Step	436.117	4	.000
	Block	436.117	4	.000
	Model	436.117	4	.000

Block 2: Method = Enter

B   Omnibus Tests of Model Coefficients

		Chi-Square	df	Sig.
Step 1	Step	14.451	1	.000
	Block	14.451	1	.000
	Model	450.567	5	.000

FIGURE 12.5   SPSS printout for model tests in hierarchical logistic regression: tubal ligation example.

predictors. In this case, the "reduced model" in the χ^2 formula for the likelihood ratio test is the model without the new predictors and the "larger model" is the model with the larger set of predictors, including new ones. The improvement likelihood ratio test, which tests the null hypothesis that the coefficient for the variable added at the last step is zero, is comparable to the F-change test in multiple regression.

As an example, suppose we had used hierarchical entry to predict tubal ligation. In the first block, we use age, number of births, and educational status as predictors. The omnibus test of this initial model, shown in panel A of Figure 12.5, yields a chi-square value of 436.117. With 4 df, this is significant at $p < .001$. In the next block we enter the variable for whether or not the woman has a child with a disability. Panel B of Figure 12.5 shows that the chi-square for this block is 14.451, which, with 1 df, is also significant at $p < .001$. This test tells us that adding the variable for having a child with a disability significantly improved the predictive power of the logistic regression model. The model chi-square in the last row of panel B is 450.567, the same value we obtained earlier when all predictors were entered simultaneously. Thus, the likelihood ratio test is a versatile test that can be used to evaluate the entire model and model improvement when predictors are added.

THE HOSMER-LEMESHOW TEST   To test the overall model, the likelihood ratio test compares the full model to the null model. An alternative is to compare the prediction model to a hypothetically "perfect" model (Tabachnick & Fidell, 2007). The perfect model is one that contains the exact set of predictors needed to duplicate the observed frequencies in the dependent variable. The full model can be tested against the perfect model in several ways, but the various approaches all involve computing differences between observed and expected frequencies. The test of this type most often used is called the **Hosmer-Lemeshow test,** and is available as an option in SPSS.

The Hosmer-Lemeshow test involves ordering cases based on their predicted probability values on the dependent variable. Then the cases are divided into 10 groups, which are sometimes called *deciles of risk*. The first group or decile has an estimated probability on the outcome variable below .10, while those in the 10th decile have estimated probabilities of .90 or higher. As an example, the first student in Table 12.2, with an estimated probability of .98 of completing graduate school, would be in the 10th decile; the second student, with an estimated probability of .27, would be in the 3rd decile. The frequency of cases in each decile, for those with a code of 1 versus 0 on the outcome variable, can be arrayed in a 2×10 contingency table.

The Hosmer-Lemeshow test evaluates how well observed frequencies versus expected frequencies agree over the entire range of probability values. The expected frequencies are obtained from the model. If the model is a good one, then most of the participants with an actual outcome coded 1 are in the higher deciles of risk, and most with an actual outcome coded 0 are in the lower deciles.

The Hosmer-Lemeshow test is a chi-square test that computes the difference between observed (O) and expected (E) frequencies for each cell of the 2×10 matrix. As in the traditional chi-square statistic described in Chapter 8, the statistic is the sum of the $(O - E)^2/E$ values for the 20 cells. With this test, a *nonsignificant* chi-square is desired. A nonsignificant result indicates that the model being tested is not reliably different from the perfect model. In other words, nonsignificance supports the inference that the model adequately duplicates the observed frequencies at the various levels of the outcome.

Panel C of Figure 12.4 shows that in our tubal ligation example, the Hosmer-Lemeshow chi-square value was 151.747, which was statistically significant ($p < .001$). This suggests that the model is significantly different from a hypothetically perfect model, and is not a good fit to the data. Given the earlier significant results for the likelihood ratio test, this result seems anomalous. One of the problems with the Hosmer-Lemeshow test is that the value of the statistic is sensitive to sample size. With a large sample, as we have in the tubal ligation example, the test statistic can be large even when the model fits well, because the value of chi-square is proportional to sample size.

Having too small a sample is also problematic for the Hosmer-Lemeshow test, and it is sometimes recommended that the test not be used if the sample size is less than 400. Also, the expected number of events in most of the 20 (2×10) groups should exceed five, and no group should have an expected value less than 1. The test may also not be appropriate if you have a small number of categorical predictors. The statistic cannot be used when there are a small number of distinct predicted probabilities, because in this situation it would not be possible to create the deciles of risk. Thus, although this test is often advocated as the appropriate test of model fit in logistic regression, Norušis (2008) has noted that "the Hosmer-Lemeshow statistic provides useful information about the calibration of the model, but it must be interpreted with care" (p. 351).

Example of the Hosmer-Lemeshow test:

Dougherty and Hunziker (2009) used logistic regression to study predictors of implantable cardioverter defibrillator (ICD) shocks during the first year after implantation. Their predictive model included three significant predictors: history of COPD, history of congestive heart failure, and ventricular tachycardia at the time of ICD implant. The Hosmer-Lemeshow test indicated that the model was a good fit to the data ($\chi^2 = 0.52, p = .77$).

Tests of Individual Predictors

It is also possible to test the significance of individual predictor variables in the logistic regression model, just as the t-statistic is used to test the significance of individual predictors in multiple regression. The statistic that is often used in logistic regression is the **Wald statistic,** which when squared is distributed as a chi-square. When the predictor variable has 1 degree of freedom, the squared Wald statistic is as follows:

$$\left[\frac{b}{SE_b}\right]^2$$

where b = the logistic regression coefficient
SE_b = the standard error of b

Figure 12.6 shows the SPSS parameter estimates in the logistic regression model for predicting tubal ligation with all four predictors. The logistic regression equation for predicting the logit for a woman's decision to have a tubal ligation is the constant (-4.087) plus the b coefficients times the value of each respective predictor. The output shows the Wald statistic associated with each predictor variable. The value for the first predictor, number of births, is 118.522, which is highly significant at $p < .001$.

A Wald statistic is computed both for the overall educational attainment variable (2.885) and for each of the two education categories for which indicator variables were created. For the contrast of not having a high school degree compared to having a college education (*edstat1*), the Wald statistic is 1.634, which is not significant at $p = .201$. In fact, none of the education effects is statistically significant. This suggests the possibility of dropping educational attainment from the model, unless there is a reason for wanting to ensure that educational attainment is statistically controlled.

All remaining predictors in this model are statistically significant at $p < .001$. Odds ratios are also shown in this panel under the heading Exp(B), together with the 95% *CI* around the odds ratio. The results suggest that in this population of mothers, having a child with a disability increases the odds of having had a tubal ligation by 40.6%, with other factors controlled. Older women and those who had a larger number of live births are also significantly more likely to have had a tubal ligation.

Variables in the Equation

		B	S.E.	Wald	df	Sig.	Exp(B)	95.0% CI for EXP(B) Lower	Upper
Step 1[a]	Births	.277	.025	118.522	1	.000	1.320	1.255	1.387
	Age	.074	.006	180.240	1	.000	1.077	1.065	1.088
	Edstat			2.885	2	.236			
	Edstat(1)	.133	.104	1.634	1	.201	1.142	.932	1.401
	Edstat(2)	.179	.106	2.870	1	.090	1.196	.972	1.472
	Chdisabl	.341	.089	14.573	1	.000	1.406	1.180	1.674
	Constant	−4.087	.212	370.165	1	.000	.017		

[a]Variable(s) entered on step 1: BIRTHS, AGE, EDSTAT, CHDISABL

FIGURE 12.6   SPSS printout for parameter estimates in the logistic regression equation.

The Wald statistic has some problematic features that should be considered in deciding how to evaluate individual predictors. When the absolute value of the b coefficient is large, the standard error is too large, which in turn produces a Wald statistic that is small and can lead to Type II errors. If the Wald statistic leads you to retain the null hypothesis for a coefficient that is large, an alternative way to test the predictor is to enter that variable in a later block and to use the improvement likelihood ratio test to determine the significance of its contribution. In fact, the likelihood-ratio improvement test is considered superior to the Wald test under most circumstances (Tabachnick & Fidell, 2007), but it does require more effort.

OTHER ISSUES IN LOGISTIC REGRESSION

This section provides some brief comments about a few additional topics relating to logistic regression. Advanced textbooks such as those by Tabachnick and Fidell (2007) or Hosmer and Lemeshow (2000) should be consulted for further guidance on this complex statistical procedure.

Classification Success

One method of assessing the success of the logistic regression model is to evaluate its ability to correctly predict the outcome for sample members whose outcome is known. Models that are highly significant (i.e., statistically reliable) are not necessarily good at classifying cases, especially if the sample size is large.

We saw earlier in our tubal ligation example that even in the absence of any predictors, 63.3% of the cases would be correctly classified simply by classifying all women as not having had the procedure (Figure 12.3). The full model with all sample members resulted in correctly classifying 65.1% of the cases, as shown in Figure 12.7, which is a modest 1.8 percentage point improvement.

In predicting important clinical outcomes, an improvement this small may seem discouraging. However, even though the overall improvement was modest, the improvement was substantial for predicting who would have a tubal ligation. In the null model, 100% of those who had had the procedure were misclassified, whereas in the new model, only 68.5% were misclassified (100% $-$ 31.5% = 68.5%). This is a very large improvement and would be noteworthy if the outcome were a clinically

Classification Table[a]

			Predicted		
			Ever Had Tubal Ligation		
	Observed		No (0)	Yes (1)	Percentage Correct
Step 1	Ever Had Tubal Ligation	No (0)	2017	366	84.6
		Yes (1)	946	435	31.5
		Overall Percentage			65.1

[a]The cut value is .500.

FIGURE 12.7   SPSS printout for classification table with full model.

vital outcome, such as mortality or presence of a disease. The cost, of course, is a higher percentage of misclassifications for those *without* the targeted outcome, but in some situations, this cost might be acceptable.

Effect Size

Researchers often want to know the magnitude of the relationship between the outcome and the set of predictors in the model. Statisticians have put considerable effort into developing an effect size index for logistic regression that is analogous to R^2 in multiple regression, but there is no widely accepted overall effect size index for logistic regression. The main problem is that R^2 in multiple regression can be interpreted as the percentage of variance in the dependent variable explained by the predictors. The variance of a dichotomous outcome variable, however, depends on its distribution. For example, variance is at a maximum for a 50–50 split on the outcome, and the more uneven the split, the smaller the variance. Despite difficulties in achieving a good analog to least squares-based R^2, several logistic R-squared measures have been proposed, and these are sometimes called **pseudo R^2.** These indexes should be reported as approximations to an R^2 obtained in least-squares regression rather than as the percentage of variance explained.

One effect size index in logistic regression is the **Cox and Snell R^2.** This statistic uses a formula that involves the ratio of likelihood indexes for the null model and the model being tested. This index is computed in SPSS, but is considered problematic because it cannot achieve a maximum value of 1.00. A second statistic, called the **Nagelkerke R^2** is a modification that was introduced so that the value could achieve the full range from .00 to 1.00. Panel B of Figure 12.4 (p. 319) indicates that in our tubal ligation example, the Cox and Snell R^2 was .113 and the Nagelkerke R^2 was .154. The Nagelkerke R^2 is the most frequently reported of the pseudo R^2 indexes.

Another effect size option is to save the predicted probabilities for each case from the logistic regression analysis and to use these values in bivariate analyses that yield effect size statistics (Tabachnick & Fidell, 2007). For example, a correlation coefficient (r) can be computed between the predicted probability value and the actual outcome, and r can be interpreted as the effect size index. As another alternative, a t test can be run using the dichotomous outcome variable as the grouping variable and predicted probabilities as the dependent variable. The analysis could then be used to compute the effect size index d, which we discussed in Chapter 6.

TIP: *For individual predictors, the odds ratio provides a direct measure of effect size. The closer the odds ratio is to 1, the smaller the effect. The odds ratio is often used as the measure of effect size in meta-analyses.*

Sample Size

As was true for least-squares regression, there are two ways of approaching sample size needs for logistic regression. One involves the ratio of cases to predictors, and the other involves a power analysis.

To achieve stability in the parameter estimates, there should be a sufficient number of cases for each predictor in the model, including any interaction terms. Recommendations range from 10 to 20 cases per predictor. We would suggest at least 15 cases per predictor, but 20 or more is preferable. Maximum likelihood estimation relies on large-sample asymptotic normality, which means that the stability of the estimates declines when the sample size is inadequate in relation to the number of predictors.

Power analysis in logistic regression is complex. In multiple regression, we used R^2 as the effect size index coupled with number of predictors to estimate sample size needs. As we have seen, however, there is no straightforward analog of R^2 in logistic regression. Moreover, with a dichotomous outcome variable as well as dichotomous predictors, power varies in relation to how close the distributions are to a 50–50 split. We were unable to locate any Internet resource offering free power analysis software for logistic regression (although Internet resources are constantly being added). Several commercial vendors do, however, offer such tools.

As a crude approximation of sample size needs, one could estimate sample size based on the relationship between the outcome and a single predictor variable—preferably, to be conservative, an important predictor that is expected to have the most modest relationship to the outcome. Methods for such a power analysis were described in earlier chapters. Another crude estimate could be obtained by using the procedures described in the previous section of using estimated probabilities to compute a d or r statistic. While these approaches are not ideal, they are likely to be better at helping to avoid a Type II error than doing nothing at all to estimate sample size needs empirically.

> **TIP:** *There are formulas for converting odds ratios into Cohen's* d *and eta-squared, which can then be used in power analyses. These formulas are described in Tabachnick and Fidell (2007) and Lipsey and Wilson (2001).*

Relative Importance of Predictors

The problems of understanding the relative importance of predictors in multiple regression apply equally to logistic regression. Making it even more difficult, neither beta weights nor semipartial correlation coefficients are generated in most logistic regression programs.

Researchers most often use the odds ratio to draw conclusions about the importance of predictors in a logistic equation. Statistically significant predictors that affect the odds of an outcome the most are interpreted as most important. Using this approach provides some insights for predictors that are categorical, but is less useful with continuous variables because they are in different measurement units.

Another solution is to compute standardized regression coefficients, which correspond to beta weights in least-squares regression. Most computer programs do not offer the calculation of standardized coefficients as an option, but one approach is to standardize predictors before the analyze and use the z scores rather than original scores in the logistic regression analysis. This approach results in parameter estimates that are standardized so that b coefficients can be more readily compared.

Assumptions in Logistic Regression

Logistic regression has gained some of its popularity because it avoids the restrictive assumptions of least-squares regression. For example, logistic regression does not assume a linear relationship between the dependent variable and the predictors, and the dependent variable does not have to be normally distributed. Moreover, there is no homogeneity of variance assumption. There are numerous examples in the nursing literature in which the researchers, facing a violation of one or more of these assumptions, opted to use logistic regression by dichotomizing a continuous outcome variable.

Example of dichotomizing a continuous outcome:

Bryanton, Gagnon, Hatem, and Johnston (2008) studied predictors of parenting self-efficacy shortly after birth and then 1 month postpartum. Their dependent variable, parenting self-efficacy, was measured using a 25-item scale and thus yielded interval-level data. They found, however, that the scores were severely negatively skewed, so they opted to dichotomize the outcome variable and use logistic rather than least-squares regression.

There are, nevertheless, a few assumptions in logistic regression. First, the error terms are assumed to be independent, which means that independent sampling is assumed. Logistic regression is not appropriate for within-subjects designs or with correlated samples such as in matched-pair designs.

A second assumption concerns linearity. Logistic regression does not require a linear relationship between the independent variables and the dependent variable, but it does assume a linear relationship between continuous predictors and the log odds of the dependent variable. When this assumption is violated, the risk of a Type II error (concluding that a relationship does not exist in the population when, in fact, it does) increases.

Unfortunately, it is not easy to check the linearity assumption in logistic regression. Many procedures have been proposed, but none is easily accomplished. If you suspect nonlinearity, the simplest approach is to divide a continuous predictor into categories. For example, in our tubal ligation example, number of births could be divided into two groups based on a median split: 1 to 3 births versus 4 or more births.

Converting a continuous variable to a categorical one throws away potentially useful information, however, and one seldom knows in advance that the linearity assumption has been violated. A strategy for testing the assumption (called a *logit step test*) is to use the continuous independent variable to create a new categorical variable with equal intervals, and then use the new variable in the logistic regression. For example, the variable *age* in our tubal ligation example could be used to create an age-category variable with 5-year intervals, which would result in six age categories. When the new variable is used in the analysis, the *b* coefficients for the six categories should increase in roughly equal linear steps if there is linearity between age and the logit for having a tubal ligation.

Problems Relating to Logistic Regression

Many of the problems discussed in the chapter on least-squares regression also apply in logistic regression. First, as in multiple regression, logistic regression performs best when measurement error is low. Predictors that are scores on a composite scale should ideally have internal consistency reliabilities of at least .80 (see Chapter 13 on internal consistency).

Multicollinearity should be avoided. As the magnitude of correlations among predictors increases, the standard errors of the logistic coefficients become inflated. Unfortunately, the SPSS logistic regression program does not produce tolerance information such as that produced in its multiple regression program. You should be on the lookout for suspiciously large standard errors for the *b* coefficients as a signal of multicollinearity. The easiest way to address multicollinearity is to eliminate a predictor that is strongly correlated with another predictor in the model.

Outliers should also be avoided in logistic regression. Outliers can be detected by examining standardized residuals for each case. In logistic regression, the *residual* is the difference between the observed probability of the dependent variable event and the predicted probability based on the model. The *standardized residual* is the residual divided by an estimate of its standard deviation. Some recommend that any standardized residual whose absolute value is greater than 2.58 be removed from the analysis or trimmed, but others use a value of 3.0 as the cutoff. In SPSS, standardized residuals (Zresid) can be requested as an option in the "Save" dialog box, or you can select the option for displaying residuals that lie outside a specified value, such as two *SD*s from the mean, which is the default.

RESEARCH APPLICATIONS OF LOGISTIC REGRESSION

Logistic regression is extremely popular among healthcare researchers for predicting clinically important outcomes. This section describes major applications of logistic regression and discusses methods of effectively displaying the logistic regression results.

The Uses of Logistic Regression

Logistic regression can be used for several purposes by nurse researchers, as described in the following section.

1. *Answering research questions*   The primary use of logistic regression is to answer questions about the relationships among research variables when the dependent variable is categorical. Logistic regression is especially useful when researchers want to estimate the probability of an event occurring, and the relative risk associated with one status on a predictor variable as opposed to another.

2. *Prediction and classification*   Logistic regression offers an excellent vehicle for making predictions about a person's classification when there is information on a set of predictor variables. Classification predictions can be important for decision making and resource management—for example, predicting which discharged patients are most in need of follow-up or projecting which patients would most benefit from a costly intervention. As an actual example, Metheny and her colleagues (2005) used logistic regression to facilitate nurses' decision making about feeding tube position. They found that several clinical variables (e.g., volume of aspirate from the feeding tube, pH of the aspirate) were accurate 81% of the time in classifying tube site (gastric versus small bowel).

3. *Validity assessments*   Instruments are sometimes developed with the specific aim of classifying people—for example, there are psychological tests that are used in the diagnosis of different types of mental illness. Logistic regression can be used as one tool for evaluating the validity of such instruments—i.e., for assessing the extent to which the instrument makes accurate classifications.

4. *Assessing bias*   In earlier chapters we discussed how *t* tests and ANOVA could be used to evaluate various types of bias, such as selection bias, nonresponse bias, or attrition bias. These assessments involve comparing groups (e.g., those who continue in a longitudinal study versus those who drop out) in terms of various background characteristics one variable at a time. Logistic regression can be used to assess whether the groups can be reliably differentiated on the basis of a set of characteristics taken as a whole. In effect, this involves an effort to model the bias—for example, to model the attrition process or the selection process. When multivariate techniques such as logistic regression are used and no biases are detected, the conclusion that results are unbiased is more compelling than when a series of univariate tests is used.

The Presentation of Logistic Regression in Research Reports

Like all other multivariate statistics, results from logistic regression almost always require the use of tables because of the complexity of the analyses and the wealth of information they yield. Often, two or more tables are needed—for example, when classification is an important research objective and it is deemed important to present the classification table.

A summary table for a simultaneous logistic regression analysis normally includes the following information in the main body: names of the predictors, logistic regression coefficients (and perhaps their standard errors), and the odds ratio for each predictor. Additional information might include the Wald statistic and its significance for each predictor, and confidence intervals around each odds ratio. The title of the table usually indicates the name of the outcome whose probability is being predicted. Sample size should be specified, either in a footnote or in the title. Finally, the value, significance level, and name of the overall model test (e.g., either the likelihood ratio test or the Hosmer-Lemeshow test) should be indicated.

An example of a logistic regression table is presented in Table 12.3, which summarizes the results from the tubal ligation example. This table lists the four predictors, followed by their associated b-weights and standard errors. The table also displays the Wald statistic associated with each predictor, the odds ratios, and the 95% CIs around the odds ratios. At the bottom of the table, information is provided about the omnibus model chi-square statistic (the likelihood ratio test), Nagelkerke R^2, and the percent correctly classified with the model. A footnote provides information about the reference category for the educational attainment variable. Finally, the table title specifies the dependent variable, and provides sample size information.

TABLE 12.3 Example of a Summary Table with Logistic Regression Results

Predictor	b (SE)	Wald	Odds Ratio	95% CI, Odds Ratio Lower	95% CI, Odds Ratio Upper
Age	.07 (.01)	180.24***	1.08	1.07	1.09
Number of births	.28 (.03)	118.52***	1.32	1.26	1.39
Educational attainment[a]		2.88			
No high school diploma	.13 (.10)	1.63	1.14	.93	1.40
Diploma or GED	.18 (.11)	2.87	1.20	.97	1.47
Has a child with a disability	.34 (.09)	14.57***	1.41	1.18	1.67
Constant	−4.09 (.21)	370.17***			

Model (likelihood ratio) chi-square = 450.57, df = 5, $p < .001$

Nagelkerke R^2 = .15

Percent correctly classified = 65.1%

[a]Reference category = A.A. or B.A. degree

*** = $p < .001$

Logistic Regression Results Predicting the Probability of a Tubal Ligation ($N = 3,764$)

The following paragraph is an example of how these results could be described in the text:

> Logistic regression was used to estimate the probability of having had a tubal ligation in this sample of low-income mothers. Four predictor variables—the woman's age, number of births, educational attainment, and whether she had a child with any type of disability—were used in the analysis, with simultaneous entry of predictors. As shown in Table 12.3, the overall predictive model was statistically significant (likelihood ratio chi-square = 450.57 [5] $p < .001$). With the exception of educational attainment, the independent variables were all significant in predicting the likelihood of a tubal ligation. Older women and those with more births were significantly more likely than younger women and those with fewer births to have had a tubal ligation. The odds of having a tubal ligation was 41% higher among women who had a child with a disability (OR = 1.41) than among women without a disabled child. Although the overall model and three predictors were statistically significant, the classification results indicated modest success, with an overall rate of correct classification of 65.1%. The overall effect size was also modest, with Nagelkerke R^2 equal to .15.

Research Example

This section describes an interesting nursing study that used logistic regression analysis. The researchers' summary table provides a good example of how multiple outcomes can be presented in a single table.

Study: "The effects of hospitalization on multiple units" (Kanak et al., 2008)

Study Purpose: The purpose of this study was to examine the effects of hospital patients' relocations to multiple care units during a hospital stay on a broad range of healthcare outcomes. The researchers noted that transfers to different hospital units are usually done to provide patients with the appropriate type and level of care, but that multiple transfers could adversely affect the quality of health care.

Methods: The data for this study were extracted from a large database created in a study of nursing outcomes effectiveness. The dataset was constructed with clinical and administrative records data from inpatient units in a large academic medical center. The sample for the study consisted of 7,851 hospitalized patients aged 60 years or older. The independent variable was the number of hospital units on which a patient resided during an acute hospitalization. A variety of clinically important outcomes were the dependent variables in the study. The dichotomous outcomes included whether or not the patient: (a) had a nosocomial infection acquired after hospital admission; (b) had a fall; (c) died during hospitalization; (d) was discharged to any location other than home; (e) had a medication error; and (f) had any adverse occurrence during hospitalization.

Analysis: Logistic regression analysis was used to assess the effect of multiunit residence during hospitalization on the dichotomous clinical outcomes. For the purposes of these analyses, number of units of hospitalization was defined as a categorical variable with four levels: 1 unit, 2 units, 3 or 4 units, or 5 or more units. To more clearly examine the relationship between number of units and the outcomes, several variables relating to patient acuity were statistically controlled: principal medical diagnosis, coded as 1 of 16 diagnostic categories; presence or absence of 30 comorbid medical conditions; and a measure of illness severity, with ratings from 1 (mild) to 4 (severe/extreme).

Results: All dichotomous outcomes, except patient mortality, were significantly associated with number of hospital units. Table 12.4 summarizes logistic regression results for three of the dichotomous outcomes. (The full model with control variables is not shown in this table; only parameter estimates for the primary independent variable are presented.) Being hospitalized on multiple units was associated with higher risk of negative outcomes, and risk increased with the number of units. For example, even after controlling for diagnosis and severity of illness, the odds of acquiring a nosocomial infection in the hospital were more than five times greater among those who had resided on 5 or more units than among those on a single unit (OR = 5.56). The risk was lower as

TABLE 12.4 The Effect of Number of Hospitalization Units During a Hospital Stay on Selected Clinical Outcomes (N = 7,851)[a]					
Number of Hospital Units[b]	**b**	**SE**	**Wald χ^2**	**p**	**OR**
Outcome 1: Nosocomial Infection[c]					
≥ 5 units (n = 1,058)	1.72	.21	66.2	<.001	5.56
3–4 units (n = 1,629)	1.05	.22	23.9	<.001	2.87
2 units (n = 2,726)	.46	.23	4.0	.046	1.59
Outcome 2: Medication Error[c]					
≥ 5 units (n = 1,058)	1.35	.15	86.4	<.001	3.87
3–4 units (n = 1,629)	.69	.15	22.6	<.001	1.99
2 units (n = 2,726)	.24	.15	2.6	.105	1.27
Outcome 3: Experienced a Fall[c]					
≥ 5 units (n = 1,058)	.89	.18	24.5	<.001	2.43
3–4 units (n = 1,629)	.58	.17	11.9	<.001	1.99
2 units (n = 2,726)	−.28	.17	2.6	.106	.76

[a]In the overall logistic model, the following variables were statistically controlled: medical diagnosis, comorbid medical conditions, and severity of illness.

[b]The category for 1 hospital unit (n = 2,438) was used as the reference category in these analyses.

[c]The Wald chi-square statistic for the overall "number of units" variable was statistically significant at $p < .001 (df = 3)$ for all outcomes.

Abridged and adapted from Kanak et al. (2008), Table 4.

the number of units declined, but was still 59% more likely for those who were on two units.

Conclusions: The authors noted the importance of nurses in coordinating the care that patients receive across inpatient units, and the need to develop and implement strategies to mediate the negative consequences associated with movement to different units.

Summary Points

- **Logistic regression** is a multivariate technique for predicting a categorical dependent variable; **binary logistic regression** is used when the outcome is dichotomous and when the goal is to predict the probability of one outcome or event occurring versus another.
- Logistic regression uses **maximum likelihood estimation (MLE)** rather than least-squares estimation and has less stringent assumptions than analyses using the general linear model (GLM), such as discriminant analysis. MLE estimates the parameters that are most likely to have generated the observed data.
- Logistic regression develops a model for estimating the *odds* that an event will occur—the ratio of the probability that it will occur to the probability that it will not. The dependent variable is transformed to be the natural log of the odds, which is called a **logit.** The logit is predicted from a combination of predictors, weighted by logistic coefficients, plus a constant.
- For each predictor, the logistic regression analysis yields an *odds ratio* (OR), which is the factor by which the odds change for a unit change in the predictor. The odds ratio is a measure of comparative risk—the odds of an event given one condition, versus the odds of the event given an alternative condition.
- **Predicted probabilities** based on the logistic regression equation can be used to classify cases—that is, to predict whether an event or outcome will or will not occur.
- Dependent variables in binary logistic regression are typically dummy-coded variables with the code 1 assigned to the event or outcome of interest, and 0 to others.
- Predictor variables can be continuous, dichotomous, or categorical. Categorical variables can be

specified such that different types of contrasts are possible (e.g., by means of *indicator coding* or *deviation coding*). Interaction terms can also be used as predictors.

- Predictors can be entered into the regression equation simultaneously, hierarchically, or in a stepwise fashion. Stepwise entry can involve either forward selection or backward elimination of predictors.

- Tests of statistical significance are available for testing the overall regression model and individual predictors. There are several alternatives for both types of test.

- The most often-reported statistic for testing the overall model is a chi-square statistic from a **likelihood ratio test** (sometimes called a **goodness-of-fit test**). The test involves the **likelihood index**, which represents the probability of the observed results; it is usually reported as -2 times the log of the likelihood ($-2LL$). The omnibus test of the model is the difference between $-2LL$ for the model being tested and $-2LL$ for the *null model*, that is, the logistic model without any predictors and only a constant term.

- An alternative method of testing the goodness of fit of the model is to compare the model with a hypothetically perfect model, using the **Hosmer-Lemeshow test.** With this test, *non*significance is desired because it indicates that the model being tested is not significantly different from a hypothetically perfect one.

- The **Wald statistic** is often used to assess the significance of individual predictors in the logistic model, although the likelihood ratio test, which can be used to test model *improvement* when predictors are added to the model in blocks, is often preferable.

- There is no equivalent to multiple regression's R^2 statistic, but statisticians have devised several **pseudo R^2** indexes to summarize overall effect size for logistic regression. The most widely reported is the **Nagelkerke R^2** which approximates the traditional R^2 statistic but which does not, strictly speaking, indicate the proportion of variance that predictors explain in the outcome variable.

- Although logistic regression does not have the restrictive assumptions of GLM procedures, it is assumed that continuous predictor variables have a linear relationship to the log odds of the dependent variable. It is a difficult assumption to test, but one option is to use the *logit step test,* which involves converting continuous variables to equal-interval categorical ones and then seeing whether the progression of *b* coefficients is linear.

Exercises

The following exercises cover concepts presented in this chapter. Exercises in Part A that are indicated with a dagger (†) can be checked against answers in Appendix C. Exercises in Part B involve computer analyses using the datasets for this textbook, and answers and comments are offered on this book's Web site.

PART A EXERCISES

† **A1.** In Table 12.2, students were classified as completing versus not completing a graduate program based on a cutpoint of .50 in the estimated probabilities. What percentage of cases would be correctly classified if the cutpoint were .40? What types of misclassifications would this cutpoint produce?

† **A2.** What is the logistic regression equation for predicting the probability of having a tubal ligation, based on information shown in Figure 12.6?

A3. Based on either your clinical knowledge or on a brief literature search, what variable would you recommend adding to improve the prediction of a woman's decision to have a tubal ligation? How would you measure or construct that variable?

† **A4.** In the example at the end of the chapter (the study by Kanak et al.), could the researchers have used a continuous variable for number of units? Why do you think they used a four-category variable to represent this independent variable? Is there evidence in Table 12.4 that the linearity assumption would have been violated if a continuous variable had been used?

PART B EXERCISES

† **B1.** For these exercises, you will be using the SPSS dataset Polit2SetB. The analyses will focus on predicting the probability that a woman is in good-to-excellent health versus fair-to-poor health, which is coded 1 versus 0, respectively, on the variable *health*. Begin by looking at results for the odds ratio when there is only one predictor of good health—whether or not the woman currently smokes cigarettes (*smoker*). First, run the SPSS crosstabs-based risk analysis (see Chapter 4). In the Analyze ➜ Descriptives ➜ Crosstabs dialog box, use *smoker* as the Row variable and *health* as the Column variable. In the Cells dialog box, select Observed frequencies and Row

and Column percentages. In the Statistics dialog box, select Chi-square and Risk. Then click Continue and OK to run the analysis, and answer these questions: (a) What percent of women in this sample smoked? What percent of women said they were in fair or poor health? (b) What percent of smokers versus nonsmokers described themselves as being in good to excellent health? (c) Is the bivariate relationship between smoking status and health statistically significant? (d) What is the odds ratio in this analysis? What is the 95% *CI* around the OR? (e) What does the odds ratio mean?

† **B2.** In this exercise, use the Logistic regression program in SPSS rather than Crosstabs to look at the bivariate relationship between *health* and *smoker*. In the Analyze ➜ Regression ➜ Binary Logistic dialog box, move *health* into the Dependent slot and move *smoker* into the Covariate slot. Click the Options pushbutton and in the next dialog box select CI for exp(B), 95%. Then run the analysis and answer the following questions, focusing on the Block 1 panels labeled Omnibus Test of Model Coefficients and Variables in the Equation: (a) For the overall model in which the probability of being in good health was predicted based on women's smoking status, was the model statistically significant? What was the value of the model chi-square statistic? (b) What is the value of the odds ratio obtained through logistic regression (this appears in a column labeled Exp(B))? (c) What is the 95% *CI* around the odds ratio? (d) How do these results compare to those obtained in the Crosstabs analysis (i.e., for chi-square, the odds ratio, and the 95% *CI*)?

† **B3.** In this next exercise, we will use five predictors to predict the probability of good health (*health*) in a standard logistic regression: The predictors include smoking status (*smoker*) and four additional predictors, which include the woman's age (*age*), whether or not she is currently employed (*worknow*), her body mass index (*bmi*), and how much stress she has been experiencing (*stressed*). In the opening logistic regression dialog box (Analyze ➜ Regression ➜ Binary Logistic), move *health* into the Dependent slot, and move the five predictors into the slot for Covariates. Click the Options pushbutton and in the next dialog box select Hosmer-Lemeshow goodness of fit, Casewise listing of residuals, and CI for Exp(B), 95%. Then click Continue and OK to run the analysis and answer the following questions: (a) In the null model, what percent of the cases were correctly classified? Comment on the nature of the misclassifications. (b) In the null model, what was the odds ratio for being in good-to-excellent health? (c) What is the value of the likelihood ratio chi-square statistic for the omnibus test of the model? Was this statistically significant? (d) What was the value of $-2LL$ for the full model? Using this information and the value of the model chi-square statistic, compute the value of $-2LL$ for the null model. (e) What were the values of the pseudo R^2 statistics? (f) What was the value of the Hosmer-Lemeshow chi-square test? Was this value statistically significant? What does this suggest?

(g) What percentage of cases was correctly classified with the full model? Comment on the degree of improvement over the null model. (h) Based on the Wald statistics, which independent variables were significantly predictive of the women's health status? (i) Interpret the meaning of the OR for *age* in this analysis. (j) Interpret the meaning of the OR for *worknow*. (k) According to the Casewise listing panel, how many cases were outliers that exceeded the criterion of 2.58 (absolute value)? Were these cases correctly classified?

† **B4.** In this next exercise, we will again use five independent variables to predict the probability of good health (*health*), but instead of using *bmi* as a continuous variable, we will use the variable *bmicat,* which classifies the women based on BMI values as normal weight, overweight, obese, or morbidly obese. In the opening logistic regression dialog box, put *health* into the Dependent slot, and move *smoker, bmicat, stressed, worknow,* and *age* into the slot for Covariates. Click the Categorical pushbutton and move *bmicat* into the slot for Categorical Covariates, leaving the default options of indicator coding using the last category (morbidly obese) as the reference group. Click the Options pushbutton and select Hosmer-Lemeshow goodness of fit and CI for Exp(B), 95%. Then click Continue and OK to run the analysis and answer the following questions: (a) How many new variables were created to be predictors for the *bmicat* variable? How were morbidly obese women coded on these new variables? How many cases were classified as morbidly obese? (b) What do the results suggest about the goodness of fit of the overall model, using both the likelihood ratio and the Hosmer-Lemeshow tests? (c) What was the value of the Nagelkerke R^2 in this analysis? How does this compare to the value obtained in Exercise B3 when the continuous *bmi* was used as a predictor? (d) What percentage of cases was correctly classified in this analysis? Compare the classification success obtained here with that obtained using the continuous BMI variable (Exercise B3). (e) Which independent variables were significant predictors of good health? (f) Comment on the pattern of odds ratios for the *bmicat* variables. What does the pattern suggest about the assumption of linearity between the original BMI values and the logit for being in good-to-excellent health?

B5. Select another variable in the Polit2SetB dataset that you might hypothesize as a predictor of good health in this population of women. Run another logistic regression, entering the new predictor in a second block (use the Next button on the opening dialog box to get a new screen for a second block of variables). Examine the Block 2 information to see if the new variable significantly improved the model. Also examine whether adding your new predictor resulted in *non*significance for any predictor in the Block 1 model.

B6. Using output from one of the previous three exercises (B3 through B5), create a table to summarize key results of the analyses. Then write a paragraph summarizing the findings.

13

Factor Analysis and Internal Consistency Reliability Analysis

Similar to many multivariate procedures described thus far, **factor analysis** involves the formation of linear combinations of variables. It is different from most other multivariate procedures, however, because factor analysis is used primarily to evaluate the structure of a set of variables, particularly in the development and testing of new scales. This chapter deals exclusively with a type of factor analysis that has come to be known as **exploratory factor analysis (EFA).** Another type—**confirmatory factor analysis (CFA)**—uses more complex modeling and estimation procedures and is not covered in this introductory statistics textbook.

Factor analysis is exceedingly complex mathematically, and so we present only an overview. For more detailed information, a particularly good resource for healthcare researchers is the book by Pett, Lackey, and Sullivan (2003), as well as that by Tabachnick and Fidell (2007).

BASIC CONCEPTS FOR FACTOR ANALYSIS

Factor analysis is used to illuminate the underlying dimensionality of a set of measures—that is, to shed light on how variables cluster together as unidimensional constructs that are of theoretical interest. For example, if we administered 50 questions relating to people's methods of coping with stress, we might determine through factor analysis that there are four distinct coping styles. Factor analysis would provide information on which of the 50 questions "belong together" on the four dimensions of coping. Researchers often have a priori ideas about which items go together to capture a unidimensional concept, but their hunches are not always consistent with participants' responses to the items. Factor analysis provides an empirical way to identify the underlying dimensionality of a set of measures.

Factor analysis reveals the structure of a set of variables by analyzing intercorrelations among them. The underlying dimensions identified in a factor analysis are called **factors.** A factor is a hypothetical entity—a *latent variable*—that is assumed to underlie the concrete measures administered to study participants.

Mathematically, a factor is a linear combination of variables in a data matrix. A raw data matrix consists of scores on k variables for N subjects. A factor could be defined by the following equation:

$$F_1 = b_1X_1 + b_2X_2 + \ldots b_kX_k$$

where
$F_1 =$ a factor score for Factor 1
$k =$ number of original variables
b_1 to $b_k =$ weights for each k variable
X_1 to $X_k =$ values on the k variables

Factor analysis solves for the b weights (called **factor loadings**) to yield **factor scores** for major dimensions underlying the original measures.

Most researchers perform factor analysis when they are developing a scale for use in subsequent research. In our example of 50 items tapping coping styles, the ultimate goal might be to understand the clinical or demographic characteristics of people with different coping styles. In this situation, the factor scores would be the dependent variables, and individual characteristics would be the independent variables. As another example, we might want to determine if a certain coping style was better than others in alleviating presurgical stress; here, coping style would be the independent variable and stress would be the dependent variable. Factor analysis thus can be viewed as a data reduction technique. Rather than having 50 variables to use as independent or dependent variables (i.e., the original items), factor analysis reduces the set to four new variables. Thus, factor analysis is important as a data management strategy that can contribute to analytic and conceptual parsimony.

Factor Matrices

Matrices play an important role in factor analysis and, indeed, matrix algebra is required in the factor analytic solution. The process begins with the original data matrix (subjects × variables). Many of the operations performed in factor analysis involve manipulations of the correlation matrix (variables × variables, across subjects).

One of the products of a factor analysis is a **factor matrix,** which arrays the original variables along one dimension and factors along the other. There are several important types of factor matrix, as we discuss later in this chapter. For now it is important to know that the entries in a factor matrix are factor loadings that convey information about the relationship between the original variables and the underlying factors.

TABLE 13.1 Hypothetical Factor Matrix for Six Aptitude Tests

Tests	Factor I	Factor II	Communality (h^2)
A	.84	.21	.75
B	.90	.24	.87
C	.74	.13	.56
D	.17	.73	.56
E	.22	.80	.69
F	.27	.91	.83
Eigenvalue	2.21	2.12	4.33
Explained Variance	36.8%	35.3%	72.1%

Table 13.1 shows a hypothetical example of a factor matrix. Let us suppose that the variables listed in the left-hand column represent six different aptitude tests (A through F) that were administered to a sample of students. Factors I and II are empirically derived factors that might represent, for example, verbal aptitude (Factor I) and quantitative aptitude (Factor II).

Factors loadings can (except in certain cases we discuss later) be interpreted in much the same fashion as correlation coefficients. They can range in value from -1.00 through zero for no correlation to $+1.00$. The first entry in the matrix in Table 13.1 indicates a strong positive correlation between Test A and Factor I (.84). Tests A, B, and C have high loadings on Factor I, while the loadings for Tests C, D, and E on the first factor are more modest—they are all less than .30. Conversely, the first three tests have modest loadings on Factor II, while the last three tests have loadings of .73 or greater on this factor. We would interpret the factors by trying to conceptualize what it is that Tests A, B, and C have in common that they do *not* have in common with Tests D, E, and F. In our example, the Tests A, B, and C might be vocabulary, reading comprehension, and sentence completion tests, respectively, all of which have a strong verbal component. The three other tests might be geometry, math computation, and problem solving tests—all of which have a quantitative component.

Table 13.1 has two other types of useful information. The **communality** is a measure of a variable's *shared* variance, sometimes referred to as **common factor variance.** Communality is sometimes labeled h^2, as it is in Table 13.1. The communalities of the original variables in the analysis are equal to the sums of squares of the factor loadings for those variables. Thus, for Test A, the communality is $(.84)^2 + (.21)^2 = .75$.

Common factor variance of a particular variable indicates the variance that it shares in common with other variables. The variability of each of the six tests in Table 13.1 can be expressed as follows:

$$V_{\text{Total}} = V_{\text{CommonFactor}} + V_{\text{Specific}} + V_{\text{Error}}$$

where
V_{Total} = total variance
$V_{\text{CommonFactor}}$ = common factor variance (h^2)
V_{Specific} = variance specific to the variable
V_{Error} = error variance

Using Test A as the example, all of the variance in students' scores on Test A consists of variance that Test A has in common with the other five tests, plus variance that is specific to Test A, plus error variance (e.g., the unreliability of the test). Across the two factors, then, 75% of the variance in Test A is common factor variance, while the remaining 25% is **unique variance,** which is partly specific variance and partly error variance. Table 13.1 indicates that Test F has the highest proportion of common factor variance (.83), while Tests C and D have the lowest (.56). The main problem of factor analysis is the allocation of the total common factor variance of a variable (h^2) to the different factors.

Below the listing of the six tests in Table 13.1 is a row labeled eigenvalue. An **eigenvalue** is the sum of the squared loadings for a specific factor. For Factor I, the eigenvalue is $(.84)^2 + (.90)^2 + (.74)^2 + (.17)^2 + (.22)^2 + (.27)^2 = 2.21$. An eigenvalue is an index of how much variance in the factor solution is explained by a given factor. In this example, the eigenvalues for both factors are about the same (2.21 and 2.12), indicating that both verbal and quantitative aptitude account for a comparable percentage of variance in the six test scores. The exact amount of variance is shown in the bottom row, 36.8% for Factor I and 35.3% for Factor II. Together the two factors account for 72.1% of the total variance in the six tests.

Requirements and Assumptions for Factor Analysis

Factor analysis uses a correlation matrix as its starting point, and thus the assumptions underlying the use of correlations should be kept in mind. Each pair of variables in a factor analysis should be linearly correlated; curvilinear relationships degrade the analysis. The factor analytic solution is enhanced when the variables are normally distributed, but the solution may be interesting and worthwhile even when normality is not attained for all variables. The discussion in Chapter 9 regarding influences on the value of correlation coefficients (e.g., the presence of outliers, a restricted range of values, curvilinear relationships, and so on) should be kept in mind because things that affect correlations also affect factor analytic solutions.

The variables in a factor analysis are generally measured on a scale that is interval or ratio, or on an ordinal scale that approximates interval properties (such as individual Likert-type items). The variables can be entire scales or tests (as in our example of factor analyzing scores on six aptitude tests) or, more typically, individual items (as in the example of analyzing 50 items that measured methods of coping with stress).

Phases in Factor Analysis

Factor analysis is often described as a two-step process (factor extraction and factor rotation, which we describe subsequently), but factor analysis typically involves many phases with several iterations and feedback loops. The complexity arises from the fact that factor analysis involves a number of semisubjective decisions, which are usually evaluated by testing alternatives.

The first step in the factor analysis involves transforming the raw data matrix into a correlation matrix and undertaking some preliminary actions to assess whether, in fact, factor analysis makes sense. If intercorrelations are too low, for example, it may not be sensible to proceed. Thus, researchers should take steps to ensure that the correlation matrix is factorable, to determine if there are missing data problems that need to be resolved, and to ascertain that the sample size is adequate.

The next phase, **factor extraction,** focuses on determining the number of factors that are needed to adequately capture the variance in the set of variables. There are many different approaches to factor extraction, and there are a number of different criteria that can be used to determine the appropriate number of factors. The product from this phase of analysis is an **unrotated factor matrix.**

Factor extraction seeks to maximize variance, but does not result in readily understandable results. Thus, the next phase of factor analysis involves transforming the original factors so that the results are more interpretable, through a process called **factor rotation.** As with factor extraction, there are alternative methods of factor rotation. The result of this phase of the analysis is a **rotated factor matrix.** The factor matrix in Table 13.1 was a rotated one.

The next phase typically involves interpreting, evaluating, and refining the factors. Researchers decide how many factors to extract and rotate, and select methods to extract and rotate them. Typically, these decisions must be evaluated to see if alternatives result in a better and more interpretable solution. Interpretation is a key activity in a factor analysis.

Once the extraction and rotation have been finalized and interpretation has been achieved, factor scores for use in subsequent analyses can be computed for each case. As with the other phases, the researcher has some options with regard to the computation of factor scores. Thus, although factor analysis is widely used and respected, its myriad options for key decisions, the lack of clearcut criteria for decision making, and the importance of interpretation make it different from other statistical procedures described in this book.

EVALUATION OF FACTORABILITY

Before undertaking a factor analysis, researchers should do a preliminary evaluation to establish that a factor analysis makes sense. This involves looking at descriptive information for the variables in questions—both univariate description (e.g., are the variables severely skewed?) and bivariate description (are correlations between variables linear?). This section covers several relevant issues for a preliminary assessment.

Sample Size

To avoid capitalizing on small random differences in the magnitude of the correlation coefficients, the sample size for a factor analysis should be large. Sample sizes of at least 300 are usually advisable. Moreover, there should be at least 10 cases per variable, and an even greater case-to-variable ratio is desirable. Thus, if there are 50 items being factor analyzed, the sample should ideally be at least 500, if not larger.

> **TIP:** *Factor analytic solutions almost always require replication. If it is possible to replicate within a single study, this opportunity should be pursued. Thus, with 20 variables and a sample of 500 cases, one alternative is to randomly divide the sample in half, perform a factor analysis with the first subsample, and then cross-validate the results through a factor analysis of the second. If the two analyses reveal similar factor structures, the results will be compelling. Confirmatory factor analysis, which uses maximum likelihood estimation, is often used to test hypotheses about the comparability of factor structure in different samples.*

Having a large overall sample does not necessarily provide a sufficient basis for factor analysis if there are large amounts of missing data. The correlation matrix for factor analysis should be based on a *rectangular matrix* of data values—that is, there should be a valid value on every variable for every person in the analysis. A correlation matrix based on *pairwise deletion* of missing values, with coefficients based on a varying number of cases, should not be used in factor analysis. If there are missing values for some people, either the missing values should be estimated or the cases should be deleted (*listwise deletion*).

If there are, say, 25 variables in the analysis, there is a strong likelihood that some people will have missing data on at least one of them. The removal of all cases with a missing value may result in a sample that is too small for a factor analysis. Thus, an early first step in factor analysis is to evaluate the extent of missing data. With a large sample and small number of missing values, the factor analysis can proceed using listwise deletion. If missing values are sporadic and sample size is marginal, a missing values replacement strategy can be pursued. If missing values are extensive, however, factor analysis may not be appropriate.

> **TIP:** *SPSS has an option for replacing missing values in its factor analysis program, but it is not always desirable to select this option. We discuss missing values in Chapter 14.*

Assessment of Correlations and Sampling Adequacy

A basic requirement for a factor analysis is that there should be a number of sizeable correlations between variables in the matrix. If correlations among the variables are low, it does not make sense to search for an underlying construct that captures what the variables have in common—the analysis may well indicate that there as many different factors as there are original variables.

Inspection of the magnitude of coefficients in the correlation matrix provides preliminary clues about factorability. If the correlation matrix consists mainly of correlation coefficients that are nonsignificant or with an absolute value less than .30, there is probably nothing to factor analyze. If some variables have particularly low correlations with other variables, they should probably be dropped from the analysis. Some recommend that the *average* of the correlations be .30 or higher.

On the other hand, if correlations are too high, problems with multicollinearity may occur. If there are variables with intercorrelations greater than .80, some should be dropped. It is not just that highly correlated variables are redundant—the problem is that very high correlations in the matrix can result in an unstable solution.

> **TIP:** *The correlation matrix should also be inspected to see if the signs on the correlation coefficients make sense from a conceptual point of view— that is, are there positive correlations between items that you think are conveying similar meaning, and negative correlations between items with opposite meanings? This is an issue we discuss in a later section.*

Computer programs for factor analysis offer many diagnostic tools for evaluating factorability in terms of magnitude of intercorrelations and **sampling adequacy,** which refers to the adequacy of sampling *variables*. One such tool is **Bartlett's test of sphericity,** which tests the null hypothesis that the correlation matrix is an *identity matrix*—one in which correlations among the variables are all zero. If this null hypothesis cannot be rejected, factor analysis is not appropriate. Significance on Bartlett's test supports further evaluation of the factorability of the data. However,

KMO and Bartlett's Test

Kaiser-Meyer-Olkin Measure of Sampling Adequacy		.791
Bartlett's Test of Sphericity	Approx. Chi-Square	3162.796
	df	55.000
	Sig.	.000

FIGURE 13.1   SPSS printout for evaluating factorability.

this test is highly influenced by sample size (number of participants), and so the test is almost always significant.

A more important tool is the **Kaiser-Meyer-Olkin (KMO) test,** a measure of sampling adequacy that compares the magnitudes of correlation coefficients to the sizes of partial correlation coefficients. In this context, the partial correlation coefficient between two variables is the correlation *after controlling for the effects of all other variables*. In a factorable set of data, partial correlations should be small in relation to observed correlation coefficients. The KMO measure of sampling adequacy (which can be computed for all of the variables combined, as well as for each variable individually) can range from 0 to 1. The closer the value is to 1, the better the prospects for factor analysis. KMO values of .80 or higher are considered good, and those in the .70s are fair. Anything below .50 is considered unacceptable for a factor analysis.

For several parts of our discussion in this chapter, we will be describing a factor analysis of 11 items that were administered to a sample of over 1,800 mothers who had a child between the ages of 2 and 6. These 11 items (listed in Figure 13.4, p. 344) measure aspects of the parent–child relationship. Respondents were asked to rate on a 0-to-10 scale the degree to which each statement was *not at all true* (0) to *completely true* (10). Figure 13.1 presents the SPSS printout for Bartlett's test and the overall KMO test for these data. This figure shows that Bartlett's test was significant ($p < .001$) and that the value of KMO (.791) is reasonably high.

KMO values for individual variables (sometimes called measures of sampling adequacy or MSA) can be found on the diagonal of the *anti-image correlation matrix*. The matrix for our example is too large to reproduce here, but KMO values ranged from a low of .695 for one item to a high of .846 for another. Once again, these values support a decision to proceed with a factor analysis.

Example of a factorability assessment:

Lerdal and colleagues (2009) factor analyzed a Norwegian translation of the 24-item Stages of Change questionnaire. Preliminary analyses were undertaken to assess the factorability of the scale. The KMO index of sampling adequacy was .863 and Bartlett's test of sphericity was statistically significant ($p < .001$). The researchers concluded that their data were amenable to factor analysis.

FACTOR EXTRACTION

A fundamental assumption in factor analysis is that underlying constructs are responsible for the correlations among the variables. The goal of the analysis is to identify these constructs. Ideally, the solution will reveal a small number of interpretable and meaningful constructs (factors) that are of substantive interest.

In the first phase of actual factor analysis, factor extraction seeks clusters of intercorrelated variables within the correlation matrix and extracts as much variance as possible from the common factors. Different statistical criteria and measurement models can be used in the factor extraction stage, and most factor analysis programs offer several alternative extraction methods.

Principal Components Analysis

A widely used method of factor extraction is the principal components method. **Principal components analysis (PCA)** differs from other factor analytic techniques in that it factor analyzes *all* variance in the observed variables, not just common factor variance. Mathematically, the issue boils down to what is placed on the diagonal of the correlation matrix prior to matrix operations, because the variance that is analyzed is the sum of the values in the positive diagonal. With PCA, all diagonal values are 1s: There is as much variance to be analyzed as there are variables in the analysis. All variance in the original variables are distributed to the factors, including unique variance and error variance for each variable.

PCA creates successive linear combinations of the observed variables. The first factor, or principal *component*, is the linear combination that accounts for the largest amount of variance, using a least-squares criterion. The second component is formed from residual correlations: It accounts for the second largest amount of variance that is uncorrelated with the first component. Successive components account for smaller and smaller proportions of total variance in the data set, and all are orthogonal to (uncorrelated with) previously extracted components. Thus, the extracted factors (components) represent independent sources of variation.

In PCA, there are as many factors as there are variables but, if the data are factorable, only the first few account for a noteworthy proportion of variance. Figure 13.2

Factor Analysis

Total Variance Explained			
	Initial Eigenvalues		
Component	Total	% of Variance	Cumulative %
1	2.955	26.859	26.859
2	1.694	15.398	42.258
3	1.089	9.899	52.156
4	.841	7.641	59.797
5	.760	6.907	66.704
6	.712	6.474	73.178
7	.694	6.310	79.488
8	.619	5.625	85.113
9	.593	5.388	90.501
10	.530	4.820	95.322
11	.515	4.678	100.000

Extraction Method: Principal Component Analysis

FIGURE 13.2 SPSS printout, total variance explained in a PCA for 11 parenting items.

presents a summary table from a PCA factor extraction of the 11 parenting items. (The figure was produced within SPSS using Analyze ➔ Data Reduction ➔ Factor; PCA is the default method of extraction.) In this analysis, 11 factors (components) were extracted. The amount of total variance explained by each component is shown in column 2 (Total), which represents initial eigenvalues for each factor. Each variable in a factor analysis is standardized to have a mean of 0 and an *SD* (and variance) of 1.0. All of the variance in the 11 original items is accounted for by the 11 factors in PCA: if we summed the eigenvalues in column 2, the total would be 11.0. To compute the proportion of variance explained by a factor, the eigenvalue associated with the factor must be divided by 11.0. For the first factor in this example, 2.955 ÷ 11.0 = .26859; that is, 26.859% of the variance in the 11 items is accounted for by the first factor, as shown in column 3. Subsequent factors account for declining percentages of variance (e.g., 15.4% for factor 2). The final column indicates the cumulative percentage of variance explained by the factor for that row, plus all preceding factors. Thus, the first three factors account for just over 52% of the variance in the 11 variables. Cumulatively, the 11 factors account for 100% of the variance in the original variables.

Example of a principal components factor extraction:

Robbins, Wu, Sikorski, and Morley (2008) used the principal components extraction method in their factor analysis of items from two scales for middle-school youth—the Adolescent Physical Activity Perceived Benefits scale (10 items) and the Adolescent Physical Activity Perceived Barriers scale (9 items). For each scale, two factors were extracted.

Factor Extraction of Common Factor Variance

Other methods of factor extraction use a different measurement model—they assume that measurement error involves both a random component and a systematic component that is not unique to individual items. Consequently, only common factor variance is factor analyzed in these other extraction methods; unique variance is excluded.

> **TIP:** *Some authors restrict the term* factor analysis *to those approaches that factor analyze common factor variance. Controversy rages among statistical experts about whether PCA or common factor variance models are preferred, but they often lead to similar conclusions.*

The **principal factors (PF) method** of extraction (sometimes called **principal-axis factoring**) is similar to PCA, and is the most popular of the common factor extraction methods. The main difference is that in the PF method, estimates of the communalities, rather than 1s, are on the diagonal of the correlation matrix. The initial communality estimates are the squared multiple correlation coefficients for the specified variable, with all other variables in the correlation matrix as the predictors. R^2, as we have seen, is an index of shared variance among variables and thus is a reasonable proxy for common factor variance. The communalities are repeatedly re-estimated from the factor loadings in an iterative fashion until there are only negligible changes in the communality estimates. As with principal components, the goal of a PF extraction is to extract the largest possible amount of variance with successive factors.

Example of a principal axis factoring:

Looman and Farrag (2009) used principal axis extraction in their factor analysis of items in an Arabic translation of the Social Capital Scale, a measure of a person's investment in relationships. The scale was used in a study of parental social capital as a possible protective factor for child health. The researchers extracted four factors that accounted for 53% of the variance.

The **alpha factor method** assumes that the variables in a particular factor analysis are a sample from a hypothetical universe of potential variables. The main concern of alpha factoring is the reliability of the common factors. Cronbach's alpha is the most widely used index of the internal consistency reliability of a measure—we discuss this statistic later in this chapter. In alpha factoring, the communalities are estimated in an iterative process that maximizes coefficient alpha for the factors.

Another option is **maximum likelihood extraction,** which uses the estimation approach discussed in Chapter 12. This method estimates population values for the factor loadings through a process that maximizes the likelihood of yielding a sample with the observed correlation matrix from the population. Again, an iterative algorithm is used to arrive at the factor solution.

Other lesser-used methods of factor extraction include **image factoring, unweighted least squares (Minres) factoring,** and **generalized least squares factoring.** Although there may be sound substantive or methodologic reasons for preferring one method over another, it has typically been found that when there are a fairly large number of variables in the data set and a large sample of participants, differences in factor extraction solutions tend to be small.

Number of Factors to Extract

In performing a factor analysis, researchers make decisions about the number of factors to extract, rotate, and score. There are two competing goals in making the decision. The first is to maximize explained variance. The greater the number of factors, the greater the percentage of variance explained. We can see in Figure 13.2 that we can account for 100% of the variance in the 11 items by using 11 factors—but we would then have as many factors as variables, nullifying the value of the factor analysis. The competing goal is parsimony: The fewer the factors, the more parsimonious is the factor solution in describing the dimensionality of the data matrix. Yet, if too few factors are extracted, the proportion of explained variance might be inadequately low and important dimensions within the data set might go unidentified. If we used only the first factor in Figure 13.2, for example, we would account for only about 27% of the variance in the data set; moreover, by using only one factor we would miss a sizeable percentage of the variance that can be accounted for by the second factor (15%). The overall goal, then, is to explain as much variance as possible using the fewest factors as is reasonable.

Researchers' decisions about number of factors to use can be based on various criteria. The simplest method is to examine eigenvalues from an initial run with principal components extraction. A factor with an eigenvalue less than 1 is not valuable. An eigenvalue in PCA represents factor variance, and so an eigenvalue lower than 1.0 is less important in accounting for variance in a factor than an original variable, all of which have a variance of 1.0. According to this criterion—sometimes called the *Kaiser-Guttman rule*—we would conclude from Figure 13.2 that there should be three factors, because factors 1, 2, and 3 have eigenvalues greater than 1.0. SPSS uses this criterion as the default.

Scree Plot for Parenting Items

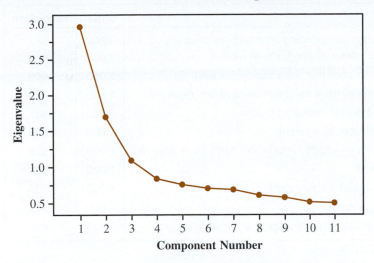

FIGURE 13.3   SPSS printout for a scree plot from a principal components analysis.

A second approach is to use a **scree test,** which plots successive eigenvalues for the factors. Figure 13.3 shows an SPSS-generated scree plot in which the eigenvalues from Figure 13.2 are graphed along the Y axis and the 11 factors are graphed along the X axis. Scree plots show declining values for the eigenvalues, consistent with the fact that each successive linear combination maximizes extracted variance. What we are looking for is a sharp discontinuity in the steep slope of the plot that separates the larger, more important factors from the smaller, less reliable factors. Expressed another way, you need to look for the point in the plot where a line drawn through the points sharply changes slope. In this example, an argument could be made that a break in the slope occurs between factors 3 and 4. This suggests again that three factors should be retained—although we can see that a two-factor solution also looks plausible.

Another criterion that is sometimes used is the proportion of variance accounted for by a factor. It has been argued that a factor is probably not important if it accounts for less than 5% of the total variance in a data matrix. In the output in Figure 13.2, nine factors meet the criterion of accounting for at least 5% of the variance—far too many factors to be useful in identifying underlying constructs and reducing the number of variables for analysis.

We can also look at the success of a three-factor solution in explaining variance in each of the original items by inspecting communalities. Figure 13.4 presents an SPSS printout (which we modified to show the wording of each of the 11 items) that shows communalities from a PCA analysis with three factors. In the column labeled Initial, the communalities are all 1s, because in PCA there are as many factors as variables, and so 100% of the variables' variability is accounted for initially by the 11 factors. When we reduce the number of factors to three, the amount of variance accounted for in each variable (its communality) is shown in the column labeled Extraction. The three factors account for a low of 38% of the variance for Item 2 (My child seems to have been harder to care for than most) to 71% of the variance for Item 9 (I am seldom annoyed or frustrated with my child). In a successful factor analysis, the communalities are large, and in this example they appear to be adequate with a three-factor solution.

A researcher's decision about the number of factors to retain and interpret is probably more critical than the decision about which factor extraction method to use.

Communalities

	Initial	Extraction
1. The best part of my day is when I'm spending time with my child.	1.000	.583
2. My child seems to have been harder to care for than most.	1.000	.379
3. There are many things my child does that really bother me a lot.	1.000	.449
4. I have given up more of my life to meet my child's needs than I expected.	1.000	.460
5. Even when tired or upset, I show my child a lot of love.	1.000	.587
6. I feel trapped by my responsibilities as a parent.	1.000	.429
7. Sometimes I lose patience with my child's attitude and don't listen anymore.	1.000	.528
8. I often feel angry with my child.	1.000	.588
9. I am seldom annoyed or frustrated with my child.	1.000	.707
10. I get a lot of joy out of being a mother.	1.000	.573
11. I've found that raising a child is much more work than pleasure.	1.000	.454

Extraction Method: Principal Component Analysis

FIGURE 13.4   SPSS printout for PCA, communalities for 11 parenting items with three extracted factors.

Yet, as we have seen in our example, different criteria can lead to different decisions. If the number of meaningful factors is not clearcut, it is usually advantageous to inspect more than one rotated factor matrix (which we discuss in the next section) to determine which solution is most sensible. It is better to begin with too many rather than too few factors, however, and to then "prune" if necessary.

> **TIP:** *Another method of deciding on number of factors involves an examination of the* **residual correlation matrix,** *which shows partial correlations between variables with the effects of the factors removed. The residual correlation matrix would be requested after a preliminary decision about number of factors has been made. If there are many sizeable residuals (coefficients greater than about .10), another factor may be desirable to account for more variance. Other decision-making strategies for number-of-factor decisions are discussed in Tabachnick and Fidell, 2007 (pp. 644–646).*

FACTOR ROTATION

Regardless of which factor extraction method is used, and regardless of how many factors are extracted, the resulting factor matrix is likely to be very difficult to interpret. For that reason, factor analysis involves a factor rotation phase that helps researchers to better understand the meaning of underlying factors. Factor rotation is performed for those factors that have met an acceptable inclusion criterion, as just described.

Factor rotation is not used to improve the quality of the mathematical fit between the variables and the factors. Rotated factors are mathematically equivalent to unrotated ones. Although factor loadings change after rotation, the communalities and percentage of variance explained remain the same. The objective with rotation is purely to improve the interpretive utility of the analysis.

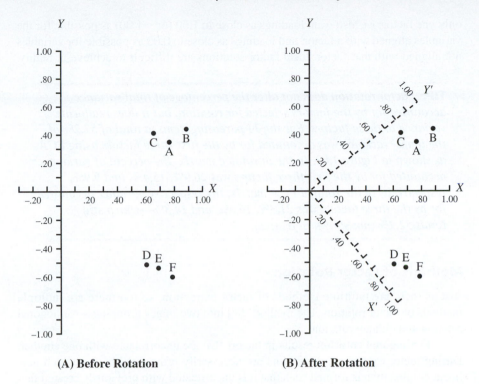

(A) Before Rotation   (B) After Rotation

FIGURE 13.5   Graphic representation of factor rotation.

Principles of Factor Rotation

Factor rotation is a conceptually complex process that can most readily be explained graphically for a situation in which there is a two-factor structure. We will use our earlier example of the six aptitude tests that yielded two factors—which we identified as verbal aptitude and quantitative aptitude—to illustrate factor rotation.

Figure 13.5 (A) shows a graph whose axes are labeled Y and X. These axes represent Factors I and II, respectively, as they are defined prior to rotation. The six dots in this two-dimensional space represent tests A through F. The unrotated factor loadings on the two factors can be read from the appropriate axis. Thus, for example, test A has a loading of about .38 on Factor I (the Y axis) and a loading of about .79 on Factor II (the X axis). As another example, test D has a loading of about −.50 on Factor I and .60 on Factor II. In this unrotated factor space, all six tests have high loadings (absolute values above .30) on both factors, making it difficult to identify their underlying dimensionality.

When the axes are rotated in such a way that the two variable clusters (A, B, and C versus D, E, and F) align more clearly with the reference axes, interpretability of the factors is enhanced. Figure 13.5 (B) shows the two axes—X′ and Y′—after rotation. With the axes turned, the factor loadings are different than they were prior to rotation. The loadings on the rotated factors are those shown in Table 13.1. For example, test A has a loading of .84 on Factor I after rotation, and a loading of .21 on Factor II. After rotation, tests A, B, and C are aligned with Factor I but not with Factor II, while tests D, E, and F are aligned with Factor II but not with Factor I. Now, by examining what tests A, B, and C have in common, and what tests D, E, and F have in common, we can infer the meaning of the factors.

The goal in rotating factors is to achieve factors that are as pure as possible. That is, we want a rotation solution such that variables have high loadings on one and only one factor; we also want loadings as close to 1.00 (or −1.00) as possible for the variables aligned with a factor, and loadings as close to 0.00 as possible for variables not aligned with that factor. Ideal factor solutions are difficult to achieve in reality.

TIP: *Factor rotation does not alter the percentage of total variance accounted for by the factors selected for rotation, but it does reallocate variance to those factors. For the 11 parenting items, a total of 52.2% of the items' variance was accounted for by the first three factors using PCA, as shown in Figure 13.2. In the unrotated matrix, the percent of variance accounted for by the first three factors was 26.9%, 15.4%, and 9.9%, respectively. In the rotated PCA matrix, the respective variance accounted for by the three factors was 21.3%, 16.6%, and 14.3%—which still totals 52.2% (not shown in figures).*

Methods of Factor Rotation

Just as there are multiple methods of factor extraction, so too there are multiple methods of factor rotation. The methods fall into two major groupings—orthogonal rotation and oblique rotation.

Orthogonal rotation results in factors that are uncorrelated with one another. During factor extraction, the factors are necessarily orthogonal because each new linear combination is formed such that it is uncorrelated with previously created factors. When factors are orthogonal they are at right angles—they are independent of one another. In Figure 13.5 (A), for example, the unrotated factors are orthogonal, and this orthogonality was maintained during rotation as shown in Figure 13.5 (B).

Oblique rotation, by contrast, results in factors that are correlated with one another. Oblique rotation allows the axes in the rotated factor space to depart from a 90° angle, thereby permitting the variables to be more closely aligned with factors. Figure 13.6 illustrates how an oblique rotation might look for the six aptitude tests. The X′ and Y′ axes are at an acute angle because they are allowed to line up more closely with the two variable clusters. Tests A, B, and C now have higher loadings on Factor I but lower loadings on Factor II than they did with orthogonal rotation. For example, test F has a loading of about .96 on Factor II, but a loading close to zero on Factor I; with orthogonal rotation, the loadings were .91 and .27, respectively.

Three major techniques, which use different statistical criteria, can be used for orthogonal rotation. The most widely used type of orthogonal rotation is **varimax rotation.** The goal of varimax rotation is to maximize the variance of the loadings within factors, across variables. The varimax method strives to minimize the number of variables that have high loadings on a factor, which facilitates interpretation. Another orthogonal method is **quartimax rotation,** which emphasizes the simplification of variables rather than factors. The goal of the quartimax method is to increase the dispersion of the loadings within the variables, across factors. **Equimax rotation** attempts to combine the goals of varimax and quartimax rotation—its goal is to simultaneously simplify factors and variables.

Example of a varimax rotation:

Yarcheski, Mahon, Yarcheski, and Hanks (2008) factor analyzed items from an existing scale that measures adolescents' interpersonal relationships, the Tilden Interpersonal Relationship Inventory. They extracted factors via PCA, and used

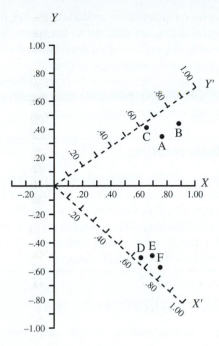

FIGURE 13.6 Oblique factor rotation.

varimax rotation. Their analysis confirmed two factors that are consistent with theories underlying the instrument—a social support factor and a conflict factor.

When oblique rotation is used, the method is usually one called **direct oblimin rotation;** another alternative in SPSS is **promax.** Oblique rotations result in both a **pattern matrix** and a **structure matrix.** A pattern matrix indicates partial regression coefficients between variables and factors, while the structure matrix indicates factor–variable correlations. With orthogonal rotation, the correlations and regression coefficients are identical, so only one factor matrix is needed to display the results. With oblique rotation, the two matrices are not the same because of correlations between factors. The pattern matrix is the one used to interpret factors. Oblique rotation also produces a **factor correlation matrix,** which displays the correlation coefficients for each factor with every other factor, like a correlation matrix.

> **TIP:** *When using direct oblimin rotation, users must specify a value for delta, which is an index that affects the amount of correlation between factors that you are willing to permit. The default for delta in SPSS is 0, which allows solutions to be moderately correlated. Negative values for delta result in nearly orthogonal rotations, while values near +1 can yield high correlations among rotated factors.*

There is some controversy regarding which rotation approach is preferable. Those who advocate the use of orthogonal rotation claim that it leads to greater theoretical clarity. The use of orthogonal rotation also makes it easier to compare factor structures across studies. Advocates of oblique rotation point out that in the real world, the underlying dimensions of a construct *are* usually correlated. For example, there is a tendency for people who have high scores on verbal aptitude tests to have higher-than-average scores on quantitative aptitude tests. Yet, oblique rotation sometimes results in peculiarities that are difficult to interpret. One approach is to use oblique rotation first and to inspect the factor correlation matrix. If the correlations are substantial, then orthogonal rotation might not make sense, but if the correlations are more modest (e.g., all under .30), then orthogonal rotation should probably be pursued. In any event, with a good, factorable data matrix, conclusions are often similar regardless of which method of rotation is used.

Example of an oblique rotation:

Maposa and Smithbattle (2008) evaluated the grandparents' version of the Grandparent Support Scale for Teenage Mothers, originally a 19-item scale to assess perceptions of grandparental actions that support or imperil a teenage mothers' care of her baby. Principal axis factoring with oblique rotation yielded two conceptually clear factors (responsive family relationships and adversarial family relationships), but resulted in the elimination of 5 of the 19 items.

INTERPRETING AND REFINING FACTORS

Once decisions about extraction method, number of factors, and rotation method have been made, the factor analysis program will produce results that require interpretation—and, often, results that suggest the need to test alternatives to help refine the factor solution.

Interpreting Rotated Factor Matrices

When orthogonal rotation is used, the rotated factor loadings are correlations between the variables and the factors. These loadings, when squared, indicate the amount of variance in a variable that is accounted for by the factor. Variables with high loadings on a factor, then, are the ones that need to be scrutinized to help identify the underlying dimension represented by the factor.

Usually loadings with an absolute value of .30 or greater are considered sufficiently large to attach meaning to them—although .40 is sometimes suggested as the cutoff value. The higher the loading, the better the variable is in capturing the essence of the factor. Loadings in excess of .70 (which means that there is at least 50% overlapping variance between the variable and the factor) are especially desirable for interpretive purposes. Ideally, there will be at least one **marker variable** in each factor. A marker variable is one that is highly correlated with one and only one factor and hence helps to define the nature of the factor. Marker variables tend to be robust—that is, they tend to load on a factor regardless of the method used to extract and rotate factors.

> **TIP:** *The process is similar for oblique rotation, although interpretation of the coefficients is less straightforward. The loading in the pattern matrix is not a correlation, but rather an index of the unique relationship between the variable and the factor (i.e., a partial regression coefficient). The coefficients in the structure matrix are correlations between variables and factors, but they are inflated by the overlap between factors. For example, a variable may correlate with one factor through its correlation with another related factor, rather than directly. For this reason, the pattern matrix is usually more interpretable than the structure matrix.*

Rotated Component Matrix[a]

	Component		
	1	2	3
4. Given up more of my life for child's needs than expected	.658		
11. Raising a child more work than pleasure	.649		
3. Many things child does bother me a lot	.618		
6. I feel trapped by responsibilities as parent	.600		
2. Child seems harder to care for than most	.586		
5. Even when tired/upset, I show child a lot of love		.764	
10. I get a lot of joy out of being a mother		.753	
1. Best part of my day spending time w/child		.748	
9. Seldom annoyed or frustrated with child			.839
8. I often feel angry with child	.380		.645
7. Sometimes lose patience w/child, don't listen	.491		.509

Extraction Method: Principal Component Analysis
Rotation Method: Varimax with Kaiser Normalization
[a]Rotation converged in five iterations.

FIGURE 13.7 SPSS printout for rotated orthogonal factor matrix: PCA with three factors.

To illustrate the interpretive process, let us assume we factor analyzed the 11 parenting items with a principal components extraction and orthogonal (varimax) rotation of three factors. SPSS output for the resulting rotated component matrix is shown in Figure 13.7. For this output, we instructed SPSS to list the items in descending order of factor loading magnitude, and to suppress printing factor loadings less than .30 so that interpretation would be easier.

The results in Figure 13.7 are far from ideal, because two items (8 and 7) have loadings greater than .30 on Factor I *and* Factor III. Yet we can begin to glean a sense of the meaning of the underlying constructs from this output. Five variables (items 4, 11, 3, 6, and 2) have high loadings on Factor I alone, and these items seem to capture something we might call *parenting stress*. For example, the item with the highest loading (.66) is item 4: "I have given up more of my life to meet my child's needs than I ever expected." Even the two items with loadings greater than .30 both on Factors I and III have content suggesting the stressful nature of the parenting role (e.g., item 8, "I often feel angry").

TIP: *When an item loads highly on two factors, researchers must decide what to do. Some researchers assign an item to one factor versus the other if the difference in loadings is at least .20 higher on the factor to which it will be assigned. In our example, this criterion would not be met for item 7 ("lose patience")—the two loadings are of similar magnitude.*

Three variables have loadings with absolute values greater than .30 on Factor II: items 5, 10, and 1. The main thrust of these items appears to concern *parental enjoyment*. For example, the item with the highest loading (.76) is item 5: "Even when I'm tired or upset I show my child a lot of love."

Three items have high loadings on Factor III: items 9, 8, and 7. This factor is more difficult to interpret, but the apparent marker variable is item 9, which has a loading of .839: "I am seldom annoyed or frustrated with my child." The other two items concern feeling angry and losing patience with the child. Perhaps these items capture a more severe level of parent–child conflict than is captured by the first factor—but this interpretation needs further exploration.

Evaluating and Refining the Analysis

If all three factors were similar to Factor II in the initial analysis—that is, if all three factors had three or more variables that clearly and strongly loaded on a single factor—we might stop at this point and conclude that we had achieved a good solution. However, given the results in Figure 13.7, it is prudent to explore other solutions. This means trying alternative methods of extraction and rotation, and examining the results with different numbers of factors. In such situations, researchers take steps to evaluate which solution yields the most parsimonious and interpretable results, or that is most consistent with an underlying theory.

In our example of 11 parenting items, the original factor solution is problematic because of multiple high loadings for two items and a strained interpretation of the third factor. We will describe efforts to achieve the best possible factor solution with our data, but steps are not necessarily in a fixed order for every problem—and we could have proceeded somewhat differently as well. Pett and colleagues (2003) offer good suggestions for proceeding with refinement of factors.

STEP 1: ALTERNATIVE FACTOR ROTATION   One possible explanation for the high loadings on multiple factors is that orthogonal rotation imposed unrealistic constraints on the ability of the two items in question (7 and 8) to clearly align with one factor. Thus, we began our exploration by rerunning the factor analysis as a PCA with direct oblimin rotation, with delta set to 0. We do not show the item-factor results because they look very similar to those obtained with orthogonal rotation: Items 7 and 8 loaded highly on both Factors I and III, for example, and the highest loading on Factor III was for item 9 ("seldom annoyed"). Moreover, we learned that the three factors, when allowed to deviate from a 90° angle, were not highly correlated with each other, as shown in Figure 13.8. The highest correlation (.23) was between Factors I and III. Thus, it does not appear that oblique rotation provides a more interpretable solution than orthogonal rotation.

STEP 2: ALTERNATIVE FACTOR EXTRACTIONS   Our next step was to explore methods of analyzing common factor variance, using different methods of factor

Component Correlation Matrix

Component	1	2	3
1	1.000	−.089	.234
2	−.089	1.000	−.112
3	.234	−.112	1.000

Extraction Method: Principal Component Analysis.
Rotation Method: Oblimin with Kaiser Normalization.

FIGURE 13.8   SPSS printout for PCA component correlation matrix for oblique rotation.

TABLE 13.2 Summary of Total Variance Explained After Extraction, Alternative Methods of Factor Extraction

Method	Sum of Squared Loadings (Eigenvalues)			Percent of Variance Explained		
	Factor I	Factor II	Factor III	Factor I	Factor II	Factor III
Principal Components	2.96	1.69	1.09	26.9	15.4	9.9
Principal Axis	2.32	1.06	.39	21.2	9.6	3.5
Maximum Likelihood	2.32	1.06	.39	21.0	9.6	3.6
Alpha	2.30	1.07	.40	20.9	9.7	3.6
Unweighted Least Squares	2.31	1.06	.39	21.1	9.6	3.5

extraction. We tried four different methods (principal axis, maximum likelihood, alpha, and unweighted least squares), and found substantial similarities among these extraction methods—but some noteworthy differences between them and PCA. Consider the information in Table 13.2, which summarizes total variance explained in the three factors whose eigenvalues were initially greater than 1, for all five factor extraction methods. Note that the top row, for PCA, is a recap of what is shown in Figure 13.2. The three factors explain less variance in the four common factor methods than in PCA—and that is to be expected because these methods ignore specific and error variance. Of particular note in this table is that Factor III accounts for under 5% of explained variance with the common factor methods, and in each case the eigenvalues (sum of the squared loadings) on this factor has sharply declined to .39.

Another important difference between PCA and the common factor methods concerned item communalities. In PCA, we found that the item with the highest communality was item 9 ("seldom annoyed"), with a communality of .707 (Figure 13.4.). Yet this variable had the *lowest* communality in the four common factor methods (not shown in figure). For example, its communality in the principal axis extraction method was only .124. This, in turn, made us suspicious of item 9—and also of Factor III. Factor III barely met the criterion for a higher-than-1 eigenvalue even in PCA (1.09), and performed weakly in the other extraction methods. These observations led us to our next set of analyses.

STEP 3: ALTERNATIVE NUMBER OF FACTORS We next examined two-factor solutions using both PCA and principal axis factoring with orthogonal rotation. Figure 13.9 shows the SPSS printout for the rotated factor matrix from the principal axis analysis. The results are more clearcut than they were previously. Seven items had high loadings on Factor I and three items had high loadings on Factor II. We can more clearly see that the first factor suggests a construct of *parenting stress* (or *parenting frustrations)* and Factor II suggests a construct of *parental enjoyment.* The item that we previously identified as potentially problematic (item 9, "seldom annoyed or frustrated") did not have high loadings on either factor.

This analysis suggests discarding item 9. Let us explore a bit further to find out what might be wrong with this item. If we think about the content of item 9, we might be surprised that it was not associated with Factor I, because it concerns frustrations

Rotated Factor Matrix[a]

	Factor 1	Factor 2
7. Sometimes lose patience w/child, don't listen	.623	
8. I often feel angry with child	.584	
3. Many things child does bother me a lot	.581	
6. I feel trapped by responsibilities as parent	.551	
2. Child seems harder to care for than most	.505	
4. Given up more of my life for child's needs than expected	.465	
11. Raising a child more work than pleasure	.397	
9. Seldom annoyed or frustrated with child		
1. Best part of my day spending time w/child		.633
5. Even when tired/upset, I show child a lot of love		.620
10. I get a lot of joy out of being a mother		.569

Extraction Method: Principal Axis Factoring.
Rotation Method: Varimax with Kaiser Normalization.
[a]Rotation converged in 3 iterations.

FIGURE 13.9 SPSS printout for rotated orthogonal factor matrix: principal axis factoring with two factors.

of parenthood—or rather, the *absence* of frustrations. We might expect the item to load on Factor I with a negative sign. For example, mothers who agree that they are *seldom* annoyed or frustrated with their child should be less likely to agree that are *often* angry with their child—these two items suggest opposite parental responses to a child. Yet, when we look at the loadings on the original Factor III in Figure 13.7, we see that the loadings for both items are in the same direction.

If we had paid closer attention to the correlation coefficients in the original matrix during the stage of evaluating factorability, we might have had early suspicions of problems with item 9. The correlations between this item and the other 10 items were all fairly low, ranging from −.02 to .32. The strongest correlation was, in fact, between "seldom annoyed" and "often angry." What could this positive correlation (.32) mean? We suspect that many respondents had conceptual difficulties with item 9—perhaps they did not see the word *seldom,* did not comprehend it, or, more likely, did not understand how to correctly respond on a "not-at-all true" to "completely true" scale to an item with a time-referencing qualifier such as "seldom." In fact, all three items in Factor III have such a qualifier—"often" in item 8 and "sometimes" in item 7. In the parlance of factor analysts, we could call the original Factor III a **method factor**—that is, a factor that captures a methodologic construct and not a substantive one. In this instance, it seems likely that this *method factor* relates to some confusion about integrating a time dimension with a true–false dimension, and that the confusion was especially acute with regard to *seldom,* a word that is not especially colloquial.

When item 9 is removed from the factor analysis, the final rotated factor matrix for the remaining 10 items with a two-factor solution looks very much like Figure 13.9, with only minor changes in loadings. The percent of variance accounted for by the two factors actually increases somewhat with item 9 removed, with two factors explaining 45.5% of the initial variance rather than 42.3%. Still, we would ideally want our factors to account for more variation in item responses. We may wish to pursue a path of further scale development—for example, adding more items with content on parental enjoyment to strengthen the second factor. Further evaluation of the two factors for use in subsequent analysis involves an assessment of internal consistency, which we describe in a later section.

Factor Scores

Researchers typically use the information from a factor analysis to create new variables. One approach is to create factor scores, which are the participants' scores on the abstract dimension defined by a factor. Factor scores are estimates of the scores participants would have received if it were possible to measure the constructs directly.

Factor scores can be obtained through factor analysis programs. Researchers who are using factor analysis results immediately as part of a substantive study (rather than as a methodological study focused on scale development) can instruct the computer to create new factor score variables for each study participant, and these variables can then be used as independent or dependent variables.

SPSS offers three methods for calculating factor scores, but they all involve assigning weights to items, multiplying the weight times the original value on each item in the factor analysis for the particular participant, and then summing to arrive at a composite score. The three methods are *regression, Anderson-Rubin,* and *Bartlett,* each of which uses somewhat different methods of solving for the factor scores. All three methods, however, result in factor scores that are standardized—that is, they all have means of 0.0 and *SD*s of 1.0. If PCA was used as the factor extraction method, all three methods yield the same factor scores—and PCA has the advantage of calculating exact scores, rather than estimates. The regression approach to estimating factor scores is perhaps the most widely used method because it results in the highest possible correlation between factors and factor scores.

In a more typical scenario, researchers use factor analysis as a tool for creating or testing multi-item scales that capture important constructs. In such situations, researchers want to measure the constructs using a method that can be replicated by others with different samples of participants. A widely used method is to create composite scales using only those items with high loadings on the factor. For example, a Parental Stress scale score would involve adding together responses to items 2, 3, 4, 6, 7, 8, and 11, which are the items with high loadings on Factor I (Figure 13.9). A Parental Enjoyment scale could be created by adding responses to items 1, 5, and 10.

If this method is adopted, attention needs to be paid to the sign of the loadings: Items with negative loadings should be reversed prior to addition. **Item reversals** can be accomplished by the following:

- If the minimum score on the item is 1 (for example, 1 = *strongly agree*, 7 = *strongly disagree*), subtract the raw score from the maximum score plus 1.
- If the minimum score on the item is 0 (for example, 0 = *not at all true* to 10 = *completely true*), subtract the raw score from the maximum score.

We did not have any negative loadings in our parenting items, but if (for example) item 11 had said that "Raising a child is more *pleasure* than *work*" (rather than "more *work* than *pleasure*") and its loading on Factor I was negative, we would need to reverse-score item 11 before summing items to calculate a total Parenting Stress score. In this example item responses were on a 0-to-10 scale, so we would subtract each original score from 10 to reverse the scoring on item 11. A person who responded 0 originally would have a score of 10 after reversal. Reverse scoring helps to ensure that all items are contributing properly to the value of the score on the construct.

INTERNAL CONSISTENCY RELIABILITY ANALYSIS

Almost invariably, researchers who perform factor analysis to create composite scales also perform a reliability analysis. And, many researchers who are simply using an existing scale to measure a construct of substantive interest also compute reliability coefficients to assess the quality of their measures. There are many different approaches to a reliability analysis (Polit and Beck, 2008; Waltz, Strickland, and Lenz, 2005), but the approach most often used to assess reliability of a multi-item scale is an evaluation of its **internal consistency reliability.**

Basic Concepts of Reliability

In an ideal world, the instruments that researchers use to measure abstract constructs would capture perfectly the variables of interest—that is, actual measurements would yield participants' **true scores** on the target constructs. In reality, virtually all scores contain **errors of measurement.** Measurement errors can occur if, for example, people complete a scale haphazardly, misrepresent their opinions, misinterpret the questions (as, perhaps, with the "seldom annoyed" item in our factor analysis example), and so on. A person's actual score on a scale is the difference between the hypothetical true score and errors of measurement.

In multi-item scales, measurement error often occurs because of inadequacies in the sample of items used in the scale. Just as larger samples tend to be more representative of a population than smaller ones, so do longer scales (those with more items) tend to be more "representative" of a hypothetical universe of all potential items measuring a construct than shorter scales. Internal consistency reliability relates to the issue of sampling adequacy of the items forming a composite scale. Indexes of internal consistency estimate the extent to which different subparts of an instrument (i.e., items) are reliably measuring the critical attribute—the extent to which items are *converging on* the underlying construct. The stronger the reliability, the stronger is the correlation between obtained scores and true scores.

Cronbach's Alpha

There are different approaches to measuring internal consistency reliability, but the most widely used method is to compute an index called **Cronbach's alpha** (or *coefficient alpha*). Like many of the statistics discussed in this book, Cronbach's alpha focuses on variability—in this case, variability of both individual items and composite scale scores. A conceptual formula for Cronbach's alpha is as follows:

$$\alpha = \frac{k}{k - 1}\left[1 - \frac{\Sigma \text{ Item variances}}{\text{Scale variance}}\right]$$

where α = Cronbach's alpha
k = number of items

The normal range of values for coefficient alpha is between .00 and +1.00. Higher values reflect better internal consistency. If you constructed a scale from random questions, you would get an alpha close to 0. If the variance of the scale is much larger than the sum of item variances—which occurs when the items are measuring the same construct and are correlated—alpha is closer to 1.0.

TIP: *Alpha coefficients are typically computed from raw item scores, but SPSS also computes a coefficient called* standardized alpha. *This coefficient is computed by first standardizing individual items to have a mean of 0 and a variance of 1. Regular and standardized alpha values usually are similar.*

For group-level comparisons, coefficients in the vicinity of .70 to .75 may be adequate (especially at the subscale level), but coefficients of .80 or greater are highly desirable. Reliability coefficients are important indicators of an instrument's quality, and high reliability is critical to success in hypothesis testing. Unreliable measures reduce statistical power and hence increase the risk of Type II errors. If data fail to support a hypothesis, one possibility is that the instruments were unreliable—not necessarily that the hypothesized relationships do not exist.

Alpha is an estimate of how much "true score" versus "error" is in the scale. In fact, we can go further and say that alpha can be directly interpreted as the proportion of true variability to total variability in scores. If, for example, coefficient alpha were .85, then 85% of the variability in obtained scores would represent true individual differences on the underlying construct, and 15% of the variability would reflect random, extraneous fluctuations. Looked at in this way, it should be clearer why scales with low internal consistency are risky to use.

Diagnostic Information in Reliability Analysis

When reliability analysis is done by computer, as it almost always is, programs provide not only the value for coefficient alpha, but also information that can be used to further understand and refine scales. In this section, we will look at some SPSS output for a reliability analysis of the parenting items used in the factor analysis example described earlier in this chapter.

The SPSS reliability program offers options for many descriptive statistics, for both items and scales. For example, item and scale means and standard deviations can be calculated, and a correlation matrix for all items can be produced. An informative piece of descriptive information is the mean of all interitem correlation coefficients. If the items are all measuring the same construct, this value should be moderate. The mean interitem correlation for the seven items on the Parenting Stress scale was .283, and the mean interitem correlation for the three items on the Parental Enjoyment scale was .366 (not shown in figures).

The reliability analysis for these two scales indicated that coefficient alpha was .725 for Parenting Stress and .632 for Parental Enjoyment. Reliability for the Parenting Stress scale is marginally acceptable, but the three-item Parental Enjoyment scale would be risky to use. Even though the average interitem correlations for this scale was reasonably high (.366), it is difficult to achieve good reliability on a scale with only three items. The reliability of this scale needs to be improved, and it should be fairly easy to do so by adding more items with relevant content.

Information that is especially interesting in a reliability analysis is the item-total statistics—that is, information about how each item relates to the total scale. For the full seven-item Parenting Stress scale, the mean scale score was 25.85 with a variance of 225.50. Figure 13.10 presents the SPSS printout for the item-total statistics for these seven items. (We used the SPSS commands Analyze ➔ Scale ➔

Reliability

Scale: Parenting Stress

Item-Total Statistics

	Scale Mean if Item Deleted	Scale Variance if Item Deleted	Corrected Item-Total Correlation	Squared Multiple Correlation	Cronbach's Alpha if Item Deleted
2. Child seems harder to care for than most	23.1736	174.797	.424	.204	.696
3. Many things child does bother me a lot	22.1851	169.455	.494	.279	.679
4. Given up more of my life for child's needs than expected	19.9471	170.726	.385	.159	.708
6. I feel trapped by responsibilities as parent	22.9041	167.522	.478	.250	.683
7. Sometimes lose patience w/child, don't listen	23.0116	173.455	.502	.313	.679
8. I often feel angry with child	23.8298	184.924	.461	.272	.692
11. Raising a child more work than pleasure	20.0198	171.979	.360	.134	.715

FIGURE 13.10 SPSS printout for reliability analysis, parenting stress items: item-total statistics.

Reliability Analysis to obtain this printout.) In this figure, the second and third column show what the scale mean and variance would be, respectively, if each item listed in column 1 were removed from the scale. The column labeled "Corrected Item-Total Correlation" presents the Pearson's r between scores on the item in the specified row and scores on the scale with the item removed. We can see that item 11 ("more work than pleasure") has the lowest item-total correlation (.360) and item 7 ("lose patience") has the highest (.502). Items that are good measures of the underlying construct should be highly correlated with the other measures, so if any of these correlations are very low, they may be good candidates to drop from the scale.

The next column ("Squared Multiple Correlation") presents additional diagnostic information about individual items. This column shows values of R^2 that are obtained when scores on each item are "predicted" from scores on all the other items. If items are capturing the same underlying construct as all the other items on the scale, this should be reflected in high values of R^2. In this example, item 11 has a relatively low value (.134), whereas item 7 has a much stronger value (.313). This pattern is consistent with the information in the previous column.

The final column is of particular interest. It presents values for what Cronbach's alpha would be if each item were deleted. For the seven-item scale, alpha was .73 (standardized alpha was also .73). Removal of *any* item would reduce alpha—for example, removal of item 2 ("child harder to care for than most") from the scale would reduce alpha from .73 to .696. Removal of item 11—the item that appears to be making the smallest contribution based on other diagnostics—would reduce alpha to .715. Researchers creating new scales for general use sometimes are willing to make small sacrifices in reduced reliability (e.g., from .73 to .72) to create a less burdensome scale. And, if the reliability analysis reveals that alpha would *increase* by discarding an item—which sometimes happens—then researchers may opt for the smaller set of items. This decision would not necessarily be a good one, though, if the scale was a widely used measure and comparisons of scale means across studies were desired.

Example of a reliability analysis:

Moser and colleagues (2009) tested the psychometric properties of an existing scale of perceived control (the Control Attitudes Scale-Revised or CAS-R) with three groups of patients with cardiac illness. Cronbach's alpha values on the eight-item CAS-R ranged from .72 in the acute myocardial infarction group to .76 in the heart failure group. The corrected item-total correlation coefficients were greater than .30 for all items, in all three patient groups.

RESEARCH APPLICATIONS OF FACTOR ANALYSIS

Factor analysis, once considered a sophisticated technique used primarily by highly experienced investigators, has come to be an analytic tool used by many researchers. Reliability analysis is even more widely used—indeed, most researchers who use multi-item scales to measure variables of interest report psychometric information from instrument development work, and also compute Cronbach's alpha with their own study data. This section focuses on major applications of factor analysis and discusses methods of reporting factor analytic and reliability results.

The Uses of Factor Analysis

Factor analysis is an important methodological and substantive tool. Although factor analysis requires researchers to make many decisions and involves some subjectivity in the decision-making and factor-interpretation process, it is an important approach to understanding and measuring constructs.

1. *Data reduction* If a researcher has multiple measures of key variables (often the dependent variables), factor analysis is a good way to streamline the primary analyses. Our earlier example of six aptitude tests that yielded two strong factors illustrates this data reduction application of factor analysis.
2. *Instrument development* A primary application of factor analysis is to develop instruments to measure constructs of interest to researchers or clinicians. Researchers often begin with a large pool of items that are derived on the basis of theory, adaptations from other instruments, or in-depth interviews. Typically, items are then reviewed by experts who evaluate the items' *content validity*, and items remaining after this review are administered to a sample of respondents. Responses are then factor analyzed to assess which items should be used to create summated scales. After appropriate psychometric analyses are performed, the scales are generally used by other researchers in subsequent investigations of the constructs.
3. *Instrument validation* Factor analysis has come to be used frequently as a method of construct validation—that is, of evaluating the extent to which the factors revealed by the factor analysis correspond to a hypothesized dimensionality of the construct. Of course, other methods of construct validation are important, but factor analysis can lend supporting evidence about the

instrument's correspondence to latent variables underlying the items. (Confirmatory factor analysis, not discussed in this book, is increasingly used for this purpose.) Factor analysis can also be used to validate previously developed instruments. This often involves factor analytic comparisons—for example, the cross-validation of a factor structure in a replication study or a confirmatory study to ascertain that the factor structure of an instrument is appropriate for different groups than the group used to develop the instrument.

The Presentation of Factor Analysis in Research Reports

When reporting the results of a factor analysis, researchers need to communicate not only the results, but also the decisions that produced them. The following aspects of the analytic procedures usually should be documented in the text of the report:

- The variables in the analysis
- The number of participants in the sample
- Any limitations that might exist and how they were addressed (outliers, missing data problems, low intervariable correlations)
- Information on sampling adequacy
- Method used to extract factors (and a rationale if an uncommon method was used)
- Criteria used to determine the number of factors
- Method used to rotate factors, and rationale for that decision
- Alternative methods of extraction and rotation that were explored
- Minimum value of loadings used to interpret factors
- Items that were deleted and the rationale for those decisions
- Method used to create factor scores, if applicable

Tables are used to summarize key results of the final factor analysis—most often, the rotated factor matrix (or, the pattern matrix for oblique rotations). The table typically lists the items, and specifies the number of factors, factor loadings, and number of cases in the analysis, at a minimum. Some researchers also present percentages of variance explained by each factor, eigenvalues, and communalities. Tables are often omitted if the factor analysis yields one strong factor.

We will use results from a factor analysis of 20 items that measure children's positive behaviors (from a real dataset) to illustrate a factor analysis presentation. Table 13.3 lists the 20 positive behavior items in the order that facilitates interpretation of the factors—not in the order items were presented to respondents. Most tables use a convention to highlight important loadings, which are usually presented to two decimal places. Here, we have bolded loadings that are greater than .40. Some authors underline important loadings, some completely omit loadings below a cutoff value (as in the SPSS printout in Figure 13.7), and others still use boxes to surround a cluster of variables loading highly on a factor. The point is to use a method that will help readers understand the basis for interpreting the factor.

The text is used to summarize methodologic decisions, to highlight the important features of the analysis, and to offer the researcher's interpretation of the factors. Here is an illustration of how the results from the factor analysis in Table 13.3 might be described in the text:

> The 20 Positive Behavior items were factor analyzed with a sample of 575 mothers, using principal components analysis for factor extraction. Preliminary analysis indicated moderately high factorability—Bartlett's test was significant at $p < .001$ and the overall value of the Kaiser-Meyer-Olkin test was .81.

TABLE 13.3 Example of a Factor Analysis Table for a Report

Variable: My Child . . .	Factor Loadings			Communality
	1	2	3	(h^2)
Is obedient, follows rules	**.76**	.32	.13	.69
Is patient if I am busy	**.73**	.05	.19	.58
Is calm, easy-going	**.70**	.39	.01	.65
Sticks with an activity	**.68**	.06	.32	.57
Is not impulsive	**.66**	.06	.08	.44
Does what I tell him/her	**.65**	.29	.17	.54
Waits his/her turn	**.61**	.32	.08	.48
Is eager to please	**.60**	.32	.23	.52
Is able to concentrate	**.53**	.28	.29	.44
Tends to give, lend, share	**.52**	.39	.18	.46
Is warm, loving	.25	**.78**	.05	.67
Is cheerful, happy	.29	**.68**	.10	.55
Is curious, exploring	.00	**.66**	.32	.54
Is helpful, cooperative	**.40**	**.58**	.30	.57
Is well-liked by children	.37	**.55**	.28	.52
Shows concern for others	.31	**.55**	.30	.48
Tries to be independent	.16	.19	**.81**	.72
Is self-reliant	.09	**.40**	**.69**	.64
Is self-assertive	.23	.06	**.67**	.51
Can find things to do on own	.23	.38	**.44**	.39
Eigenvalue	8.25	1.65	1.10	11.00
Percent of Variance Explained	41.3	8.3	5.5	55.1

NOTE: Varimax was used for factor rotation. All loadings greater than .40 are in bold.

Varimax Rotated Factor Matrix for Principle Components Analysis of 20 Positive Behavior Items for Children Ages 6–10 ($N = 575$)

Using a minimum eigenvalue of 1.0 as the extraction criterion for factors, three factors that accounted for a total of 55.1% of the variance were extracted. Communalities were fairly high, ranging from .39 to .69, as shown in Table 13.3. The three factors were orthogonally rotated using varimax. (Oblique rotation yielded virtually identical results and thus orthogonal rotation was retained because of conceptual simplicity and ease of description.) The items in Table 13.3 are ordered by size of loading to facilitate interpretation of the factor matrix.

Overall, the factor structure that emerged was reasonably clear and interpretable. The first factor, which accounted for 41.3% of the variance, had 11 items with loadings above the cutoff of .40. This factor appears to capture the child's ability to be disciplined, self-controlled, and obedient. We called this factor Self-Control. Ten of the 11 items had loadings in excess of .50 on the factor; only one ("my child is helpful, cooperative") also had a loading greater than .40 on another factor.

The second factor had seven items with loadings above .40, and six of these items had high loadings only on Factor 2. The theme of this factor involves the child's social interactions—his or her tendency to show warmth and concern for other people. We call this factor Social Competence.

Four items had high loadings on the third factor. Although this factor accounted for only 5.5% of the variance, it was relatively well defined, with a clear-cut marker variable that had a loading of .81. This factor captures a dimension of independence and self-reliance, and has been named Autonomy.

For subsequent analysis, factor scores were created by summing together scores on the items most clearly associated with the factors, with unit weighting. Thus, the sum of responses to the first block of 10 items formed scores on a Self-Control scale (Cronbach's alpha reliability = .88); the second block of six items was used to compute scores on a Social Competence scale (alpha = .86); and the third block of four items was used to compute scores on an Autonomy scale (alpha = .76).

This example illustrates a situation in which several items had fairly high loadings on more than one factor. In this case, these items were assigned to the factor (scale) with the highest factor loading.

Research Example

Detailed results from a factor analysis are most likely to be reported in the context of a methodological study focused on instrument development or instrument validation, as in this example.

Study: "Development of an instrument to assess perceived self-efficacy in the parents of infants" (Črnčec, Barnett, & Matthey, 2008).

Study Purpose: The purpose of this study was to examine the psychometric properties of a new 15-item scale to measure perceived parental self-efficacy among parents with infants—the Karitane Parenting Confidence Scale (KPCS).

Methods: The researchers administered the original 18 items to a sample of 187 Australian mothers of infants younger than 12 months of age. Response options for the 18 items of perceived parental self-efficacy were on a four-point scale of frequency: *Hardly ever, Not very often, Some of the time,* and *Most of the time.* Initial inspection of the items led the researchers to delete three items because of problems with score variability. The researchers also made an a priori decision to eliminate items if inter-item correlations exceeded .75, to avoid multicollinearity, but no items were excluded on that basis. Thus, 15 items (Table 13.4) were factor analyzed. The researchers indicated that there were no outliers, and that there were only four cases of missing item data. These missing values were replaced with item means. The factor analysis was deemed to have adequate sample size, with about 12.5 respondents per item.

Analysis: Principal components analysis was used to extract factors. There were four factors with eigenvalues greater than 1.0 in the original unrotated matrix. The researchers felt, however, that the scree test results supported a three-factor solution. After examining both three- and four-factor results, they found the three-factor results to be more interpretable. Varimax rotation was used to rotate the three factors.

Results: The three-factor solution explained 49.3% of the total variance in item responses. The large first factor explained 30.1% of the variance. Item communalities ranged from .36 to .67. Items were considered associated with factors if they had loadings of .40 or higher. Using this criterion, high loadings were found for eight items on Factor I, six items on Factor II, and two items on Factor III. One item ("confidence in establishing a sleep routine") had a loading greater than .40 on Factors I and II, but it was retained on Factor I, on which it had the higher loading, because of its "critical face validity" (p. 488). The researchers interpreted Factor I as the *Perceptions of parenting ability* subscale, Factor II as the *Perceived parenting support* subscale, and Factor III as the *Perceptions of child development* subscale. The researchers felt justified in combining scores on the three subscales into a total scale score because there were moderately high correlations between scores on the three factors and total scores, ranging from .47 for Factor III to .91 for Factor I. Cronbach's alpha for the overall scale was .81, and subscale reliabilities ranged from .44 for Factor III to .80 for Factor I.

TABLE 13.4 Varimax-Rotated Loadings, Principal Components Analysis of the Karitane Parenting Confidence Scale Items (N = 187)

Item	Questionnaire Ordering	Factor[a]		
		I	II	III
I understand what it is my baby is trying to tell me.	(5)	.73		
I know what to do when my baby cries.	(4)	.72		
I can soothe my baby when he/she is distressed.	(6)	.68		
I can settle my baby.	(2)	.67		
If my baby has a cold or fever, I am confident about handling it.	(8)	.63		
I am confident about playing with my baby.	(7)	.61		
I am confident helping my baby establish a good sleep routine.	(3)	.50	.41	
I can make decisions about the care of my baby.	(11)	.47		
I feel sure people will be there when I need support.	(15)		.71	
I feel I am doing a good job as a mother.	(14)		.70	
I am sure my partner will be there for me when I need support.	(9)		.60	
Other people think I'm doing a good job as a mother.	(14)		.55	
Being a mother is very stressful for me (reverse scored).	(12)		.55	
I am confident that my baby is doing well.	(10)			.76
I am confident about feeding my baby.	(1)			.68
Percent of variance (Total = 49.3%)		30.1	11.1	8.1
Cronbach's alpha[b]		.80	.64	.44

[a]Factor I = Parenting; Factor II = Support; Factor III = Child Development

[b]Cronbach's alpha for overall scale = .81

Adapted from Table 4, Črnčec, Barnett, and Matthey (2008).

Summary Points

- **Factor analysis** is a statistical technique used to elucidate the underlying structure and dimensionality of a set of variables. By analyzing correlations among variables, factor analysis determines which variables cluster together to reveal unidimensional constructs.

- Mathematically, factor analysis creates **factors** that are linear combinations of variables. Factor analysis begins with **factor extraction,** which involves the extraction of as much variance as possible through the successive creation of linear combinations that are orthogonal to (uncorrelated with) previously created combinations.

- A widely used factor extraction procedure is the **principal components method,** an approach that analyzes *all* variance in the variables.

- Other methods of factor extraction, which analyze **common factor variance** (i.e., variance that is shared with other variables), include the **principal factors method**, the **alpha method**, and the **maximum likelihood method.**

- Various criteria can be used to decide how many factors account for a reliable amount of variance in the data set. One criterion is to use only factors with eigenvalues greater than 1.0. An **eigenvalue** is a standardized index of the amount of variance each factor extracts. Another approach is to use a **scree test** to identify sharp discontinuities in the eigenvalues for successive factors.

- Factor extraction results in a **factor matrix** that indicates, through the **factor loadings,** the relationship between original variables and the factors.

- Across factors, the sum of the squared loadings for a given variable indicate the variable's **communality** (shared variance). Across variables, the sum of squared loadings for a given factor is the factor's eigenvalue.

- The initial factor matrix is often difficult to interpret, and so most factor analyses involve **factor rotation.** Factor rotation moves the reference axes within the factor space such that variables more clearly align with a single factor.

- **Orthogonal rotation** keeps the reference axes at right angles and results in factors that are uncorrelated. Orthogonal rotation is usually performed through a method called **varimax,** but other methods (**quartimax** and **equimax**) are also available. The product of an orthogonal rotation is a **rotated factor matrix.**

- **Oblique rotation** allows the reference axes to rotate into acute or oblique angles, thereby resulting in correlated factors. When oblique rotation is used, there are two resulting matrices: a **pattern matrix** that indicates partial regression coefficients between variables and factors, and a **structure matrix** that indicates variable-factor correlations.

- Factors are interpreted by examining the pattern and magnitude of the factor loadings in the rotated factor matrix (orthogonal rotation) or pattern matrix (oblique rotation). With orthogonal rotation, the factor loadings, when squared, indicate the proportion of variance accounted for in the variable by the factor.

- Ideally, there is one or more **marker variable**—a variable with a very high loading on one and only one factor. Loadings of .30 and higher are usually sufficiently large to be meaningful in terms of interpreting the construct that the factor represents.

- Once a factor is interpreted and labeled, researchers can create **factor scores,** which are scores on the abstract dimension defined by the factor. A common scoring method is to sum the item values for all items attributed to the specified factor.

- The **internal consistency reliability** of multi-item scales, such as those developed based on factor analysis, is most often assessed through a statistic called **Cronbach's alpha,** which is a measure of how much **true score** is present in a composite scale score. **Errors of measurement** can occur for many reasons, but one persistent problem is the inadequate sampling of items to capture the underlying dimension. Alphas of at least .80 are desirable.

Exercises

The following exercises cover concepts presented in this chapter. Appendix C provides answers to Part A exercises that are indicated with a dagger (†). Exercises in Part B involve computer analyses using the datasets provided with this textbook, and answers and comments are offered on this book's Web site.

PART A EXERCISES

† **A1.** Using information from Figure 13.4 (PCA communalities) and Figure 13.7 (factor loadings for three factors), compute the absolute values of the loadings for items 7 and 8 on Factor II.

† **A2.** With regard to Figure 13.2, indicate the equation for Component 1 that yielded the percent of variance (26.86).

† **A3.** In Table 13.4, what are the eigenvalues for Factors I through III?

A4. In a PCA of eight items, assume initial eigenvalues were: 2.83, 2.08, 1.09, .80, .42, .36, .22 , .20. Graph these values on a scree plot. How many factors do you think should be extracted and rotated?

† **A5.** Suppose that a seventh test (Test G) was added to the factor analysis graphed in Figure 13.5. This test has the following coordinates on the unrotated axes: Y ($-.40$), X (.45). Plot this test on graph (B) of this figure. What would the coordinates be on the new (rotated) reference axes? Is it more likely that Test G is a measure of verbal aptitude (Factor I) or of quantitative aptitude (Factor II)?

A6. Comment on the researchers' decisions in the research example at the end of this chapter (Črnčec et al., 2008). What, if anything, would you recommend doing differently?

PART B EXERCISES

† **B1.** For these exercises, you will be using the SPSS dataset Polit2SetC. This file contains responses to individual items on the Center for Epidemiologic Studies—Depression (CES-D) Scale. This scale presents respondents with 20 statements about their mood and feelings. They are asked to rate each item for its frequency in the prior week on the following scale: 1 (*rarely or never—less than 1 day*), 2 (*some or a little—1–2 days*), 3 (*occasionally or a moderate amount—3–4 days*), or 4 (*most or all—5–7 days*). The CES-D has been used in thousands of studies, and has undergone rigorous psychometric testing. Still, it is worthwhile to assess its dimensionality and psychometric adequacy for a population of low income minority women. Let us begin by running basic frequency information. In the file, you will find that there are 24 CESD items because four items (item 4, 8, 12, and 16) are worded positively (e.g., "I was happy,"), and so to consistently measure depression these items have to be reverse scored. We have done this for you. Run basic descriptives for the 24 variables (starting at *cesd1* and ending at *cesd20*) and

then answer the following questions: (a) Were there any items that did *not* have a full range of responses, from 1 to 4? Were there any outliers? (b) What was the range of missing data for individual items? (c) Comment on the similarity or differences in means and *SD*s across items. (d) Examine the frequency distribution information for item 4 and item 4 reversed. Does it appear that the reversal was done properly? (Note: If you will be doing the exercises in Chapter 14 on Missing Values, keep the output from this exercise for later reference.)

† **B2.** Before performing a factor analysis, do a reliability analysis for the entire 20-item scale. Click Analyze ➔ Scale ➔ Reliability Analysis. Move the 16 negatively worded CESD items and the four *reverse-coded items* into field for items. Click the Statistics pushbutton and in the next dialog box, click Descriptives for all three options (Item, Scale, Scale if Item Deleted); Inter-Item Correlations; and Summaries for Means, Variances, and Correlations. Click Continue, then OK, then answer these questions: (a) How many cases were in this analysis? Why do you think the number is so low? (b) For the 20-item CES-D scale, what is the value of Cronbach's alpha? Does this indicate adequate internal consistency? (c) What was the range of correlation coefficients between pairs of items on the CES-D? Does something about this range seem puzzling? Between which pairs of items are the correlations highest and lowest in value? (d) What was the mean inter-item correlation? (e) In the panel for Item-Total Statistics, which item had the strongest corrected item-total correlation? Which had the weakest? (f) Which item had the strongest (and weakest) squared multiple correlation? (g) Would the value of Cronbach's alpha increase if any items were deleted—and, if so, which items and by how much?

† **B3.** In this exercise, you will undertake a principal components analysis of the CES-D items, using all 20 original items (no reversed items). Go to Analyze ➔ Data Reduction ➔ Factor Analysis. Select the 20 CES-D items, being careful not to select reversed items, and move them into the box for Variables. Click the Descriptives pushbutton and in the next dialog box select Univariate descriptives and Initial solution under Statistics; and KMO + Bartlett's test and Anti-image under Correlation Matrix. Click Continue and then on the original dialog click the Extraction pushbutton. In this dialog box, select Methods ➔ Principal Components; Analyze ➔ Correlation Matrix; Display ➔ Unrotated factor matrix and Scree plot; and Extract ➔ Eigenvalues over 1. Then click Continue and select Rotation from the original dialog box. Select Method ➔ Varimax and Display ➔ Rotated solution. Click Continue and then click the Options pushbutton. Select Missing values ➔ Delete listwise and, for Coefficient Display Format, select Sorted by Size and Suppress absolute values less then .30. Click Continue, then OK to run the analysis, and then answer the following questions: (a) What was the

value of the KMO measure of sampling adequacy for the entire set of items? What does this suggest about the factorability of the items? (b) Was Bartlett's test significant? (c) Look at the anti-image correlation matrix and inspect the measures of sampling adequacy (MSA) of individual items along the diagonal. What is the lowest value—and does this support a factor analysis? (d) In terms of communalities, how many items had extraction communalities exceeding .50? Which item had the highest communality, and which had the lowest? (e) How many factors were extracted in this PCA? What percentage of variance do these factors account for? What are the eigenvalues for the extracted factors? (f) Examine the scree plot. Does the plot suggest the same number of factors as were originally extracted? (g) Looking at the unrotated factor matrix (the Component Matrix), are there items with high loadings on more than one factor? (h) Interpret the rotated component matrix. What does the pattern of loadings suggest about the adequacy of the factor solution?

† **B4.** Now you will undertake a factor analysis of the CES-D items using principal axis factoring, two factors, and oblique rotation. Proceed with the same set of variables as in Exercise B3. You can remove some of the Descriptive options (e.g., no further need for the KMO test or inspection of the anti-image matrix). Click the Extraction push-button and in this dialog box, select Methods ➜ Principal axis factoring; Analyze ➜ Correlation matrix; Display (no options); and Extract ➜ Number of factors: **2**. Then click Continue and select Rotation in the original dialog box. Select Method ➜ Direct Oblimin; Delta ➜ 0; Display ➜ Rotated solution. Click Continue and run the analysis by clicking OK. Then answer the following questions: (a) In the pattern matrix, did any item have a loading greater than .30 on both factors? (b) How many items had loadings greater than .40 on Factor I and Factor II? Were there any items that did not load on *either* factor with a loading of at least .40? (c) What would you name the factors? (d) What is the correlation between the two factors? What does this suggest about orthogonal versus oblique rotation?

† **B5.** In this exercise, run a reliability analysis for each of the two factors from the previous exercise. In the first reliability analysis, use all 16 of the negatively worded items that had loadings greater than .30 on Factor I in Exercise B4. Then, do a second analysis for the four items that had loadings greater than .30 on Factor II (you can use either the original or reversed items, it will not make a difference because all items are scored in the same direction). Use the SPSS instructions from Exercise B2 to guide you in doing this analysis. Then answer the following questions: (a) For the 16 items on the first factor, what is the value of Cronbach's alpha? How does this compare to the value from Exercise B1? (b) Could alpha be increased by eliminating any of the 16 items? If yes, which one? (c) For the four items on the second factor, what is the value of Cronbach's alpha? Should a subscale such as this one be used to measure Positive Affect? (d) Could alpha be increased by eliminating any of the four items? If yes, which one? (e) What do these analyses suggest about researchers' use of the full CES-D scale with this population?

B6. Write up a description of the results of Exercises B4 and B5, creating a table appropriate for a research report. Remember to include some basic information about factorability from Exercise B3.

14

Missing Values

Basic Concepts for Handling Missing Values
Missing Data Problems
Factors to Consider in Designing a Missing
  Values Strategy
Patterns of Missing Data
Overview of Missing Values Strategies
Deletion Methods
Imputation Methods

Missing Values Processes
Strategies for Understanding Missing Values
Addressing Missing Values Problems
Reporting Missing Values Information
Research Example
Summary Points
Exercises

The problem of missing data is the bane of many nurse researchers' efforts to produce rigorous evidence for nursing practice. It is a rare study that has no missing data, and so it is a problem with which almost all nurse researchers must contend. Data values can be missing for any number of reasons—for example, when study participants skip over questions in a questionnaire, miss a data collection appointment, refuse to continue in a study, are unable to continue because of disability or death, or move away from the study area. In some cases, missing values arise because of equipment malfunction, data entry errors, or other research-related problems.

This chapter provides some preliminary guidance about missing data strategies. We acknowledge that some of the best and most sophisticated strategies are not fully described in this introductory statistical text-book, but we offer suggested readings for further guidance on this important topic.

BASIC CONCEPTS FOR HANDLING MISSING VALUES

There have probably been more conceptual and statistical advances regarding the treatment of missing data in the past 20 years than regarding any other analytic topic of relevance to healthcare research. Many of the advances have stemmed from the seminal work of Roderick Little and Donald Rubin, who published a second edition of their groundbreaking book on missing values in 2002. In this section we discuss why this topic is so important, and what factors need to be considered in addressing it.

Missing Data Problems

The recent heightened awareness of and attention to the topic of missing data is partly a reflection of the emerging focus on evidence-based practice: The quality of the evidence can be seriously compromised when there are values missing for some study participants. One way to think about the problems that are created when there are missing values is to consider the validity framework proposed by Campbell and Cook (Shadish, Cook, & Campbell, 2002). This framework of four key aspects of validity has been used for decades as a guide for evaluating the quality of research evidence, particularly evidence that has implications for causal inferences (Polit & Beck, 2008).

When there are missing values, it means that analyses are based on fewer study participants than were in the full study sample. This, in turn, means less statistical power, which can undermine *statistical conclusion validity*—the degree to which the statistical results are accurate. Missing data can also affect *internal validity*—the degree to which inferences about the causal effect of the independent variable on the dependent variable are warranted. For example, if the most severely ill participants drop out of an experimental group at a higher rate than control group members because the intervention is too demanding, then the missing values would result in attrition bias. Such bias could make the treatment look more (or less) effective than it actually is. A high rate of dropouts in a study could also undermine *external validity*—the degree to which results are generalizable to the full population from which the full sample was recruited. Finally, missing values can have implications for *construct validity*. For example, when there are missing values on individual items in an instrument development study using factor analysis (Chapter 13), the construct may be inadequately defined.

Another way to consider the implications of missing data is to understand the effects from a statistical point of view. Reduced power (from a smaller sample size) means larger standard errors and a heightened risk of a Type II error. Biases that threaten internal validity can affect statistical estimates as well. These biases can result in Type I errors, over- or underestimation of effect size indexes, erroneous confidence intervals, underestimations of variance, and faulty regression coefficients, to name only a few statistical problems.

Some missing values strategies are better than others at addressing these statistical problems. The selection of an appropriate strategy depends on numerous factors.

Factors to Consider in Designing a Missing Values Strategy

The first defense for missing values is to make every effort to avoid the problem in designing the study and collecting the data. Strategies might include persistent follow-up, flexibility in scheduling appointments, paying incentives, using well-proven methods to track people who have moved, performing a thorough review of completed data forms prior to excusing participants, and so on. These strategies typically involve the expenditure of resources, but the payoff is well worth the effort.

Yet, a certain amount of missing data is probably inevitable in most studies. There are many different ways to address the problem of missing data and, unfortunately, there is not a "one size fits all" approach. Nor, for that matter, is there an easy formula for deciding which approach to use. We can, however, identify major factors that could affect the decision and its likelihood of success.

- *Extent of missing data:* Researchers usually handle the problem differently if there is only 1% missing data as opposed to, say, 25% missing.
- *Pattern of missing data:* It is more straightforward to deal with data that are missing in a haphazard, random fashion, as opposed to a systematic fashion that typically reflects a bias. We discuss three distinct patterns in the next section.
- *Nature of missing data:* Sometimes values are missing for only one item in a multi-item measure, and sometimes an entire variable is missing. In other situations, all data are missing for certain study participants, such as follow-up data in an intervention study or an entire wave of data in a longitudinal survey.

- *Role of the variable:* How one handles the missing data problem may depend on whether a variable is considered a primary outcome, a secondary outcome, an independent (predictor) variable, or a control variable (covariate).
- *Level of measurement of the variable:* Some strategies are best applied when the variable is measured on an interval or ratio scale, while others only make sense for nominal-level variables.

Another issue that is relevant to readers of this book is analysts' level of statistical sophistication and their access to specialized software. Some of the most highly esteemed methods are, unfortunately, technically complex and require software that is not available in all institutions. Yet every researcher, regardless of statistical skills, should be aware of methods to address missing data problems, and the possible consequences of not using the best ones.

Patterns of Missing Data

Much attention has been paid to the issue of the *pattern* of missing data. This is because the pattern of missing data is considered more important in addressing the problem than how much is missing, unless the amount missing is trivial (e.g., 1%).

To illustrate different patterns, let us use as a hypothetical example an experimental study of a smoking cessation intervention in which 25 men and 25 women are randomly assigned to an experimental group and similar numbers are assigned to a no-treatment control group. With no missing data, the grand mean for postintervention cotinine is 185.0 ng/mL. This is shown in the top row of Table 14.1.

From the point of view of "fixing" a missing data problem, the most desirable pattern is when data are **missing completely at random (MCAR).** When a variable has missing data that are MCAR, it means that the probability that the observation is missing is completely unrelated to either the value of the missing case, or the value of any other variables. If some participants in our hypothetical smoking cessation study had missing data for postintervention urinary cotinine because they had a car accident on the way to the clinic, or had a family emergency, or had moved from the area, the data would be MCAR. In this situation, the missing values are not related to urinary cotinine values, or to the value of other characteristics, such as the person's age, sex, or experimental group status. A car accident, family emergency, or residential move could have happened to anyone in the sample. The subsample with missing values is a totally random subset of the original sample. When data are MCAR, the analysis remains unbiased—although the absence of such data still results in reduced power. As shown in Table 14.1, the difference in mean value for urinary cotinine is only modestly (and nonsignificantly) different between the full 100 subjects ($M = 185.0$) and the 90 for whom full data were available ($M = 185.5$)—although, of course, this would not be known in a real study.

Data are, unfortunately, rarely missing *completely* at random, but they may be classifiable as **missing at random (MAR).** Data can be considered MAR if missingness does not depend on the value of the variable with the missing data (urinary cotinine in our example) *after controlling for another variable.* That is, in MAR, missingness is unrelated to the value of the variable itself, but it *is* related to other variables that can be identified. For example, suppose men were more likely to have missing data than women (e.g., men were less likely to keep their follow-up appointment). Thus, missingness is related to a person's gender. But suppose that, among males, the likelihood of providing follow-up data is equally likely for men with high and low cotinine levels. Within the subgroup of male participants, missingness is random. This would mean that the pattern is MAR, though not MCAR.

TABLE 14.1 Patterns of Missing Data

Study: 100 smokers randomly assigned to smoking cessation intervention: 25 men and 25 women in experimental group and 25 men and 25 women in no-treatment control group

Pattern[a]	Number at Follow-up	Reason for Missing Data	Mean Cotinine Level (ng/mL)	
			All 100 Subjects	90 Subjects
No missing	50 men, 50 women	Not applicable	185.0	—
MCAR	45 men, 45 women	Miscellaneous, at random—lab error, car accident, bad weather, residential move, family death, etc.	185.0	185.5
MAR	40 men, 50 women	Male dropouts lost interest in study. Among males (who, as a group, smoked more than women), dropping out was unrelated to cotinine values.	185.0	175.0
MNAR	40 men, 50 women	Male dropouts had resumed heavy smoking, were too embarrassed to continue in study, so dropping out *was* related to cotinine values.	185.0	165.0

[a]MCAR = Missing completely at random; MAR = Missing at random; MNAR = Missing not at random

We think that MAR was an unfortunate choice of terms, but it has become widely used and is unlikely to ever be changed. The phrase can easily cause confusion because the word *random* typically suggests the absence of bias. In this context, however, *random* does not mean that there is no risk of bias because even though men with higher versus lower cotinine levels were equally likely to drop out, *men overall had higher cotinine levels than women*. Thus, with 10 men no longer in the study, the grand mean for cotinine level based on 90 participants is lower (175.0) than it would have been if no data were missing (185.0). Thus, having data that are MAR does not mean that you can ignore the problem.

TIP: *Equally unfortunate, MAR is sometimes referred to as a pattern of* ignorable *missing values, even though it would be most unwise to* ignore *missing data of any type.*

The third classification is **missing not at random (MNAR)**, sometimes called a *nonignorable* pattern. In this case, missingness *is* related to the value of variable with missing data—and, usually, to other variables as well. In our example, suppose that the 10 men who dropped out of the study refused to provide the data specifically because they knew their cotinine values would be high—that is, the dropouts were ones who had resumed heavy smoking. When data are MNAR, there is clearly a problem, and it is a problem that is difficult to solve. In our example, the overall grand mean for the sample is 165.0 ng/mL, which is a seriously biased estimate of postintervention smoking.

In an actual study, it is difficult to ascertain which of these three missing values patterns apply, although we will offer a few suggestions for gathering suggestive evidence. Suffice it to say that missing data are least likely to be MCAR and most likely to be MAR or MNAR—the classifications that are most difficult to resolve.

TIP: *It is often helpful, in formulating a strategy, to have information about the underlying reasons for missingness. It matters, for example, whether data are missing because of a technical error (e.g., equipment malfunction) or refusals. To the extent possible, reasons for missing values should be documented.*

OVERVIEW OF MISSING VALUES STRATEGIES

There are over two dozen approaches to dealing with the problem of missing values, only some of which are covered in this book. Most approaches can be classified in one of two broad categories—*deletion* methods and *imputation* methods. (There are also sophisticated multilevel modeling techniques not covered in this introductory textbook that allow substantive analyses of certain types to proceed with missing values [e.g., Acock, 2005; Singer & Willett, 2003].)

Numerous simulation studies have been conducted in recent years to test how good a job the various methods do at "getting it right." That is, researchers have begun with a dataset without missing values, and then have systematically "created" missing values that conform to the three patterns just described, for differing amounts of missingness. Then, statistics (e.g., means, *SD*s) are computed for the full sample and the various simulated samples. In general, imputation methods (especially the more sophisticated ones) have been found to be superior to deletion methods in minimizing errors while maintaining statistical power.

Deletion Methods

Deletion methods involve removal of cases or variables with missing data. Even though deletion methods are often not the most suitable methods, they are commonly used by researchers in most fields. Three methods in the deletion category are described here.

LISTWISE DELETION   **Listwise deletion** (also called **complete case analysis**) is simply the analysis of those cases for which there are no missing data. The use of listwise deletion is based on an implicit assumption of MCAR. Researchers who use this method typically have not made a formal assessment of the extent to which MCAR is probable, but rather are simply ignoring the problem of missing data.

In our example of the smoking cessation intervention, if the researcher used listwise deletion for the situations in the last three rows of Table 14.1, mean cotinine levels would be computed for 90 study participants. As we can see, the computed mean is only a reasonably good approximation in the MCAR scenario. In the MAR and MNAR situations, if male dropouts were disproportionately in the experimental group, not only would the grand mean be wrong, but the experimental control group comparison would be biased. In other words, by ignoring missing values, the researcher might come to erroneous conclusions about the effectiveness of the intervention. Even when MCAR applies, listwise deletion can result in errors in statistical decisions because of reduced power.

TIP: *The "gold standard" for analyzing data from randomized controlled trials is to use an* **intention-to-treat analysis,** *which involves analyzing outcome data from all subjects who were randomized, regardless of whether they dropped out of the study ("once randomized, always analyzed"). Intention-to-treat (ITT) analyses are often claimed in nursing and medical RCTs, but true ITT analyses are seldom actually achieved (Polit & Gillespie, in press; Gravel, Opatrny, & Shapiro, 2007; Wood, White, & Thompson, 2004). Complete case analysis has been found to be the most frequently used approach to dealing with missing values in clinical trials.*

In many statistical programs, including SPSS, listwise deletion is the default for many types of analysis. In such a situation, the program performs the requested analysis only for those cases with nonmissing values for every variable in the analysis. Thus, one reason for the popularity of this approach is that it is simple. Although seldom the preferred method for dealing with missing values, listwise deletion might be acceptable when MCAR is a realistic assumption and when the percent of missing values is low (<5%) in a large sample of participants.

PAIRWISE DELETION   **Pairwise deletion** (also called **available case analysis**) involves omitting cases from the analysis on a variable-by-variable basis. In this approach, a case is deleted from the calculation of a statistic only when the specific variables in the analysis have any missing values. For example, in a correlation matrix with pairwise deletion, correlations are computed for cases with nonmissing values for each variable pair. This results in a correlation matrix with values of *r* that are not necessarily based on the same subset of the sample. When such correlation matrixes are the basis for further analysis, such as multiple regression or factor analysis, serious errors and interpretive problems can ensue.

Although few researchers pursue a pairwise (some call it *un*wise) deletion strategy within a correlation matrix scenario, pairwise deletion is extremely common among researchers who compare groups on multiple outcomes. For example, in the Wetta-Hall (2007) study that we used as an example of dependent-groups *t* tests in Chapter 6, the number of cases in the analyses ranged from 158 for one self-report outcome measure, to 165 for a different self-report outcome measure, to 487 for an outcome measure based on hospital records (Table 6.3). When the difference in the number of cases for different outcomes is small (e.g., 158 versus 165), it may be prudent to use listwise deletion so that the sample is consistent across outcomes—or, at a minimum, to assess whether listwise deletion changes the results, and to note that information in the report. The difference between 158 for some outcomes and 487 for another, however, should not have been ignored—the researchers should have helped readers to understand why so much data were missing and what pattern of missingness likely applied. Pairwise deletion may not lead to errors if the missing data are MCAR and the percentage missing is small, but in this example it is unlikely that the two thirds of the sample who did not complete the self-report measures was a random subset of the entire original sample.

Example of pairwise deletion with likely MCAR pattern:

Liao and colleagues (2008) studied the effect of a warm footbath on body temperatures, skin temperatures, and sleep outcomes among 15 Taiwanese elders with sleep disturbance, using a crossover design. Three cases had missing temperature values during sleep due to problems with temperature recording, and so the analysis of core body temperatures was done with only 12 participants. For other outcomes, data from all 15 participants were used.

TIP: *Within SPSS, listwise deletion is the default for some types of analyses, and pairwise is the default for others. In most cases, use the Options pushbutton to select the approach you want.*

VARIABLE DELETION **Variable deletion** involves totally eliminating a variable from consideration in the analyses. Clearly, this is not an attractive option for certain types of variables—for example, you would never use this option for primary outcome variables. Yet, in some cases throwing out a variable makes better sense than throwing out a lot of cases. If a variable is a relatively minor (secondary) outcome variable, for example, it may not be necessary to include it in final analyses. Or, if a variable is a covariate in a regression or ANCOVA analysis, it might be reasonable to drop the variable or substitute an alternative covariate. As an example, it has repeatedly been found that many people do not provide self-report information about family income—and this is especially true of those in higher and lower income brackets, which means that the missing values are MNAR. If income was envisioned as a covariate and the amount of missing data is high, perhaps another socioeconomic variable could be used as a proxy, such as educational attainment.

Variable deletion makes most sense when the amount of missing values is high. There have been several recommendations for what is considered high in this context, ranging from 15% missing to 40% missing (Fox-Wasylyshyn & El-Masri, 2005). Decisions about what to consider "high" are likely to depend on how substantively important the variable is to the study.

Example of variable deletion:

Lee, Fogg, and Menon (2008) gathered information about Korean-American women's knowledge and beliefs relating to cervical cancer and screening via telephone interviews with 189 women. Demographic variables and knowledge questions were used in a logistic regression to predict having had a Pap smear. Several predictors were dropped from the analysis (e.g., income and many knowledge questions) because of high percentages of missing values.

Imputation Methods

The most respected methods for addressing missing values are in a broad class involving **imputation methods**—that is, the "filling in" of missing values with values that are thought to be good estimates of what the values would have been, had they not been missing. An attractive feature of imputation is that it allows researchers to maintain full sample size, and thus statistical power is not compromised. The danger is that the imputations will be poor approximations to the real values, leading to biases of unknown magnitude and direction.

There are numerous imputation strategies, some of which are described here, but a basic issue is where to obtain the imputed value. Some strategies use information from other people in the sample to estimate the missing values, and others use information from the case with the missing values (i.e., from other variables) in the estimation. It has typically been found that using information from the case itself, rather than from the sample, yields better estimates.

A persistent problem with imputation, regardless of the source of the information, is that variability tends to be lower than it would have been had there been complete data. By substituting a missing value with an estimate from either the case or the sample, the overall set of values tends to be more consistent, regular, and homogeneous. Virtually all statistical analyses involve disentangling intersubject variability, and so reduced variability is inherently problematic.

MEAN AND SUBGROUP MEAN SUBSTITUTION   The oldest and possibly most widely used imputation method involves **mean substitution**—replacing a missing value with the mean of that variable, calculated from all sample members with non-missing data. In our earlier smoking cessation example (Table 14.1), the 10 people with missing values would not be removed from the analysis using mean substitution. Rather, they would all be given a cotinine value of 185.0, regardless of the pattern of missingness. Sometimes, if the distribution of values is skewed or if the measurement scale is ordinal, the median rather than the mean is used as the replacement value, and modal values are sometimes used to replace nominal-level data. These substitution decisions represents the researcher's best guess—absent any further information—about what the missing value is.

Mean substitution is, like listwise deletion, a popular method because of its simplicity—and also because some programs offer this approach as an option. For example, the SPSS factor analysis program allows missing values on individual items to be replaced by the item's mean value. Yet, even though mean substitution increases sample size and leaves variable means unchanged, it is rarely the best approach. Regardless of what the underlying pattern of missingness is, mean imputation underestimates variance—and variance is progressively underestimated as the percentage of missing values increases. This in turn can lead to a range of problems. For example, reduced variance can enhance the *apparent* precision of estimates because it artificially lowers standard errors; consequently, the probability of a Type I error can increase. But reduced variance can also decrease the magnitude of correlations and thus increase Type II errors. It is probably best to avoid mean imputation unless the percentage of missing values is *very* small and other options cannot reasonably be pursued.

A variant on mean substitution is to use the mean value for a relevant subgroup—sometimes called a **subgroup** (or *conditional*) **mean substitution**. In this situation, it is assumed that a better estimate of the missing value can be obtained by making the substitution conditional on one or more of the participants' characteristics. For example, in the second row of Table 14.1, five men and five women had missing values. Rather than replacing all missing values with 185.0, we could replace the five women's missing values with the mean cotinine level for women, and the five men's missing values with the mean cotinine level for men. This is a better option than mean substitution because the substituted values are presumably closer to the real values, and also because variance is not reduced as much. Nevertheless, conditional (subgroup) mean substitution is not a preferred approach, except when overall missingness is low.

Example of subgroup mean substitution:

de Montigny and Lacharité (2008) studied the role of nurse–parent relationships in the development of parenting self-efficacy. They tested a complex model using self-report data from a sample of about 200 Canadian parents. Missing values, which constituted less than 5% of the data, were replaced using variable means separately for mothers and fathers.

CASE MEAN SUBSTITUTION   In certain circumstances, it might be appropriate to re-place a missing value with the mean of other relevant variables from the person with the missing value. This approach has an implicit assumption that people are "internally consistent" across similar questions. The most obvious situation in which this might be appropriate is when there are missing values in a set of items that form a unidimen-sional scale. If a person skipped one item on a 10-item scale, for example, the person's mean on the nine nonmissing items would be substituted for the missing value on the 10th item. This method of imputation, which uses person-specific information to in-form the estimate, has the advantage of not throwing out data altogether (listwise dele-tion), and not assuming that a person is similar to all others in a sample or subgroup (mean substitution). Case mean substitution has been found to be an acceptable method of imputation at the item level, even compared to more sophisticated methods to be discussed later. A recent simulation study suggested that case mean substitution works reasonably well when up to 30% of item values on a scale are missing (Shrive, Stuart, Quan, & Ghali, 2006).

Example of case mean substitution:

Aroian, Hough, Templin, and Kaskiri (2008) developed and tested an Arab version of an instrument called the Family Peer Relationship Questionnaire, specifically for use with Arab immigrants. Prior to the analyses, which involved a confirmatory fac-tor analysis, missing values at the item level were imputed using the respondent's average score from the scale associated with the missing value. The researchers noted that the amount of missing data was less than 1% for any scale.

REGRESSION IMPUTATION   Another method of addressing missing data is to use **regression imputation**. This approach involves using the variable with the missing values as the dependent variable in a regression with a set of predictors (other vari-ables in the dataset) for those participants for whom there are no missing values. In essence, this process is an extension of subgroup mean substitution, using multiple variables to estimate the value that is missing rather than just one. In our example of the smoking cessation intervention, we could estimate the missing cotinine values for the 10 study participants by doing a multiple regression analysis with the 90 par-ticipants with full information, using (for example) such variables as sex, experi-mental group status, baseline smoking history, and baseline cotinine levels as predic-tors. The regression equation would then be used to "predict" the missing cotinine value for the 10 dropouts.

Researchers sometimes repeat the regression analysis multiple times to im-prove the estimates. In a second round, all cases, including ones with the imputed missing values, are included in the regression to develop a more precise regression equation. The process continues until predicted missing values become very similar from one iteration to the next (Tabachnick & Fidell, 2007).

To be successful, regression imputation relies on having a reasonably good set of predictors of the variable with missing data. Evidence suggests that regression imputation is most useful when up to 15% of missing values are MAR, or when 10% or less of missing values are MNAR (Fox-Wasylyshyn & El-Masri, 2005). Multiply iterated regression imputation is most appropriate when missing values exceed 15% to 20%.

The regression approach typically yields better estimates than mean substitution, and results in less reduction to variance. Nevertheless, regression imputation does not really add new information and does not always eliminate bias. People with the same values on the predictors will have exactly the same imputed value, which usually means lower variance on imputed values than would have been the case with the actual values. This, in turn, leads to inappropriately small standard errors and heightened risk of a Type I error.

One way to address this problem is to incorporate some error into the regression estimate, an approach sometimes called **regression with error** (Engels & Diehr, 2003) or **stochastic regression imputation** (Haukoos & Newgard, 2007). This approach incorporates uncertainty into the imputed value by adding some random error, which provides some additional variance into the imputed estimates. The SPSS program called Missing Values Analysis (MVA) offers this type of regression imputation. However, MVA is an add-on module within SPSS and is not routinely available in all SPSS systems.

Example of regression imputation:

Horgas, Yoon, Nichols, and Marsiske (2008) studied the relationship between pain and functional ability in older White and African-American adults. In their model, they planned to control for socioeconomic factors, but found that information on income was missing for 16.5% of their sample. They used regression to impute values of income.

LAST OBSERVATION CARRIED FORWARD   Several approaches, most often used in clinical trials with multiple points of data collection, involve imputing missing values for outcome variables from a person's obtained values on the same outcomes at a different point in time. In an approach called **last observation carried forward (LOCF),** a missing outcome value at, for example, time 3 would be replaced with the value of the outcome for that person at time 2. In a simple before–after design, missing values postintervention are sometimes imputed with baseline values, which is sometimes called *baseline observation carried forward* or *BOCF*.

The LOCF approach can be used with outcomes measured on any scale. For example, if the outcome variable was an obesity category (normal weight, overweight, obese, or morbidly obese), a missing value would be imputed using the category observed at the prior measurement. If the outcome were body mass index (BMI), the previous BMI would be used.

LOCF has an implicit assumption that the outcome did not change over time—an often undesirable position. Until recently, LOCF was the approach recommended by the U.S. Food and Drug Administration because it presumably offers a conservative estimate of the efficacy of a treatment. LOCF was found recently to be the most often-used method of imputing missing outcomes among RCTs reported in 10 top medical journals (Gravel et al., 2007), but it appears to be used infrequently in nursing clinical trials.

Several variations of LOCF can be used in clinical trials or in other studies involving longitudinal data collection. For example, if there are actual values for an outcome at T1, T2, and T3, then a missing value at T4 could be replaced with the mean (or median) of the person's T1 to T3 values. Or, if there are real values at T1 and T3, but a missing value at T2, the imputation might involve using an interpolated value, which assumes a consistent linear trajectory. These approaches clearly require variables measured on at least the ordinal scale.

> **TIP:** *Another strategy that is sometimes used in clinical trials when there is a dichotomous outcome is called* **worst case imputation.** *This extremely conservative approach replaces missing values with the "worst case scenario." For example, if a primary outcome in a smoking cessation intervention were resumption versus nonresumption of smoking, anyone whose outcome data were missing would be assumed to have resumed smoking. In* **best case imputation,** *the opposite would be done—those with missing values would be assumed to have the best case scenario, such as nonresumption of smoking (Haukoos & Newgard, 2007).*

Although LOCF and related approaches have had considerable popularity until recently, more sophisticated and accurate methods are now preferred.

Example of last observation carried forward:

Budin and colleagues (2008) undertook a randomized controlled trial that tested alternative interventions to promote emotional and physical adjustment among patients with breast cancer. Outcomes were measured at baseline (entry into the study); at diagnosis, i.e., when the diagnosis of breast cancer was confirmed; and at three subsequent points postsurgery. The report indicated that "if there were missing data in the diagnostic period, the value from baseline was carried forward to the diagnostic period" (p. 206). LOCF was not, however, used to impute missing values in subsequent periods.

EXPECTATION-MAXIMIZATION IMPUTATION Some of the best modern-day approaches to addressing missing values use maximum likelihood (ML) imputation. There are several different ways to obtain ML estimators, and the most common algorithm is called **expectation-maximization (EM) imputation**. EM imputation is an iterative two-step process that generates estimated values using expectation (E-step) and maximization (M-step) algorithms. In the E-step, expected values are calculated based on all complete data points. In the M-step, the procedure substitutes the expected values for the missing data obtained from the E-step, and then maximizes the likelihood function as if no data were missing to obtain new parameter estimates. These new estimates are substituted back into the E-step, and then a new M-step is performed. The two-step process continues in an iterative fashion until changes in expected values from one iteration to the next are trivial.

EM imputation is one of the missing values options available in the SPSS Missing Values Analysis module. A product of this analysis is a new dataset in which missing values are imputed with maximum likelihood values.

EM imputation is considered preferable to all previously discussed methods of imputation. It produces unbiased estimates for MCAR and estimates with modest bias for MAR (although small samples can lead to biased ML estimates). The problem of reduced standard errors does, however, persist using EM imputation.

Example of EM imputation:

Musil, Warner, Yobas, and Jones (2002) used EM imputation in a simulation, using data from their longitudinal study on stress and health in older adults. They created a dataset with missing data (MAR) on items from the Center for Epidemiological Studies Depression scale (CES-D). They found that the EM algorithm produced estimates of missing values that were close to the original values.

MULTIPLE IMPUTATION Imputation using EM is an important advance over more traditional approaches, but it is flawed primarily because, like other imputation methods we have reviewed, it involves *single imputation*. A single value is imputed and substituted for the missing value. All methods of single imputation tend to underestimate standard errors and thus overestimate the level of precision. Single imputation treats the imputed values as if they were true, and does not address a fundamental issue—the *uncertainty* of the estimate.

To obtain more accurate estimates of the standard errors and *p* values, and to deal with the issue of uncertainty, an approach called **multiple imputation (MI)** has been developed and is quickly becoming the "gold standard" approach to handling missing data that are MAR. Despite a growing consensus about the advantages of MI, its use is not yet widespread, in part because of its complexity but also because software for using this approach has been limited. Only as this book was being completed did MI become available within the SPSS Missing Value Analysis module, in SPSS version 17.0.

Computationally, MI is enormously complex, but it is conceptually fairly straightforward. MI is essentially a three-step process (Figure 14.1). First, each missing value is replaced with plausible estimates using MLE, and a new dataset with imputed values is created. The imputations are redone *m* times, and a new dataset is created each time. Because an element of randomness is introduced in developing the imputations, the *m* estimates for the missing values are all different. In the second step, the desired substantive analysis (e.g., ANCOVA, logistic regression) is undertaken *m* times, once for each new dataset with imputed values. In the

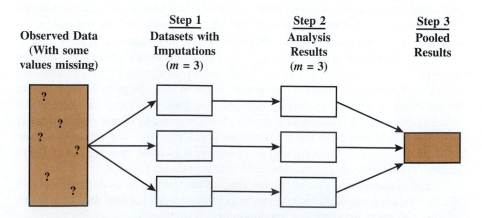

FIGURE 14.1 Schematic representation of multiple imputation, with *m* = 3.

third and final step, the results from the *m* analyses are pooled and average parameter estimates are obtained. The pooling takes into account the variation among the *m* analyses (between-imputation variation), and variation within each analysis (within-imputation variation). The MI process, including a discussion of MI models and estimation algorithms, has been nicely described for nonstatisticians by Patrician (2002).

The MI procedure uses available data to predict a participant's missing values, given his or her observed values on other variables. In datasets with many variables, the selection of variables to use in predicting the missing values clearly is critical to the success of the imputation. It has been shown that, when imputing values for a predictor variable or covariate, it is preferable to include the outcome variable in the prediction model, even though this may seem like "a self-fulfilling prophecy" (Moons, Donders, Stijnen, & Harrell, 2006).

The number of imputations needed to achieve a satisfactory solution depends on various factors—most importantly the amount of missing data. Three to five replications are usually sufficient when missingness does not exceed 20% (Little & Rubin, 2002). Iterations should continue as long as the imputations continue to produce significantly different estimates.

TIP: *ML estimates in EM and multiple imputation assume MAR, yet this is an assumption that is unlikely to be precisely satisfied in most cases. It has been argued, however, that in many realistic applications, departures from MAR are probably not large enough to invalidate the results of a MAR-based analysis (Schafer & Graham, 2002).*

The advantages of MI are noteworthy. The procedure has been found repeatedly in simulation studies to yield the best estimations of missing values, especially in comparison to crude imputation methods like mean substitution. Appropriate statistical inferences can be drawn from an analysis of MI datasets, and there is no loss in statistical power. Both internal and external validity are safeguarded against biases stemming from nonresponse. MI is also a versatile imputation procedure. It has been found useful for imputing predictors, covariates, and outcomes; it is appropriate for items in multi-item scales as well as complete variables. Continuous and dichotomous nominal-level variables can be imputed by MI. (Dichotomous variables imputed under a normal model must be rounded to the nearest category.)

The major disadvantage of MI has been that its use has been constrained by the limited availability of suitable software, but that situation is changing. Another issue is that MI solutions are not unique. Two researchers using MI with the same dataset might get somewhat different results. However, MI results can be saved by any given researcher and the imputations can be used in many different analyses.

TIP: *Even for those without access to the new SPSS MVA module, MI is available through a program called NORM, which can be obtained free of charge over the Internet (http://www.stat.psu.edu/~jls/misoftwa.html).*

Multiple imputation has been described extensively in several nursing papers (e.g., Kneipp & McIntosh, 2001; Patrician, 2002; McCleary, 2002), and its use in nursing studies is just beginning to emerge.

Example of multiple imputation:

Koniak-Griffin and a team of researchers (2008) evaluated a theory-based HIV prevention program for Latino adolescent mothers and their partners. Data were collected at baseline and at 3-month and 6-month follow-ups for couples in the treatment group or a comparison group. Couples with no follow-up data were dropped from the sample, but other missing data were imputed using MI.

MISSING VALUES PROCESSES

In this section we offer some concrete suggestions for how to proceed with efforts to "fix" missing data problems, using examples from an actual dataset. Most of this discussion does not involve the SPSS Missing Values Analysis module, even though this module includes important tools, because this module is not universally available (for example, it is not included in the student version of SPSS). However, we do discuss a few features of SPSS MVA, using version 16.0.

Strategies for Understanding Missing Values

Earlier in this chapter, we indicated that developing a missing values strategy depended on various factors. Some of the information would be immediately known, such as whether the variable was an item in a scale or a full variable, what the measurement level of the variable was, and whether the variable was envisioned as a predictor or a primary or secondary outcome variable. What is usually *not* known without further investigation is how much data are missing, and the pattern of missingness.

AMOUNT OF MISSING DATA It is easy to examine how much data are missing from a dataset on a variable-by-variable basis by simply running frequency distributions—although it is important to keep in mind participants for whom the frequency distribution is relevant. As an example, let us consider the 11 items on parenting that we factor analyzed in Chapter 13 (items are listed in Figure 13.4). Figure 14.2 (A) shows the SPSS output for the first two items (obtained through Analyze ➜ Descriptive Statistics ➜ Frequencies) for all mothers in the sample ($N = 3,960$). We might be alarmed to see that valid data were obtained for only 1,859 women for the first item—a rate of missingness of 53%. This number grossly exaggerates our problem, however, because the questions were administered only to women with a child between the ages of 2 and 6. Panel B of Figure 14.2 shows the amount missing

A	**Full Sample ($N = 3960$)**			B	**Relevant Subsample ($N = 1911$)**		
	Statistics				**Statistics**		
		1. Best part of my day spending time w/child	2. Child seems harder to care for than most			1. Best part of my day spending time w/child	2. Child seems harder to care for than most
N	Valid	1859	1858	N	Valid	1859	1858
	Missing	2101	2102		Missing	52	53
	Mean	8.8230	2.6690		Mean	8.8230	2.6690
	Std. Deviation	1.93110	3.45674		Std. Deviation	1.93110	3.45674
	Minimum	.00	.00		Minimum	.00	.00
	Maximum	10.00	10.00		Maximum	10.00	10.00

FIGURE 14.2 SPSS frequency information for full sample (A) and relevant subsample (B).

for the subsample of 1,911 women with an age-appropriate child. For the first item, data were missing for 52 women, a rate of missingness of 2.7%.

By inspecting variable-by-variable missing values, we can see whether it might be sensible to delete an entire variable. For the 11 items, the number of missing values among the 1,911 women ranged from 52 (item 1) to 71 (item 9), which translates to 2.7% to 3.7% missing. This does not suggest the need to drop a variable. You can look at frequency distributions to learn the range of missing values for all variables of interest. If you have access to the MVA module in SPSS, this information is produced in a single descriptive table.

Another issue is missingness within a case. Would we want, for example, to factor analyze the data for a person who was missing 10 out of the 11 items? We cannot make decisions about whether to drop a case or impute missing values without knowing how much data are missing for individual participants.

If you do not have access to the Missing Values Analysis module of SPSS, you can learn about extent of missingness for individual participants by creating a new variable (sometimes called a *flag*) that represents a count of how many of the variables of interest are missing for each person. In our example, among women who answered all 11 questions, the value on this new variable would be 0; women who answered 9 of the 11 questions would have a value of 2. Figure 14.3 presents the SPSS frequency distribution printout for the variable we created (through the Transform ➜ Count Values command) to count missing values for the 11 parenting items. This printout shows us that 5.7% of the women had at least one missing value (100% – 94.3% with 0 missing), 96.4% had no more than two missing, and 2.6% had either 10 or 11 missing.

In illustrating factor analysis in the previous chapter, we used listwise deletion and ran the analysis with 1,803 cases. If we had chosen the option within the SPSS factor analysis program to use mean substitution, the analysis would have been done on all 1,911 cases. Given that 45 women had no data at all on any of the 11 items, however, it would not be sensible to impute values for individual items for these women for a factor analysis. In such a situation, it would probably make most sense to use case mean substitutions for the 40 women with only one or two missing items,

Number of missing values, Parenting items

		Frequency	Percent	Valid Percent	Cumulative Percent
Valid	0	1803	94.3	94.3	94.3
	1	31	1.6	1.6	96.0
	2	9	.5	.5	96.4
	3	4	.2	.2	96.7
	4	1	.1	.1	96.7
	5	2	.1	.1	96.8
	6	1	.1	.1	96.9
	7	1	.1	.1	96.9
	8	11	.6	.6	97.5
	10	3	.2	.2	97.6
	11	45	2.4	2.4	100.0
	Total	1911	100.0	100.0	

FIGURE 14.3   SPSS printout, frequencies for newly created "missing items" variable.

and to use listwise deletion for the women with more than two items missing. In sub-sequent analyses involving the full Parenting Stress and Parenting Enjoyment scales as independent or dependent variables, scale scores could be imputed for those with missing values.

> **TIP:** *There are no strict guidelines for how many missing items in a scale make it imprudent to impute item values, although 30% has been suggested. Our advice is to forego imputation when more than 25% of the items are missing. In this example with 11 items, two missing values per case (18%) is probably the most that should be imputed.*

In the SPSS MVA module, it is easy to examine the amount of missingness in different *combinations* of missing values. The output with 11 variables (the parenting items) is unwieldy, and so we illustrate with a different example from the same dataset, using data for children aged 2 to 6. Let us suppose that we wanted to test the relationship between children's weight in pounds (the dependent variable) and their food security/hunger status in a multiple regression analysis, holding constant other characteristics. The food security variable was created through the mothers' responses to a series of questions about their family's eating patterns. The child's food security variable is coded 1 if there is food security and 0 if the child is either in hunger or on a reduced quality diet. Our analysis will also include data on the child's age, gender, number of siblings, and the mother's health rating of the child (1 = excellent to 5 = poor). In the MVA descriptive statistics table (Figure 14.4), we learn that there are no missing data for the child's age, gender, or number of siblings. Missingness was low for the child's health rating ($n = 7$) and food security status ($n = 5$), but 158 mothers (8.3%) either did not know or refused to report their child's weight.

The MVA "Tabulated Patterns Table" for the three variables with missing data is shown in Figure 14.5. In SPSS, the default is to show only those patterns that are present for at least 1% of the cases, but we used a lower threshold (0.1%) so that all patterns of missingness would be displayed. This table shows that 1,753 cases (91.7%) had no missing values on any of the six variables, 151 cases (7.9%) had missing values for weight only, two cases (.1%) had missing values for both weight

MVA

Univariate Statistics

	N	Mean	Std. Deviation	Missing Count	Missing Percent	No. of Extremes[a] Low	No. of Extremes[a] High
Weight	1753	45.4963	13.82701	158	8.3	2	73
Health	1904	1.83	1.008	7	.4	0	0
Age	1911	4.6049	1.08312	0	.0	0	0
Siblings	1911	2.81	1.404	0	.0	0	213
FoodSec	1906			5	.3		
Gender	1911			0	.0		

[a]Number of cases outside the range (Q1 – 1.5*IQR, Q3 + 1.5*IQR).

FIGURE 14.4 SPSS MVA printout: descriptive statistics table.

Tabulated Patterns

Number of Cases	Missing Patterns[a]						Complete if...[b]	Weight[c]	Age[c]	Siblings[c]	Gender[d]	
	Age	Siblings	Gender	FoodSec	Health	Weight					Female	Male
1753	Age	Siblings	Gender	FoodSec	Health	Weight	1753	45.4963	4.5881	2.78	907	846
151						X	1904	.	4.7815	3.16	76	75
2					X	X	1906	.	5.0000	2.00	1	1
5				X	X	X	1911	.	5.0000	3.40	3	2

Patterns with less than .1% cases (2 or fewer) are not displayed.

[a]Variables are sorted on missing patterns.
[b]Number of complete cases if variables missing in that pattern (marked with X) are not used.
[c]Means at each unique pattern.
[d]Frequency distribution at each unique pattern.

FIGURE 14.5 SPSS MVA printout: tabulated patterns table.

and the health rating, and five cases (.3%) had missing cases for all three variables (marked with Xs). The column labeled "Age" shows the mean age for the cases in the pattern for a particular row. For example, for the 1,753 cases with no missing values, the mean age was 4.5881, and for the 151 cases with only weight missing, the mean age was 4.7815. The last two columns show the number of girls and boys in the various patterns. The relationship between missingness and other case characteristics is an important area to explore in trying to understand if missing values are MCAR or not.

MVA can also be used to examine patterns of missingness within *cases,* which may eliminate the need to create a missing values flag. Figure 14.6 shows a small portion of the MVA output for the cases with missing values on more than one variable (the full table lists every case with at least one missing value). Figure 14.6 indicates that case number 992 had a missing value of 7 (the code for a refusal) for the child's health rating and a missing values code of 997 (also a refusal) for the child's

MVA

Missing Patterns (cases with missing values)

Case	# Missing	% Missing	Missing and Extreme Value Patterns[a]					
			Siblings	ChildAge	ChildSex	Chfoodsec	ChHealth	ChildWgt
992	2	33.3				−	7	997
45	2	33.3				−	7	997
1213	3	50.0	+			S	8	998
1796	3	50.0				S	8	998
1779	3	50.0	+			S	8	998
1296	3	50.0				S	7	997
1911	3	50.0				S	8	998

− indicates an extreme low value, while + indicates an extreme high value. The range used is (Q1 − 1.5*IQR, Q3 + 1.5*IQR).

[a] Cases and variables are sorted on missing patterns.

FIGURE 14.6 SPSS MVA printout: missing patterns—cases with missing values.

weight. The last entry in the table, for case number 1911, had three missing values: systems-missing (S) for the food security variable, code 8 (don't know) for the child health rating, and code 998 (don't know) for child's weight. Although this MVA table can be extremely helpful, the use of a missing values indicator may be preferable when the number of variables is large (as, for example, our 11 parenting items) or when the sample size is large.

RELATIONSHIPS AND PATTERNS OF MISSINGNESS   There are two reasons for analysts to explore the relationship between missingness and other variables in the dataset. The first is to shed light on whether or not the missing data are MCAR. If missing values are systematically related to other variables, then they are not MCAR—they are either MAR or MNAR, although it is difficult to know for sure which of the two patterns apply. A second reason to examine patterns of missingness is to understand the nature and extent of any biases for interpretive purposes. If, for example, control group members drop out of a study at a higher rate than those in the experimental group, then the missing outcome values indicate attrition bias that should be reported and taken into consideration in discussing study results.

For those without access to SPSS's Missing Values Analysis, the procedure for exploring relationships with missingness is fairly straightforward, but requires a bit of effort. The first step is to create a dummy variable indicating whether or not each case has a real data value or a missing value on the target variable. As an example, let us create a missing values indicator for the variable in our dataset with considerable missing data, children's weight. Using the Compute command in SPSS, we created the variable *misswate* and set it to 0 if the mother reported her child's weight and 1 if the data are missing. Next, we can use *t* tests and chi-square tests to see whether having missing data on weight is systematically related to other characteristics of the child or the mother.

Table 14.2 summarizes results from a series of *t* tests. (A similar table can be created within the MVA module without needing to create a missing values indicator variable.) The bottom row of Table 14.2 indicates that those with versus those without missing values on child's weight are not significantly different in terms of the child's health rating, child height, mother's body mass index, and monthly household income. However, mothers who did not report their child's weight had significantly older children ($p = .024$) and significantly more children in their households ($p = .002$).

TABLE 14.2 Comparison of Cases With and Without Missing Values for Child's Weight, on Various Child and Mother Characteristics

	Child/Maternal Characteristics					
	Child's Age	Child's Health Rating	Child's Height (in.)	No. of Siblings	Mother's BMI	Monthly HH Income
# Weight Present	1753	1753	1336	1753	1703	1593
# Weight Missing	158	151	27	158	142	133
Mean (Present)	4.59	1.82	39.97	1.78	27.48	$1344.06
Mean (Missing)	4.79	1.89	37.74	2.15	28.58	$1200.17
t	−2.259	−.758	1.564	−3.168	−.181	1.739
df	1909	1902	1361	1909	1843	1724
p (2-tail)	.024	.448	.118	.002	.857	.082

> **TIP:** *With small samples, you will need to be careful not to be guided by significance levels alone. The* t *tests for the missingness indicator may lack sufficient power to reveal real differences that exist. When the means look different even though* p *values are greater than .05, it may be a good idea to compute an effect size index such as Cohen's* d *to consider the magnitude of the effect of missingness.*

A series of chi-square analyses were also run to see if weight-missingness was related to categorical variables (not shown). We found that missingness was unrelated to the child's gender, race, food security status, or hospitalization within the prior year, or to the mother's current marital status. However, missingness was significantly related to the mother's education. Mothers who had not completed high school were significantly more likely to have missing child weight information ($p = .005$), and women who had post–high school education were significantly less likely to have this missing information ($p = .004$).

The results of these analyses provide a lot of important information. First, the various significant relationships strongly support the inference that the missing data are not MCAR. If the data were missing completely at random, it is unlikely that there would be so many significant (and interpretable) relationships. Second, the analyses also offer some modest suggestive evidence that the missing values are MAR rather than MNAR. For example, if women had a tendency to refuse to provide information about their children's weight because of embarrassment about the weight value itself (a situation that would lead to MNAR), one might expect to find a significant difference on the mother's own body mass index value (for which there was relatively little missing data). However, missingness on children's weight was not related to the mother's BMI. This suggests that weight data are not missing *because of* the children's weight—which would be an MNAR situation. Although we would ideally want a pattern that is MCAR, this is almost never the case, so any supporting evidence that the missing values are MAR rather than MNAR is encouraging. A third important result is that missingness on weight (our dependent variable in our substantive analysis) was not significantly related to our primary independent variable (food security status).

> **TIP:** *In the SPSS MVA module, there is a significance test called* **Little's MCAR test,** *which appears as a footnote to EM means tables. When the test is significant, you can reject the null hypothesis that the missing value is MCAR—although you would not know for sure if it was MAR or MNAR. In our example, the test was significant at* p $= .007$—*which is not surprising, given the many significant* t *test and chi-square results.*

In conclusion, we have learned that the dependent variable for our substantive analysis, the child's weight, is missing for about 8% of the children, and that the missing data are probably MAR. Next, we must make decisions about what to do about this situation.

Addressing Missing Values Problems

Once analysts have learned something about the amount and pattern of missing values for their analyses, they can formulate and implement a plan. Although one always hopes for an MCAR situation so that the results will be unbiased, the reality is

TABLE 14.3 Comparison of Alternative Missing Values Strategies for Child's Weight

	Method of Imputation				
	None (Listwise Deletion)	Mean Substitution	Subgroup Mean Substitution (Sex)	Regression (via SPSS Compute)	EM (via SPSS MVA)
N	1753	1904	1904	1904	1904
Mean weight, imputed missing values (N = 151)	—	45.50	45.52 (M_{Male} = 46.36 M_{Female} = 44.69)	46.43	46.38
SD, imputed values	—	0.00	0.84	5.95	5.93
Mean weight, full sample	45.50	45.50	45.50	45.57	45.57
SD, full sample	13.83	13.27	13.28	13.37	13.49
R^2, predicting weight in substantive analysis[a]	.185	.170	.171	.198	.197
b weight, child food security variable	−1.530	−1.417	−1.441	−1.415	−1.382
Significance of child food security variable	.023	.023	.021	.022	.026

[a]Child's weight regressed on child's food security status, controlling for child's age, gender, health rating, and number of siblings in household.

that MAR or MNAR will most often apply. This means that statistical estimates are likely to be biased, but the goal is to use a strategy that keeps bias to a minimum. Uncorrected missing values can also lead to biased estimates of important parameters, and will reduce statistical power.

EXAMPLE OF ALTERNATIVE IMPUTATIONS If you do not have access to the MVA module in SPSS (which can simultaneously impute missing values for several variables), you may want to consider using more than one strategy of dealing with missing values. In our example, there were a handful of cases that had missing values for weight, food security, and the health rating (Figure 14.5). Given our large sample size, it seems acceptable to drop those seven cases, which represent only 0.4% of the sample. Dropping all cases with missing values, however, would result in a loss of over 8% of the sample, and so we will impute the missing values for the 151 cases in which only weight was missing. The use of multiple strategies within a single investigation is not uncommon, as we will see in the research example in the next section.

Table 14.3 presents information about various imputation strategies for the missing weight variable. The first column shows that, using listwise deletion with 1,753 cases, the mean and SD for the child's weight are 45.50 and 13.83, respectively. Mean substitution, which involved replacing all 151 missing with 45.50 did not change the mean, but it lowered the SD to 13.27. Subgroup mean imputation, which imputed 46.36 for the missing values of boys and 44.69 for the missing values of girls, did not change the overall sample mean, and did little to improve the deflated SD.

If you are doing imputations without the aid of specialized missing values software, regression imputation is likely to be the best bet in many situations, such as in our current example. For regression imputation, we used data from the 1,753 cases with complete weight data to regress the child's weight on three variables: gender, age, and number of siblings. We chose these predictors because they were significantly correlated with weight, and also because *none of these variables had any missing values themselves.* The result of this regression analysis was the following equation:

$$Weight' = 20.909 + 5.377\,(age) + 1.794\,(gender) - .342\,(number\ of\ siblings)$$

The equation was then used to "predict" (impute) the weight of children with missing weight information, using the SPSS Compute command. Table 14.3 shows that with our calculated regression imputation, the mean weight for the sample was 45.57, and the *SD* of 13.37 was larger than with mean or subgroup mean substitution.

> **TIP:** *If regression is used in the SPSS MVA module, missing values are imputed for **all** quantitative values in the analysis, based on predictors that are declared as quantitative rather than categorical. The SPSS regression imputation procedure adds the residual of a randomly selected case to each estimate, which helps to address deflated variability. In our example, the mean child weight with regression-imputed values via SPSS's MVA was 45.55, very close to our value of 45.57, and the SD was 13.46.*

The bottom three rows of Table 14.3 show some results for the substantive multiple regression in which we addressed the question: Is a child's food security status related to his or her weight, once age, gender, health, and family size are controlled? (This regression analysis is analogous to an ANCOVA with four covariates.) For each scenario, we found a significant relationship: Net of the statistically controlled characteristics, children with a reduced quality diet or hunger weighed significantly more than children who were food secure (presumably because their diets tended toward foods that are less expensive and nutritious, but more caloric).

It is important to realize that we do not know which of these analyses does a better job of representing the truth. In our example, we would have reached the same conclusion about the food security–weight relationship regardless of how we handled the missing values—probably because the very large sample size gave considerable stability to the estimates. With a smaller sample—which is usually the case in nursing studies—results could well be different. Even in our example, the values for R^2 ranged from .170 (mean substitution) to .198 (regression imputation).

If you have access to special missing values software such as SPSS's MVA, you should probably pursue either EM imputation or multiple imputation, especially if there is evidence that the pattern of missingness is not MCAR. The results from the EM imputation using MVA in SPSS Version 16.0 are shown in the far right column of Table 14.3. As this table shows, the full sample mean with EM-imputed missing values was 45.57 and the *SD* was 13.49. The EM results in this particular example were quite close to the regression results.

SENSITIVITY ANALYSES   In many situations, it may be crucial to conduct **sensitivity analyses** in which the consequences of alternative missing values strategies are explored. Table 14.3 displays, in effect, the results of a sensitivity analysis. We tested whether our conclusions about the relationships between children's weight and their food security status would be different using alternative missing values strategies. In our case they did not—and this in itself lends credence to the results.

Sensitivity analyses are especially important when there are missing values on primary outcomes in a clinical trial. If an intervention has been found to be effective in trials in which there are missing values (which is usually the case), it can be persuasive to demonstrate that the intervention's effects were found under the most conservative estimates (e.g., LOCF or "worst case" imputation), and with less conservative estimates, for example, via multiple imputation or "best case" imputation.

As another example of a sensitivity analysis, researchers whose analyses involve group comparisons and who have a slightly different number of cases for different outcomes should consider running their analyses both listwise and pairwise to see if the results change when the same people are used for all tests.

Example of a sensitivity analysis:

Chen and colleagues (2008) examined the effects of a simplified Tai-Chi exercise program on the physical health of elders in long-term care facilities. They collected data from a single group who received the intervention at seven points in time—three pretests prior to the intervention and four posttests after the intervention began. Missing data were imputed using last observation carried forward, followed by a series of sensitivity analyses to test the adequacy of the imputations.

Reporting Missing Values Information

The majority of nursing studies do not mention missing values at all. One can sometimes infer that pairwise deletion was used (for example, when tables show statistical information for varying numbers of participants), but readers should not have to make guesses about the researchers' missing data strategy.

If there are no missing values at all, researchers should state this in their Method section, preferably in the subsection on data analysis. If values are missing, researchers should include a paragraph to explain the missing values situation and the researchers' approach to the problem. The report should indicate the extent of missing values, for example, by stating the range of missingness on important variables. The presumed pattern of missingness (MCAR, MAR, or MNAR) should be reported, together with evidence supporting the inference. Biases relating to missingness, as evidenced from t tests or chi-squared analyses comparing those with versus those without missing values, should be reported. Then, the strategy or strategies that were used to address missing values should be described, together with the results of any sensitivity analyses. If thresholds were used to make decisions, these should also be reported. For example, if variables were discarded when more than a certain percentage of the cases had missing information, that threshold should be stated.

> **TIP:** *In intervention studies, it is advisable to include a flow chart such as those suggested in the Consolidated Standards of Reporting Trials or* **CONSORT guidelines***, which have been adopted by major medical and nursing journals, such as* Nursing Research. *CONSORT guidelines include a template for a flow chart to track participants through a clinical trial, from eligibility assessment through analysis of outcomes. One explicit goal of the flow chart is to indicate participant loss over time, for each study group. Although these materials were specifically designed for use with RCTs, many aspects of it can be productively applied to any quantitative study. Further information about the CONSORT guidelines is available at www.consort-statement.org.*

The Discussion section of a report should also provide an interpretation of the effect of the missing values problem on the results. Research evidence can best be trusted when missing values have been appropriately handled, and when researchers take potential biases into account in drawing conclusions about the evidence from their data.

Research Example

Researchers rarely report the level of detail about missing values in their reports that we have recommended. This may partially reflect page constraints in journals, but may also be the result of "benign neglect" of this important issue. Here is an example of an article with fairly good coverage of the missing values situation.

Study: "Factors influencing diabetes self-management in Chinese people with type 2 diabetes" (Xu, Toobert, Savage, Pan, & Whitmer, 2008).

Study Purpose: The purpose of this study was to test a complex model of the effects of individual and environmental factors on diabetes self-management among patients with type 2 diabetes in Beijing China.

Methods: The researchers gathered cross-sectional data from a convenience sample of 201 Chinese adults during outpatient visits at one of China's largest hospitals. The researchers distributed self-administered questionnaires to eligible patients. The questionnaires incorporated six psychosocial scales, a demographic form, and questions about diabetes history. The six multi-item scales measured variables conceptualized as affecting diabetes self-management (e.g., diabetes knowledge, diabetes self-efficacy, social support, and beliefs in treatment effectiveness).

Missing Data Analysis: The principal analyses involved a sophisticated test of a theoretical model using structural equations modeling. Prior to their substantive analyses, the researchers addressed missing values problems. The amount of missing data varied considerably across variables, from a low of 0.5% to 6.0% (the paper did not indicate whether missingness was at the item or variable level). According to the report, the pattern of missingness was MAR. For variables with missing values in the 0.5% to 2.5% range, mean substitution was used to impute missing values. For variables with 2.5% or more missing values, the missing values were imputed via regression. Therefore, all cases and all variables were used in the substantive analyses.

Results: The researchers found that, in their final model, a patient's belief in treatment effectiveness and their diabetes self-efficacy were the proximal factors affecting a patient's ability to self-manage their diabetes. Diabetes knowledge, social support, and provider communication had an indirect effect on self-management, through the effects of self-efficacy and beliefs about treatment effectiveness.

Summary Points

- **Missing values** are a pervasive problem in research, and can threaten the validity of the study.
- Various factors must be considered in developing a missing values strategy, including the role and type of variables with missing data in the analysis, the extent of missingness, and, of particular importance, the pattern of missingness.
- There are three basic missing values patterns. The first, and most desirable, is **missing completely at random (MCAR)**, which occurs when cases with missing values are just a random subsample of all cases in the sample. When data are MCAR, analyses remain unbiased, although power is reduced.
- Data can be considered **missing at random (MAR)** if missingness is related to other variables—but *not* related to the value of the variable that has the missing values. This pattern is perhaps the most prevalent pattern of missingness in clinical research.
- The third pattern is **missing not at random (MNAR)**, a pattern in which the value of the variable that is missing is related to its missingness. This is often found for such variables as income. In actual studies, it is often difficult to distinguish the MAR and MNAR pattern.
- The two primary approaches to addressing missing values are **deletion methods** (in which missing

values are removed from subsequent analyses) or **imputation methods** (in which the missing values are estimated and substituted for the missing codes).

- Deletion methods include **listwise deletion** (*complete case analysis*) in which cases with missing values are dropped; **pairwise deletion** (*available case analysis*) in which cases with missing values are dropped on an analysis-by-analysis basis; and **variable deletion,** in which an entire variable is removed. The latter may make sense when the variable has a considerable amount of missing data and it is not critical to the analysis. Most computer programs use either listwise or pairwise deletion as the default.
- Imputation methods involve taking information from other sample members, or from the case with missing values, to estimate what the value would have been had it not been missing. A general problem is that variance is lower with imputed values than it would have been with complete data.
- Until recently **mean substitution** (replacing missing values with the mean for the sample or a subgroup) was widely used. Its virtues are ease and simplicity, but this method is no longer considered a good strategy. **Case mean substitution** (imputing a mean from other variables within the case) can, however, be profitably used to impute values of items in a multi-item scale.
- **Regression imputation** involves using complete cases to "predict" what the missing value would have been, based on other variables in the dataset. Variability remains underestimated using regression, and so a more sophisticated approach

(**regression with error**) adds random error into the imputed values.

- The approach most often used to impute values for outcome variables in randomized controlled trials is **last observation carried forward** (**LOCF**), which imputes the missing outcome using the previous measurement of that same outcome. A variation involves substituting the mean of all previous measurements.
- **Expectation-maximization** (**EM**) **imputation** is a two-step process that uses maximum likelihood imputation. It is preferred to most other methods, and is available in a special module of SPSS that offers Missing Values Analysis (MVA).
- **Multiple imputation** (**MI**) is the current "gold standard" for addressing missing values problems, but has not often been used because of its complexity and the limited availability of appropriate software, although that situation is changing. MI addresses a fundamental issue—the uncertainty of any given estimate—by imputing several (*m*) estimates, each of which has an element of randomness introduced. Results across the *m* imputations are later pooled.
- Researchers should examine the patterns and extent of missingness in developing a missing values strategy. A useful approach is to use **senstivity analyses** to understand how alternative strategies affect the substantive results.
- Research reports should contain descriptions about the amount and pattern of missing values in the analyses, and steps researchers took to address the problem.

Exercises

The following exercises cover concepts presented in this chapter. Appendix C provides answers to Part A exercises that are indicated with a dagger (†). Exercises in Part B involve computer analyses using the datasets provided with this textbook, and answers and comments are offered on this book's Web site.

PART A EXERCISES

† **A1.** The following table shows actual data values on the seven items used to create the Parenting Stress scale in our factor analysis of 11 parenting items (Chapter 13) for five mothers. Each case has a missing value, coded 99. Impute values to replace the missing values, using case mean substitution.

2. Child Hard to Care For	3. Many Things Bother Me	4. Given Up a Lot for Child	6. Trapped by Parenthood	7. Lose Patience with Child	8. Often Feel Angry with Child	11. More Work than Pleasure
0	1	10	99	0	0	10
0	0	3	0	0	99	4
99	2	10	1	0	1	0
4	2	0	3	99	1	10
5	4	99	0	0	0	5

A2. For the five items in Exercise A.1 with missing values, the item means for all cases for whom data were available are as follows:

Item	2	4	6	7	8
Mean	2.66	5.91	2.93	2.80	2.00
N	1857	1840	1841	1842	1845

Write a brief statement about whether you think that mean substitution or case mean substitution would be preferred for the five cases with a missing value, based on the information you obtained in Exercise A1. Provide a rationale for your answer.

† **A3.** Using the guideline we suggested in a Tip (p. 380), would it be advisable to impute missing values for two items on the Parenting Stress *subscale*?

† **A4.** Manually impute the missing child weight values, using the regression equation presented in the textbook, for children with the following values on the predictor variables:

Age (yrs)	Gender (0 = female, 1 = male)	No. of siblings	Weight (pounds)
5	1	7	?
6	1	3	?
3	1	4	?
5	0	4	?
4	0	4	?

A5. Look at a recent issue of a nursing research journal, such as *Nursing Research, Journal of Advanced Nursing,* or *Research in Nursing & Health*. How many of the quantitative studies had any reference to missing values? Did any article discuss patterns and amounts of missingness? What methods were used to address missing values?

PART B EXERCISES

† **B1.** For these exercises, you will be using the SPSS dataset Polit2SetC. We will begin by looking at individual responses to items on the Center for Epidemiologic Studies—Depression (CES-D) Scale. For a description of these 20 items, refer to Exercise B1 in Chapter 13. If you did Exercise B1 in Chapter 13 and have kept your output, you can answer the questions here without redoing any analyses. Otherwise, run frequency distributions for the 20 items (*cesd1* to *cesd20*), ignoring the four items that were reverse coded. Then, answer the following questions: (a) What was the range of missing data for individual items, in terms of numbers and percentages? (b) Which item had the least missing data? (c) Which item had the most missing data? (d) How would you describe the "typical" amount of missing data for these 20 items?

† **B2.** Now we will look at how many missing values individual participants had for these 20 CES-D items. To do this, we need to create a new variable (we will call it *misscesd*) that is a count of how many values are missing for each person. Select Transform ➡ Count Occurrences of Values Within Cases. In

the Target Variable field, enter *misscesd;* you can add a descriptive label such as "Number of missing CESD items." Then move the 20 individual CES-D items into the field labeled Numeric Variables. Click the Define Values pushbutton to get to the next dialog box. In the section labeled "Value," select System- or user-missing, then click the Add button. Click Continue, then OK. Next, run a frequency distribution and descriptive statistics for the new *misscesd* variable, and use the output to answer the following questions: (a) How many women answered all 20 items? (b) How many women answered none of the 20 items? (c) What percent of cases had missing values on more than half of the items? (d) What was the mean, median, and modal number of missing items? (e) If we used the standard of imputing missing values only for items with no more than 25% of the items missing, for how many cases would we impute missing values? If we then computed CES-D scales scores, for what percent of the cases would we not be able to compute a CES-D score?

† **B3.** In the situation such as the one we have with missing CES-D items, we would recommend case mean substitution for cases with five or fewer missing values, but achieving this through SPSS commands is tedious, particularly for scales with 20 items such as the CES-D. With small samples, it is likely to be simpler to manually fill in case-mean imputed values. We will guide you through the imputation of a single missing item to illustrate the process. We will do this for item 9, the one with the highest percentage of missing values. Select Transform ➡ Compute Variable, which will create a new variable. (We could have imputed the missing values into the original *cesd9* variable, but it is often wise to create a new variable and to preserve the original in case you make a mistake in the imputation process.) Enter a name for the Target Variable, such as *newcesd9*. To set the new variable equal to old CES-D values, enter *cesd9* in the field for Numeric Expression. Then click OK. Next, go back to the Compute Variable dialog box, leaving *newcesd9* as the Target Variable. In the Numeric Expression field, you need to tell the computer to add the values of the other 19 items and divide by 19, to set *newcesd9* equal to the person's mean for all other items. For the CES-D scale, we need to use the four reverse-coded items to get the appropriate value. Here is the command to insert in the Numeric Expression field:

$$(cesd1 + cesd2 + cesd3 + cesd4rev + cesd5 + cesd6 + cesd7 + cesd8rev + cesd10 + cesd11 + ces12rev + cesd13 + cesd14 + cesd15 + ces16rev + cesd17 + cesd18 + cesd19 + cesd20)/19$$

Next, click the If (optional case selection) button, which brings up a new dialog box. Select "Include if case satisfies condition." Type in the following in the blank field: MISSING (cesd9), then click Continue and OK. This will impute a value for *newcesd9* only for those cases with a missing value—all others will have the original data. Now, run frequencies and descriptive statistics for both *cesd9* and *newcesd9* and answer the following questions. (a) How many cases were missing for the *newcesd9* variable? (b) For how many cases were imputations performed? (c) Why do you think imputations were not done for all missing cases? (d) Did the mean value change for the new variable, compared to the original? How about the *SD*? (e) What was the range of values for just the new imputed values? (You will need to glean this information by comparing the frequency distributions for *cesd9* and *newcesd9*.)

† **B4.** The Polit2SetC dataset includes the variable *cesd,* which is a total CES-D score for cases with nonmissing values, plus cases for whom missing values were imputed using case mean substitution. (The imputation was done only for cases that had no more than five missing values.) Looking at the output for Exercise B2, how many cases should have a CES-D score? Confirm that your answer corresponds to what is in the dataset by running descriptive statistics on *cesd.* (Note that CES-D scores were computed by adding together all item values with appropriate item reversals, and then subtracting 20. This is because the original CES-D scale uses codes of 0, 1, 2, and 3, rather than 1, 2, 3, and 4. It is desirable to have scores on the same scale as the original because cutoff scores are used to establish whether a person is at risk or at high risk of clinical depression.)

† **B5.** We will next explore patterns of missingness for the CES-D scale score. First, create a missing values indicator variable, which we will call *cesdstat*. Select Transform ➜ Compute Variable, and enter *cesdstat* into the slot for Target Variable. Set the new variable equal to 1 by entering the number 1 into the Numeric Expression field, then click OK. Then, click Compute Variable again, enter the number 2 in the Numeric Expression field, and click the If pushbutton. In the next dialog box, click "Include if case satisfies condition," and then enter the following: cesd ≥ 0 AND cesd ≤ 60. This will set the value of the new *cesdstat* variable to 2 for those cases that have a valid value, which is between 0 and 60. Then click Continue and OK. (The values can be labeled by clicking the Variable View tab at the bottom of the screen—for example code 2 could be labeled, *Has a CESD score*.) Check that this new *cesdstat* variable has been properly created by running a frequency distribution. How many cases were coded 1 and how many were coded 2? Does this correspond to what you learned in Exercise B4?

† **B6.** Next, we will run a series of statistical tests to see if missingness is related to other characteristics of the women in this sample, beginning with *t* tests. Select Analyze ➜ Compare Means ➜ Independent Samples T Test. Move the following quantitative variables into the Test Variable list: Age at the time of the interview; Age at first birth; # of children living in HH past month; Family income, all sources; Number of types of abuse of 4 mentioned; SF-12 Physical Health Component Score; and SF-12 Mental Health Component score. Then, enter *cesdstat* as the Grouping Variable and click the Define Groups pushbutton. Enter the value 1 for Group 1 and the value 2 for Group 2, then click Continue. Click the Options pushbutton and make sure that Missing Values is set to: Exclude cases analysis by analysis (i.e., pairwise deletion for these tests of missing versus nonmissing CES-D values). Then click Continue and OK to run the analysis. Answer the following questions based on the output: (a) We know from the previous exercise that there are no missing values for the new variable *cesdstat*. What is the extent of missing values for other variables in these analyses? (b) Looking at the column labeled Sig. (2-tailed) in the Independent Samples Test table, were there any significant differences between women who did and did not have a CES-D score for any variables in the analysis? If so, for which variables?

† **B7.** We will continue to test whether missingness on the CES-D scale is related to mothers' characteristics, this time with chi-square tests to test differences in proportions on categorical variables. Select Analyze ➜ Descriptive Statistics ➜ Crosstabulations. Use *cesdstat* as the column variable, and the following variables as row variables: race/ethnicity, educational attainment, current employment status, and marital status. Select the chi-square test as the statistics option, and request observed column percentages in the Cells option. Answer the following questions based on the output: (a) What is the extent of missing values for the four variables in these analyses? (b) Were there significant differences between women who did and those who did not have a CES-D score on any of the variables in these analyses? (c) Based on our findings in Exercise B6 and B7, would you infer that the pattern of missingness is MCAR, MAR, or MNAR?

B8. If you have access to the SPSS Missing Values Analyses, run the MVA with the same set of variables and use Little's MCAR test to see if you reach different conclusions based on the results of that test than you did based on results from Exercises B6 and B7.

† **B9.** With only 3.8% missing values on the CES-D scale in a very large sample, we might well use listwise deletion for any further substantive analyses with the *cesd* variable. As an exercise, however, we will impute missing values on the CES-D total scale using regression analysis. We will restrict the regression to two predictors that are significantly correlated with CES-D scores, but that have minimal missing values themselves: educational attainment and current employment status. (Other variables with low levels of missing data—age, race/ethnicity, and number of children—were not significantly correlated with CES-D scores; you could verify this yourself.) Use the instructions in Chapter 10 for running a standard multiple regression, with *cesd* as the dependent variable and educational attainment and current employment status as the independents. Then answer the following questions: (a) How many cases were used in this regression analysis? (b) What was the value of *R*? (c) Was the overall model statistically significant? (d) Was educational attainment significant, once current employment was controlled? (e) Was current

employment status significant with educational attainment controlled? (f) Interpret what the *b* weights mean in terms of scores on the CES-D. (g) What is the regression equation for imputing missing values on *cesd*?

† **B10.** Using the answer to Exercise B9 (g), impute missing CES-D scores. First, create a new CES-D variable so that any possible mistakes do not affect the original scores. With the Compute Variable command, set the new variable (e.g., *newcesd*) equal to the original, *cesd*. Then, do another Compute Variable, and set *newcesd* equal to the predicted value from the regression equation. Click the If pushbutton and select "Include if case satisfies condition," and then enter: MISSING (cesd). This will result in imputations only for cases with missing CES-D scores (and nonmissing values for education and current employment status). Click continue, then OK. Then run descriptive statistics (within the Frequencies program) for both *cesd* and *newcesd* and answer the following questions: (a) Look at the Polit2SetC dataset in Data view and find the values for the *newcesd* variable. Case 17 originally had a missing value for *cesd*. What is the imputed value for this case on the *newcesd* variable? (b) How many cases have valid CES-D scores for the *newcesd* variable? (c) In an earlier exercise, we learned that there were missing values on current employment status for two women. What would explain why there are not two missing values for *newcesd*? (d) Are the means for *cesd* and *newcesd* the same? (e) Are the *SD*s for the two variables the same?

B11. If you have access to the Missing Values Analysis module in SPSS, impute the missing values for *cesd* using expectation maximization. Compare the means and *SD*s obtained through regression and EM.

REFERENCES

Methodological and Statistical References

Acock, A. C. (2005). Working with missing values. *Journal of Marriage and Family, 67,* 1012–1028.

American Psychological Association. (2001). *Publication manual of the American Psychological Association* (5th ed.). Washington, DC: Author.

Barnett, V., & Lewis, T. (1994). *Outliers in statistical data* (3rd ed.). New York: John Wiley & Sons.

Braitman, L. (1991). Confidence intervals assess both clinical significance and statistical significance. *Annals of Internal Medicine, 114,* 515–517.

Cohen, J. (1988). *Statistical power analysis for the behavioral sciences* (2nd ed.). Hillsdale, NJ: Lawrence Erlbaum Associates.

Cohen, J., Cohen, P., West, S., & Aiken, L. (2003). *Applied multiple regression/correlation analysis for the behavioral sciences* (3rd ed.). Mahwah, NJ: Lawrence Erlbaum Associates.

Conover, W. J. (1999). *Practical nonparametric statistics* (3rd ed.). New York: Wiley.

Cooper, H. (2010). *Research synthesis and meta-analysis* (4th ed.). Thousand Oaks, CA: Sage Publications.

DeVellis, R. F. (2003). *Scale development: Theory and application* (2nd ed.). Thousand Oaks, CA: Sage Publications.

DiCenso, A., Guyatt, G., & Ciliska, D. (2005). *Evidence-based nursing: A guide to clinical practice.* St. Louis, MO: Elsevier Mosby.

Engels, J. M., & Diehr, P. (2003). Imputation of missing longitudinal data: A comparison of methods. *Journal of Clinical Epidemiology, 56,* 968–976.

Few, S. (2004). *Show me the numbers.* Oakland, CA: Analytics Press.

Field, A. (2005). *Discovering statistics using SPSS* (2nd ed.). Thousand Oaks, CA: Sage Publications.

Fox-Wasylyshyn, S., & E1-Masri, M. (2005). Handling missing data in self-report measures. *Research in Nursing & Health, 28,* 488–495.

Gravel, J., Opatrny, L., & Shapiro, S. (2007). The intention-to-treat approach in randomized controlled trials: Are authors saying what they do and doing what they say? *Clinical Trials, 4,* 350–356.

Gravetter, F., & Wallnau, L. (2008). *Essentials of statistics for the behavioral sciences* (6th ed.). Belmont, CA: Wadsworth Publishing Co.

Grbich, C. (2007). *Qualitative data analysis: An introduction.* Thousand Oaks, CA: Sage Publications.

Hair, J., Black, W., Babin, B., & Anderson, R. (2009). *Multivariate data analysis* (7th ed.) Englewood Cliffs, NJ: Prentice Hall.

Haukoos, J., & Newgard, C. (2007). Missing data in clinical research—Part I: An introduction and conceptual framework. *Academic Emergency Medicine, 14,* 662–668.

Hosmer, D. W., & Lemeshow, S. (2000). *Applied logistic regression* (2nd ed.). New York: John Wiley.

Jaccard, J., & Becker, M. A. (2001). *Statistics for the behavioral sciences* (4th ed.). Belmont, CA: Wadsworth Publishing Co.

Kneipp, S., & McIntosh, M. (2001). Handling missing data in nursing research with multiple imputation. *Nursing Research, 50,* 384–389.

Lipsey, M., & Wilson, D. (2001). *Practical meta-analysis.* Thousand Oaks, CA: Sage Publications.

Little, R., & Rubin, D. (2002). *Statistical analysis with missing data.* (2nd ed.). New York: John Wiley.

McCall, R. B. (2000). *Fundamental statistics for behavioral sciences* (8th ed.). Belmont, CA: Wadsworth Publishing.

McCleary, L. (2002). Using multiple imputation for analysis of incomplete data in clinical research. *Nursing Research, 51,* 339–343.

Melnyk, B. M., & Fineout-Overholt, E. (2005). *Evidence-based practice in nursing and healthcare: A guide to best practice.* Philadelphia: Lippincott Williams & Wilkins.

Miles, M. B., & Huberman, A. M. (1994). *Qualitative data analysis: An expanded sourcebook* (2nd ed.). Thousand Oaks, CA: Sage.

Moons, K., Donders, R., Stijnen, T., & Harrell, F. (2006). Using the outcome for imputation of missing predictor values was preferred. *Journal of Clinical Epidemiology, 59,* 1092–1101.

Musil, C., Warner, C., Yobas, P., & Jones, S. (2002). A comparison of imputation techniques for handling missing data. *Western Journal of Nursing Research, 24,* 815–829.

Norušis, M. J. (2008). *SPSS 16.0: Statistical procedures companion*. Upper Saddle River, NJ: Prentice Hall.

Nunnally, J., & Bernstein, I. H. (1994). *Psychometric theory* (3rd ed.). New York: McGraw-Hill.

Olobatuyi, M. (2006). *A user's guide to path analysis*. Lanham, MD: University Press of America.

Patrician, P. (2002). Multiple imputation for missing data. *Research in Nursing & Health, 25,* 76–84.

Pett, M., Lackey, N., & Sullivan, J. (2003). *Making sense of factor analysis: The use of factor analysis for instrument development in health care research.* Thousand Oaks, CA: Sage Publications.

Polit, D. F., & Beck, C. T. (2008). *Nursing research: Generating and assessing evidence for nursing practice* (8th ed.). Philadelphia: Lippincott Williams & Wilkins.

Polit, D. F., & Gillespie, B. (in press). The use of the intention-to-treat principal in nursing clinical trials, *Nursing Research.*

Polit, D. F., & Sherman, R. (1990). Statistical power in nursing research. *Nursing Research, 39,* 365–369.

Sackett, D. L., Straus, S. E., Richardson, W. S., Rosenberg, W., & Haynes, R. B. (2000). *Evidence-based medicine: How to practice and teach EBM* (2nd ed.). Edinburgh, Scotland: Churchill Livingstone.

Schafer, J., & Graham, J. (2002). Missing data: Our view of the state of the art. *Psychological Methods, 7,* 147–177.

Shadish, W., Cook, T., & Campbell, D. (2002). *Experimental and quasi-experimental designs for generalized causal inference.* Boston: Houghton Mifflin Co.

Shrive, F., Stuart, H., Quan, H., & Ghali, W. (2006). Dealing with missing data in a multi-question depression scale: A comparison of imputation methods. *BMC Medical Research Methodology, 6,* 57.

Singer, J., & Willett, J. (2003). *Applied longitudinal data analysis.* New York, NY: Oxford University Press.

Sprent, P., & Smeeton, N. (2007). *Applied nonparametric statistical methods* (4th ed.). Boca Raton, FL: Chapman and Hall.

Tabachnick, B. G., & Fidell, L. S. (2007). *Using multivariate statistics* (5th ed.). Boston: Allyn & Bacon.

Wallgren, A., Wallgren, B., Persson, R., Jorner, U., & Haaland, J. (1996). *Graphing statistics & data: Creating better charts.* Thousand Oaks, CA: Sage Publications.

Waltz, C. F., Strickland, O. L., & Lenz, E. R. (2005). *Measurement in nursing and health research* (3rd ed.). New York: Springer Publishing Co.

Wood, A., White, I., & Thopson, S. (2004). Are missing data adequately handled? A review of published randomized controlled trials in major medical journals. *Clinical Trials, 1,* 368–376.

Zimmerman, D. W. (2001, April). The effect of selection of samples for homogeneity on Type I error rate. *Interstat.* Retrieved June 9, 2009 from http://interstat .statjournals.net

References for Nursing Studies Cited as Examples

Al-Kandari, F., & Thomas, D. (2008). Adverse nurse outcomes: Correlation to nurses' workload, staffing, and shift rotation in Kuwaiti hospitals. *Applied Nursing Research, 21,* 139–146.

Aroian, K., & Hough, E., Templin, T., & Kaskiri, E. (2008). Development and psychometric evaluation of an Arab version of the Family Peer Relationship Questionnaire. *Research in Nursing & Health, 31,* 402–416.

Barnett, T., Li-Yoong, T., Pinikahana, J., & Si-Yen, T. (2008). Fluid compliance among patients having haemodialysis: Can an educational programme make a difference? *Journal of Advanced Nursing, 61,* 300–306.

Bekhet, A., Zauszniewski, J., & Wykle, M. (2008). Milieu change and relocation adjustment in elders. *Western Journal of Nursing Research, 30,* 113–129.

Bennett, J., Young, H., Nail, L., Winters-Stone, K., & Hanson, G. (2008). A telephone-only motivational intervention to increase physical activity in rural adults. *Nursing Research, 57,* 24–32.

Bryanton, J., Gagnon, A., Hatem, M., & Johnston, C. (2008). Predictors of early parenting self-efficacy. *Nursing Research, 57,* 252–259.

Bu, X., & Wu, Y. B. (2008). Development and psychometric evaluation of the instrument: Attitude toward patient advocacy. *Research in Nursing & Health, 31,* 63–75.

Budin, W., Hoskins, C., Haber, J., Sherman, D. W., Maislin, G., Cater, J., et al. (2008). Breast cancer: Education, counseling, and adjustment among patients and partners. *Nursing Research, 57,* 199–213.

Carruth, A., Browning, S., Reed, D., Skarke, L., & Sealey, L. (2006). The impact of farm lifestyle and health characteristics. *Nursing Research, 55,* 121–127.

Certain, H., Mueller, M., Jagodzinski, T., & Fleming, M. (2008). Domestic abuse during the previous year in a sample of postpartum women. *Journal of Obstetric, Gynecologic, & Neonatal Nursing, 37,* 35–41.

Cha, E., Kim, K., & Burke, L. (2008). Psychometric validation of a condom self-efficacy scale in Korean. *Nursing Research, 57,* 245–251.

Chang, S., Wung, S., & Crogan, N. (2008). Improving activities of daily living for nursing home elder persons in Taiwan. *Nursing Research, 57,* 191–198.

Chaplin, R., Jedynak, J., Johnson, D., Heiter, D., Shovelton, L., & Garrett, N. (2007). The effects of valerian on the time course of emergence from general anesthesia in Sprague-Dawley rats. *AANA Journal, 75,* 431–435.

Chen, K. M., Lin, J., Lin, H., Wu, H., Chen, W., Li, C., & Lo, S. (2008). The effects of a Simplified Tai-Chi Exercise Program (STEP) on the physical health of older adults living in long-term care facilities: A single group design with multiple time points. *International Journal of Nursing Studies, 45,* 501–507.

Cho, J., Holditch-Davis, D., & Miles, M. (2008). Effects of maternal depressive symptoms and infant gender on the interactions between mothers and their medically at-risk infants. *Journal of Obstetric, Gynecologic, & Neonatal Nursing, 37,* 58–70.

Choi, M., Phillips, L., Figueredo, A., Insel, K., & Min, S. (2008). Construct validity of the Korean women's abuse intolerance scale. *Nursing Research, 57,* 40–50.

Corless, I., Voss, J., Nicholas, P., Bunch, E., Bain, C., Coleman, C., et al. (2008). Fatigue in HIV/AIDS patients with comorbidities. *Applied Nursing Research, 21,* 116–122.

Črnčec, R., Barnett, B., & Matthey, S. (2008). Development of an instrument to assess perceived self-efficacy in the parents of infants. *Research in Nursing & Health, 31,* 442–453.

de Montigny, F., & Lacharité, C. (2008). Modeling parents and nurses' relationships. *Western Journal of Nursing Research, 30,* 743–758.

Dougherty, C. M., & Hunziker, J. (2009). Predictors of implantable cardioverter defibrillator shocks during the first year. *Journal of Cardiovascular Nursing, 24,* 21–28.

Eastwood, J., Doering, L., Roper, J., & Hays, R. (2008). Uncertainty and health related quality of life 1 year after coronary angiography. *American Journal of Critical Care, 17,* 232–242.

Ellett, M., Beckstrand, J., Flueckiger, J., Perkins, S., & Johnson, C. (2005). Predicting the insertion distance for placing gastric tubes. *Clinical Nursing Research, 14,* 11–27.

Elliott, A., Horgas, A., & Marsiske, M. (2008). Nurses' role in identifying mild cognitive impairment in older adults. *Geriatric Nursing, 29,* 38–47.

Evangelista, A., & Sims-Giddens, S. (2008). Gender differences in discipline of nurses in Missouri. *Western Journal of Nursing Research, 30,* 501–514.

Fick, D., Mion, L., Beers, M., & Waller, J. (2008). Health outcomes associated with potentially inappropriate medication use in older adults. *Research in Nursing & Health, 31,* 42–51.

Fredland, N., Campbell, J., & Han, H. (2008). Effect of violence exposure on health outcomes among young urban adolescents. *Nursing Research, 57,* 157–165.

Gance-Cleveland, B., Mays, M., & Steffen, A. (2008). Association of adolescent physical and emotional health with perceived severity of parental substance abuse. *Journal for Specialists in Pediatric Nursing, 13,* 15–25.

Gies, C., Buchman, D., Robinson, J., & Smolen, D. (2008). Effect of an inpatient nurse-directed smoking cessation program. *Western Journal of Nursing Research, 30,* 6–19.

Good, M., & Ahn, S. (2008). Korean and American music reduces pain in Korean women after gynecologic surgery. *Pain Management Nursing, 9,* 96–103.

Groth, S. W. (2008). The long-term impact of adolescent gestational weight gain. *Research in Nursing & Health, 31,* 108–118.

Holditch-Davis, D., Merrill, P., Schwartz, T., & Scher, M. (2008). Predictors of wheezing in prematurely born children. *Journal of Obstetric, Gynecologic, & Neonatal Nursing, 37,* 262–273.

Horgas, A., Yoon, S., Nichols, A., & Marsiske, M. (2008). The relationship between pain and functional disability in black and white older adults. *Research in Nursing & Health, 31,* 341–354.

Im, E. O., Chee, W., Guevara, E., Lim, H., & Shin, H. (2008). Gender and ethnic differences in cancer patients' needs for help: An Internet survey. *International Journal of Nursing Studies, 45,* 1192–1204.

Kanak, M. F., Titler, M., Shever, L., Fei, Q., Dochterman, J., & Picone, D. (2008). The effects of hospitalization on multiple units. *Applied Nursing Research, 21,* 15–22.

Kennedy-Malone, L., Fleming, M. E., & Penny, J. (2008). Prescribing patterns of gerontological nurse practitioners in the United States. *Journal of the American Academy of Nurse Practitioners, 20,* 28–34.

Kim, H. S., & Song, M. (2008). Technological intervention for obese patients with type 2 diabetes. *Applied Nursing Research, 21,* 84–89.

Koniak-Griffin, D., Lesser, J., Henneman, T., Huang, R., Huang, X., Tello, J. *et al.* (2008). HIV prevention for adolescent mothers and their partners. *Western Journal of Nursing Research, 30,* 724–742.

Kowalski, S., & Bondmass, M. (2008). Physiological and psychological symptoms of grief in widows. *Research in Nursing & Health, 31,* 23–30.

Lauver, D. R., Worawong, C., & Olsen, C. (2008). Health goals among primary care patients. *Journal of the American Academy of Nurse Practitioners, 20,* 144–154.

Lee, E., Fogg, L., & Menon, U. (2008). Knowledge and beliefs related to cervical cancer and screening among Korean American women. *Western Journal of Nursing Research, 30,* 960–974.

Lerdal, A., Moe, B., Digre, E., Harding, T., Kristensen, F., Grov, E., et al. (2009). Stages of change—continuous measure (URICA-E2): Psychometrics of a Norwegian version. *Journal of Advanced Nursing, 65,* 193–202.

Leung, A., DeAngelis, D., Hurwitz, J., Simpson, E., Oestricher, J., Ing, E., et al. (2007). Surgical waiting times for ocular and periocular cancer patients in Toronto. *Canadian Journal of Opthalmology, 42,* 826–831.

Li, Y., Scott, C., & Li, L. (2008). Chinese nursing students' HIV/AIDS knowledge, attitudes, and practice intentions. *Applied Nursing Research, 21,* 147–152.

Liao, W. C., Chiu, M. J., & Landis, C. (2008). A warm foot-bath before bedtime and sleep in older Taiwanese with sleep disturbance. *Research in Nursing & Health, 31,* 514–528.

Liu, H. E. (2008). Changes of satisfaction with appearance and working status for head and neck tumour patients. *Journal of Clinical Nursing, 17,* 1930–1938.

Liu, H., Feurer, I., Dwyer, K., Speroff, T., Shaffer, D., & Pinson, C. E. (2008). The effects of gender and age on health-related quality of life following kidney transplantation. *Journal of Clinical Nursing, 17,* 82–89.

Looman, W. S., & Farrag, S. (2009). Psychometric properties and cross-cultural equivalence of the Arabic Social Capital Scale. *International Journal of Nursing Studies, 46,* 44–53.

Mak, S. S., Yeo, W., Lee, Y., Mo, K., TRse, K., Tse, S., et al. (2008). Predictors of lymphedema in patients with breast cancer undergoing axillary lymph node dissection in Hong Kong. *Nursing Research, 57,* 416–425.

Maposa, S., & Smithbattle, L. (2008). Preliminary reliability and validity of the grandparent version of the Grandparent Support Scale for Teenage Mothers (GSSTM-G). *Journal of Family Nursing, 14,* 224–241.

McInerney, P., Nicholas, P., Wantland, D., Corless, I., Ncama, B., Bhengu, B., et al. (2007). Characteristics of anti-tuberculosis medication adherence in South Africa. *Applied Nursing Research, 20,* 164–170.

McMillan, S., Tofthagen, C., & Morgan, M. (2008). Relationships among pain, sleep disturbances, and depressive symptoms in outpatients from a comprehensive cancer center. *Oncology Nursing Forum, 35,* 603–611.

Metheny, N., Schnelker, R., McGinnis, J., Zimmerman, G., Duke, C., Merritt, B., et al. (2005). Indicators of tubesite during feedings. *Journal of Neuroscience Nursing, 37,* 320–325.

Miller, S. K., Alpert, P., & Cross, C. (2008). Overweight and obesity in nurses, advanced practice nurses, and nurse educators. *Journal of the Academy of Nurse Practitioners, 20,* 259–265.

Missildine, K. (2008). Sleep and the sleep environment of older adults in acute care settings. *Journal of Gerontological Nursing, 34,* 15–21.

Morrison-Beedy, D., Carey, M., Feng, C., & Tu, X. (2008). Predicting sexual risk behaviors among adolescent and young women using a prospective diary method. *Research in Nursing & Health, 31,* 329–340.

Moser, D., Riegel, B., McKinley, S., Doering, L., Meischke, H., Heo, S., et al. (2009). The Control Attitudes Scale-Revised: Psychometric evaluation in three groups of patients with cardiac illness. *Nursing Research, 58,* 42–51.

Nakagami, G., Sanada, H., Konya, C., Kitagawa, A., Tadaka, E., & Matsuyama, Y. (2007). Evaluation of a new pressure ulcer preventive dressing containing ceramide 2 with low frictional outer layer. *Journal of Advanced Nursing, 59,* 520–529.

Nannini, A., Lazar, J., Berg, C., Barger, M., Tomashek, K., Cabral, H., et al. (2008). Physical injuries reported on hospital visits for assault during the pregnancy–associated period. *Nursing Research, 57,* 144–149.

Nyamathi, A., Nahid, P., Berg, J., Burrage, J., Christiani, A., Aqtash, S., et al. (2008). Efficacy of nurse case-managed intervention for latent tuberculosis among homeless subsamples. *Nursing Research, 57,* 33–39.

Oostrom, J., & van Mierlo, H. (2008). An evaluation of an aggression management training program to cope with workplace violence in the healthcare sector. *Research in Nursing & Health, 31,* 320–328.

Park, H. J., Jarrett, M., Cain, K., & Heitkemper, M. (2008). Psychological distress and symptoms are related to severity of bloating in women with irritable bowel syndrome. *Research in Nursing & Health, 31,* 98–107.

Park, J. H., Lee, W., & Chung, H. (2008). Incidence and risk factors of breast cancer lymphoedema. *Journal of Clinical Nursing, 17,* 1450–1459.

Peterson, U., Bergstrom, G., Samuelsson, M., Asberg, M., & Nygren, A. (2008). Reflecting peer-support groups in the prevention of stress and burnout: Randomized controlled trial. *Journal of Advanced Nursing, 63,* 506–516.

Polit, D. F., & Beck, C. T. (2008). Is there gender bias in nursing research? *Research in Nursing & Health, 31,* 417–427.

Rew, L., Grady, M., Whittaker, T., & Bowman, K. (2008). Interaction of duration of homelessness and gender on adolescent sexual health indicators. *Journal of Nursing Scholarship, 40,* 109–115.

Robbins, L., Wu, T., Sikorski, A., & Morley, B. (2008). Psychometric assessment of the Adolescent Physical Activity Perceived Benefits and Barriers Scales. *Journal of Nursing Measurement, 16,* 98–112.

Rungreangkulkij, S., & Wongtakee, W. (2008). The psychological impact of Buddhist counseling for patients suffering from symptoms of anxiety. *Archives of Psychiatric Nursing, 22,* 127–134.

Salamonson, Y., Everett, B., Koch, J., Andrew, S., & Davidson, P. (2008). English-language acculturation predicts academic performance in nursing students who speak English as a second language. *Research in Nursing & Health, 31,* 86–94.

Schumacher, K., Stewart, B., Archbold, P., Caparro, M., Mutale, F., & Agrawal, S. (2008). Effects of caregiving demand, mutuality, and preparedness on family caregiver outcomes during cancer treatment. *Oncology Nursing Forum, 35,* 49–56.

Shin, H., Kim, K., Kim, Y., Chee, W., & Im, E. (2008). A comparison of two pain measures for Asian American cancer patients. *Western Journal of Nursing Research, 30,* 181–196.

Shishani, K. (2008). Chronically ill adults' educational needs on self-medication. *Applied Nursing Research, 21,* 54–59.

Skybo, T., & Buck, J. (2007). Stress and coping responses to proficiency testing in school-age children. *Pediatric Nursing, 33,* 413–418.

Soundy, A., Taylor, A., Faulkner, G., & Rowlands, A. (2007). Psychometric properties of the 7-Day Physical Activity Recall Questionnaire in individuals with severe mental illness. *Archives of Psychiatric Nursing, 21,* 309–316.

Toffolo, S. R., Furtado, R., Klein, A., Watanabe, S., Andrade, L., & Natour, J. (2008). Measurement of upper limb ulcers in patients with systemic sclerosis. *Nursing Research, 57,* 84–92.

Tullai-McGuinness, S. (2008). Home healthcare practice environment: Predictors of RN satisfaction. *Research in Nursing & Health, 31,* 252–260.

Vadlamudi, R., Adams, S., Hogan, B., Wu, T., & Wahid, Z. (2008). Nurses' attitudes, beliefs and confidence levels regarding care for those who abuse alcohol. *Nurse Education in Practice, 8,* 290–298.

Walker, S., Pullen, C., Hertzog, M., Boekner, L., & Hageman, P. (2006). Determinants of older rural women's activity and eating. *Western Journal of Nursing Research, 28,* 449–468.

Webb, M. (2008). Focus groups as an intervention for low-income African American smokers to promote participation in subsequent intervention studies. *Research in Nursing & Health, 31,* 141–151.

Weis, K., Lederman, R., Lilly, A., & Schaffer, J. (2008). The relationship of military imposed marital separations on maternal acceptance of pregnancy. *Research in Nursing & Health, 31,* 196–207.

Welch, C., Miller, C., & James, N. (2008). Sociodemographic and health-related determinants of breast and cervical cancer screening behavior, 2005. *Journal of Obstetric, Gynecologic, & Neonatal Nursing, 37,* 51–57.

Wetta-Hall, R. (2007). Impact of a collaborative community case management program on a low-income uninsured population in Sedgwick County, KS. *Applied Nursing Research, 20,* 188–194.

Winkelman, C., Norman, D., Maloni, J., & Kless, J. (2008). Pain measurement during labor: Comparing the visual analog scale with dermatome assessment. *Applied Nursing Research, 21,* 104–109.

Woods, D. L., Kovach, C., Raff, H., Joosse, L., Basmadjian, A., & Hegadoren, K. (2008). Using saliva to measure endogenous cortisol in nursing home residents with dementia. *Research in Nursing & Health, 31,* 283–294.

Xu, Y., Toobert, D., Savage, C., Pan, W., & Whitmer, K. (2008). Factors influencing diabetes self-management in Chinese people with type 2 diabetes. *Research in Nursing & Health, 31,* 613–625.

Yarcheski, A., Mahon, N., Yarcheski, T., & Hanks, M. (2008). Psychometric evaluation of the Interpersonal Relationship Inventory for early adolescents. *Public Health Nursing, 25,* 375–382.

Yip, Y., Sit, J., Fung, K., Wong, D., Chong, S., Chung, L., et al. (2007). Impact of an arthritis self-management programme with an added exercise component for osteoarthritic knee sufferers on improving pain, functional outcomes, and use of health care services. *Patient Education & Counseling, 65,* 113–121.

GLOSSARY

Absolute frequencies. The count of the number of cases with a given score value.

Absolute risk. The proportion of people in a group who experienced a specified outcome, usually expressed as a negative outcome.

Absolute risk reduction (ARR). The difference between the absolute risk in one group (e.g., those exposed to an intervention) and the absolute risk in another group (e.g., those not exposed); sometimes called the *risk difference* or *RD*.

Absolute value. The value of a number regardless of its positive or negative sign (e.g., the absolute value of -10, symbolized as $|-10|$, is 10).

Adjusted means. The mean values of the dependent variable for different groups, after removing the effects of covariates through multiple regression or ANCOVA.

Adjusted R^2. The squared multiple correlation coefficient adjusted for sample size and number of predictors to give a more accurate estimate of relationships in the population; also known as *shrunken R^2* and sometimes symbolized as $\widetilde{R}^2$.

Alpha (α). (1) In tests of statistical significance, the level designating the established risk of committing a Type I error; (2) an index used to evaluate internal consistency reliability called *Cronbach's alpha* or *coefficient alpha*.

Alpha factor method. A method of factor analysis that analyzes common factor variance and strives to maximize Cronbach's alpha (internal consistency reliability) for the factors.

Alternative hypothesis. In hypothesis testing, a hypothesis different from the null hypothesis; often symbolized as H_1; the alternative hypothesis is usually the actual research hypothesis.

Analysis. A method of organizing data in such a way that research questions can be answered.

Analysis of covariance (ANCOVA). A statistical procedure used to test mean group differences on a dependent variable, while controlling for one or more confounding variables, or a preintervention measure of the outcome variable (covariates).

Analysis of variance (ANOVA). A statistical procedure for testing mean differences among three or more groups by comparing the variability between groups to the variability within groups.

Assumption. In statistical analysis, characteristics of the data presumed to be true for the purpose of the analysis being performed, a violation of which can invalidate the results.

Asymmetric distribution. A distribution of data values that is skewed, i.e., that has two halves that are not mirror images of the each other.

Attenuation. The reduction in a correlation coefficient attributable to measurement error.

Attrition bias. The bias resulting from the loss of participants during the course of a study, which can alter the composition of the sample initially drawn.

Available case analysis. Analysis based on cases with non-missing data on a selective (pairwise) basis, involving the deletion of cases with missing data only when one variable is paired with another variable that has missing data.

Bar graph. A graphical presentation of a frequency distribution for a categorical variable, representing values of the variable on one axis and frequencies or percentages on the other.

Bartlett's test of sphericity. A statistical test used in multivariate analyses (e.g., factor analysis) that tests the null hypothesis that the correlation matrix is an identity matrix (one in which all correlations are zero).

Bartlett's test of Wilks' lambda (λ). In canonical analysis, a significance test used to evaluate whether an R_c (or a set of R_cs) is significantly different from zero.

Beta (β). (1) In statistical testing, the probability of committing a Type II error; (2) in multiple regression, a standardized coefficient indicating the relative weight of a predictor variable expressed as a standardized z score in the regression equation.

Between-subjects test. A statistical test that is appropriate for research designs in which separate (independent) groups of people are being compared (e.g., men versus women); also called a test for independent groups.

Bias. An influence that distorts the results and undermines study validity.

Bimodal distribution. A distribution of values with two peaks (high frequencies).

Binary logistic regression. A regression procedure that uses maximum likelihood estimation to estimate the odds of an event occurring; the analysis examines relationships between independent variables and a binary (dichotomous) outcome variable.

Binomial distribution. A probability distribution for a dichotomous variable.

Bivariate descriptive statistics. Statistics used to analyze the empirical relationship between two variables.

Bivariate normal distribution. A distribution of two variables (X and Y) such that scores on X are normally distributed for each value of Y, and vice versa.

Bonferroni correction. A correction used to correct the significance level, usually following post hoc tests or tests of different dependent variables with the same sample; the correction involves dividing the desired alpha by the number of tests performed (e.g., for $\alpha = .05$ and 3 tests, the corrected alpha would be .017).

Box *M* test. A statistical test used to test the homogeneity of a variance–covariance matrix, an assumption underlying several multivariate analyses.

Boxplot. Also called a *box-and-whisker plot,* a convenient way of graphically portraying key aspects of a distribution of values; the lower quartile (Q_1) and upper quartile (Q_3) are the edges of the "box;" and the "whiskers" indicate the values that are *not* outliers, defined in relation to the interquartile range (*IQR*).

Canonical analysis. A multivariate statistical procedure for examining the relationship between two *sets* of variables, such as two or more independent variables and two or more dependent variables.

Canonical correlation coefficient (R_c). The index summarizing the magnitude of the correlation between pairs of canonical variates in canonical analysis.

Canonical variate. In canonical analysis, the composite formed by a linear combination of independent variables or dependent variables.

Canonical weight. In canonical analysis, the standardized weights associates with each independent and dependent variable, analogous to beta weights in multiple regression.

Case mean substitution. An approach to dealing with missing values that involves imputing a missing value with the mean of other relevant variables from the person with the missing value (e.g., using the mean of nine nonmissing items on a scale to impute the value of the 10th item, which is missing).

Categorical variable. A variable that has discrete categories, such as a nominal-level variable (e.g., a person's marital status).

Causal modeling. The development and statistical testing of hypothesized causal relationships among phenomena.

Causal relationship. A relationship between two variables such that one variable (the "cause") determines the presence/absence or value of the other (the "effect").

Ceiling effect. The effect of having scores at or near the highest possible value, which can constrain the amount of upward change possible and also tends to reduce variability in a variable.

Cell. The intersection of a row and column in a table with two or more dimensions.

Central limit theorem. A statistical principle stipulating that (a) the larger the sample, the more closely the sampling distribution of the mean will approximate a normal distribution; and (b) the mean of a sampling distribution is equal to the population mean.

Central tendency. An index that comes from the center of a distribution of scores, describing what is a "typical" value; the three most common indices of central tendency are the mode, the median, and the mean.

Change score. The score value obtained by subtracting scores on a variable at one point in time from scores on the same variable measured at an earlier point in time.

Chi-square goodness-of-fit test. A statistical test used in several contexts to determine the fit of the data to hypothesized population values or a hypothesized model.

Chi-square test of independence. A statistical test used to assess whether a relationship exists between two categorical variables in a contingency table; symbolized as χ^2.

Class interval. A grouping of data on a continuous variable into a subset of values, which makes the data easier to interpret when displayed in a grouped frequency distribution.

Cochran's *Q* test. A nonparametric test for population differences in proportions, used for within-subjects designs when the dependent variable is dichotomous.

Code. A numerical value assigned to a variable according to a set of rules to represent a status on that variable (e.g., for gender, code 1 for males, code 2 for females).

Coefficient alpha. See *Cronbach's alpha.*

Coefficient of determination. An index indicating the proportion of variance in the dependent variable accounted for or explained by independent variables, more commonly referred to as r^2 or R^2.

Cohen's *d*. The effect size index that summarizes the magnitude of differences between two group means, expressed in pooled standard deviation units; sometimes called the *standardized mean difference* or *SMD.*

Common factor variance. A measure of the variance that two or more measures share in common; also referred to as *communality.*

Communality. A measure of a variable's shared variance in the context of a factor analysis; also referred to as *common factor variance* and sometimes symbolized as h^2.

Complete case analysis. Analysis based only on cases with nonmissing data for all variables, i.e., using listwise deletion as the method of dealing with missing values by eliminating cases with any missing data.

Compound symmetry. An assumption in repeated measures analyses, stipulating the homogeneity of within-treatment variances and homogeneity of covariance between pairs of within-treatment levels.

Confidence interval. The range of values within which a population parameter is estimated to lie at a specified level of probability; abbreviated *CI.*

Confidence level. The estimated probability that a population parameter lies within a given confidence interval.

Confidence limits. The upper and lower boundaries of a confidence interval.

Confirmatory factor analysis (CFA). A factor analysis, based on maximum likelihood estimation, designed to confirm a hypothesized measurement model.

Confounding variable. An extraneous variable that confounds the relationship between the independent and dependent variables and that should ideally be controlled either in the research design or through statistical procedures.

Construct validity. The degree to which an instrument truly measures the construct under consideration.

Contingency table. A two-dimensional table that displays a crosstabulation of the frequencies of two categorical variables.

Continuous variable. A variable that can take on an infinite range of values between two points on a continuum (e.g., height).

Control. The process of holding constant possible influences on the dependent variable under investigation.

Control group. Participants in an experiment (clinical trial) who do not receive the experimental intervention and whose performance provides a baseline against which the effects of the treatment can be measured.

Correlation. A bond between variables, wherein variation in one variable is related to variation in the other.

Correlation coefficient. An index that summarizes the magnitude and direction of a relationship between two variables; correlation coefficients typically range from $+1.00$ (for a perfect positive relationship) through .00 (for no relationship) to -1.00 (for a perfect negative relationship).

Correlation matrix. A two-dimensional display showing the correlation coefficients between all combinations of variables of interest.

Covariance. A measure of the joint variance of two variables, computed by summing the cross products of each variable's deviation scores and dividing by degrees of freedom; when each covariance is divided by the standard deviations of the two variables, the result is Pearson's r.

Covariate. A variable that is statistically controlled (held constant) in analysis of covariance; the covariate is typically an extraneous, confounding influence on the dependent variable or a pretest measure of the dependent variable.

Cox and Snell R^2. One of several pseudo R^2 statistics used as an overall effect size index in logistic regression, analogous to R^2 in least-squares multiple regression, but lacking the ability to truly capture the proportion of variance explained in the outcome variable.

Cramér's V. An index describing the magnitude of relationship between nominal-level data, typically used when the contingency table to which it is applied is larger than 2×2.

Criterion-related validity. The extent to which scores on an instrument are correlated with an external criterion.

Critical region. The area in the sampling distribution representing values that are "improbable" if the null hypothesis is true.

Cronbach's alpha. A reliability coefficient that indicates how much the items on a scale are measuring the same underlying dimension, thus a measure of internal consistency; also referred to as *coefficient alpha*.

Cross products. The multiplication of deviation scores for one variable by the deviation scores for the second; used in the calculation of covariances and correlations.

Crossover design. An experimental design in which participants are exposed to more than one condition or treatment, in random order.

Crosstabulation. The calculation of a two-dimensional frequency distribution for two categorical variables (e.g., gender—male/female—crosstabulated with smoking status—smoker/nonsmoker); the results are typically presented in a contingency (crosstabs) table.

Cross-validation. The process of verifying the validity of the results of an analysis done with one subset of the sample by replicating the analysis with a second subset from the same sample.

Cumulative relative frequency. In a frequency distribution, the percentage of cases with a given score value, combined with percentages for all those values that preceded it.

Curvilinear relationship. A relationship between two continuous variables such that, when plotted in a scatterplot, a curve rather than a straight line is formed.

d. See *Cohen's d*.

Data. The pieces of information obtained in a study.

Data analysis. The systematic organization and synthesis of research data, and the testing of hypotheses with those data.

Data analysis plan. The overall plan for the analysis of research data that serves as a guide to answering the research questions and interpreting the results.

Data cleaning. The preparation of data for statistical analysis by performing checks to ensure that the data are accurate and internally consistent.

Data matrix. A two-dimensional array of data (subjects $\times$ variables).

Data transformation. An alteration of the raw research data, often designed to put them in a form that can be meaningfully analyzed.

Dataset. The total collection of data on all variables for the entire research sample.

Default. In statistical computer packages, the analysis automatically performed or the option automatically used, unless a specific alternative request is made to override it.

Degrees of freedom (df). A concept used in tests of statistical significance, referring to the number of components that are free to vary about a parameter (e.g., by knowing a sample mean, all but one value would be free to vary).

Deletion methods. A broad class of methods used to address missing values problems by deletion of cases or variables.

Dependent groups *t* test. A statistical test for comparing group means when people in the groups being compared are the same (e.g., a before-after comparison) or are paired (e.g., husbands and wives).

Dependent variable. The variable that is hypothesized to depend on or be caused by another variable (the independent variable); also called the *outcome variable*.

Descriptive statistics. Statistics used to describe and summarize data (e.g., means, percentages, standard deviations).

Deviation score. A score computed by subtracting an individual score value from the mean of the distribution of scores.

Dichotomous variable. A variable having only two values or categories (e.g., gender).

Direct oblimin rotation. In factor analysis, the most widely used method of oblique rotation of factors following factor extraction.

Directional hypothesis. A hypothesis that makes a specific prediction about the nature and direction of the relationship between two variables.

Discrete variable. A variable that has a finite number of values between any two points.

Discriminant analysis. A statistical procedure used to predict group membership or status on a categorical (nominal-level) variable on the basis of two or more independent variables, using least-squares estimation.

Discriminant function. In discriminant analysis, a linear combination of independent variables formed to maximally separate groups.

Discriminant score (*D* score). The predicted value from a discriminant analysis equation, used as a basis for classifying cases into groups.

Dummy coding. A method of coding categorical variables into dichotomous variables, using codes of 0 and 1 to represent the presence or absence of an attribute (e.g., married = 1, not married = 0); results in dummy (indicator) variables.

Duncan's multiple-range test. A post hoc test used following a significant ANOVA to test differences between all possible pairs of means.

Dunn procedure. A procedure involving the post hoc comparison of all possible pairs of groups following a significant overall test (e.g., the Mann-Whitney *U* test or Friedman test), using a Bonferroni correction to adjust the level of significance.

Durbin-Watson statistic. A statistical test used to detect nonindependence of errors of prediction in a regression analysis.

Effect coding. A way of coding categorical variables for multivariate analysis that uses 1, 0, and −1 to designate categories.

Effect size. A statistical expression of the magnitude of the relationship between two variables, or the magnitude of the difference between groups on an attribute of interest.

Eigenvalue. The value equal to the sum of the squared weights for a linear composite (e.g., a factor in factor analysis), indicating how much variance in the solution is explained.

Epsilon. A correction factor for addressing violations of the sphericity assumption in repeated measures analyses; two formulas for epsilon are the Greenhouse-Geisser epsilon and Huynh-Feldt epsilon.

Errors of prediction. The differences between the actual values of a dependent variable and the predicted values in a regression analysis; the portion of the dependent variable not explained by the predictor variables; also called the *residuals*.

Estimation procedures. The procedures used in inferential statistics to estimate a population parameter on the basis of sample data.

Eta-squared. A statistic calculated (often in connection with ANOVA), to indicate the proportion of variance in the dependent variable explained by the independent variables, analogous to R^2 in multiple regression; computed by dividing the sum of squares between groups by the total sum of squares.

Evidence-based practice. A practice that involves making clinical decisions on the best available evidence, with evidence that is from disciplined research and thus is often supported through statistical analysis.

Expectation-maximization (EM) imputation. A sophisticated single-imputation process that generates an estimated value for missing data in two steps (an expectation or E-step and a maximization or M-step), using maximum likelihood estimation.

Expected frequency. The number of observations that would be expected in a cell of a contingency table if the null hypothesis were true, that is, if the two variables in the table were unrelated.

Experimental group. The participants in a clinical trial who receive the experimental treatment or intervention.

Exploratory factor analysis. A factor analysis undertaken to determine the underlying dimensionality of a set of variables, most often using least-squares estimation.

External validity. The degree to which results from a study can be generalized to settings or samples other than those used in the research.

Extraneous variable. A variable that confounds the relationship between the independent and dependent variables and that should ideally be controlled either in the research design or through statistical procedures.

***F* ratio.** The statistic obtained in several statistical tests (e.g., ANOVA) in which variation attributable to different sources (e.g., between groups and within groups) is compared.

Factor. In factor analysis, a linear combination of variables in a data matrix that captures an underlying dimension or latent variable.

Factor analysis. A statistical procedure for reducing a large set of variables into a smaller set of variables (factors) with common characteristics or underlying dimensions.

Factor correlation matrix. In factor analysis with oblique rotation, the factor $\times$ factor matrix that shows the correlations among the factors.

Factor extraction. The first major phase of a factor analysis, which involves the extraction of as much variance as possible through the successive creation of linear combinations of the variables in the analysis.

Factor loading. In factor analysis, the b weight associated with a variable on a given factor.

Factor matrix. A matrix produced in factor analysis that has variables on one dimension and factors on the other.

Factor rotation. The second major phase of factor analysis, during which the reference axes for the factors are rotated such that variables more clearly align with a single factor.

Factor score. A person's score on a latent variable (factor).

Factorial design. An experimental design in which two or more independent variables are simultaneously manipulated, permitting an analysis of the main effects of the independent variables, plus the interaction effects.

Fisher's exact test. A statistical procedure used to test the significance of the difference in proportions, used when the sample size is small or cells in the contingency table have no observations.

Fisher's least significant difference (*LSD*) test. A post hoc test, also known as the *protected t test*, used following a significant ANOVA to test differences between all possible pairs of means; *LSD* is an acronym for least significant difference.

Floor effect. The effect of having scores at or near the lowest possible value, which can constrain the amount of downward change possible and also tends to reduce variability in a variable.

Frequency distribution. A systematic array of data values (usually from the lowest to the highest), together with a count of the number of times each value was obtained.

Frequency polygon. A graphic display of a frequency distribution, in which dots appear above score values on the X axis to indicate frequency on the Y axis, and are connected by a straight line.

Friedman test. A nonparametric analog of ANOVA, used to test differences in a paired-groups or repeated measures situation when there are three or more sets of observations.

General linear model (GLM). A flexible statistical linear model that encompasses a broad class of statistical techniques (e.g., t test, analysis of variance, multiple regression), and that uses the least squares criterion for estimating parameters.

Goodness-of-fit test. See *chi-square goodness-of-fit test*.

Grand mean. The overall mean for a set of scores, for all groups.

Greenhouse-Geisser epsilon. A widely used correction factor for addressing violations of the sphericity assumption in repeated measures analyses.

Grouped frequency distribution. A frequency distribution in which score values are clustered into sets (class intervals); used to facilitate interpretation of the distribution when the range of values is wide.

Heterogeneity. The degree to which objects are dissimilar with respect to some attribute (i.e., characterized by high variability).

Heteroscedasticity. A property describing the variability of two variables (X and Y) such that for different values of X the variability of the Y scores differs; the opposite of homoscedasticity.

Hierarchical multiple regression. A multiple regression analysis in which predictor variables are entered into the equation in ordered steps that are specified by the analyst; sometimes called *sequential regression*.

Histogram. A graphic presentation of frequency distribution data on two axes, in which bars are used to indicate the number or percentage of times each score value occurs.

Homogeneity. The degree to which objects are similar (i.e., characterized by low variability).

Homogeneity of regression assumption. In ANCOVA and MANCOVA, the assumption that the covariate has the same relationship with the dependent variable in every group being compared.

Homogeneity of variance assumption. The assumption in several statistical tests that the variance of the groups being compared is equal in the populations.

Homogeneity of the variance–covariance matrix assumption. The multivariate analog of the assumption of homogeneous variances for multiple dependent variables, evaluated through the Box M test.

Homoscedasticity. A property describing the variability of two variables (X and Y) such that for each value of X the variability of the Y scores is about the same and vice versa; the opposite of heteroscedasticity.

Hosmer-Lemeshow test. A test used in logistic regression to evaluate how well observed frequencies of predicted probabilities corresponding to expected frequencies in an ideal model over the range of probability values, as arranged in deciles; a good fit between the observed and the hypothetically perfect model is indicated by *lack* of statistical significance.

Hotelling's trace criterion. A statistical index used in MANOVA and other multivariate tests to evaluate the significance of group differences.

Huynh-Feldt epsilon. A widely used correction factor for addressing violations of the sphericity assumption in repeated measures analyses.

Hypothesis testing. The application of inferential statistics in which sampling distributions are used to make objective, probabilistic decisions about the acceptance or rejection of null hypotheses.

Imputation methods. A broad class of methods used to address missing values problems by estimating (imputing) the missing values.

Independent groups *t* test. A statistical test for comparing group means when people in the groups being compared are not the same and are independent (e.g., men versus women).

Independent variable. The variable that is the hypothesized cause of or influence on the dependent variable.

Indicator variable. A variable created by coding categorical variables into dichotomous variables, using codes of 0 and 1 to represent the presence or absence of an attribute (e.g., married = 1, not married = 0); also called a *dummy variable.*

Inferential statistics. Statistics that rely on the laws of probability to help researchers draw conclusions about whether relationships and characteristics observed in a sample are likely to occur in the population.

Intention-to-treat analysis. An approach to analyzing data from all subjects in a randomized controlled trial, regardless of whether or not they dropped out of the study, to ensure the integrity of random assignment.

Interaction effect. The effect of two or more independent variables acting in combination (interactively) on a dependent variable.

Intercept. The point at which a regression line intercepts (crosses) the Y axis when the value on the X axis is zero; also called the *constant* and often symbolized as *a.*

Internal consistency reliability. The type of reliability that concerns the degree to which the subparts of an instrument (e.g., items) are all measuring the same attribute or construct.

Internal validity. The degree to which it can be inferred that an observed outcome was *caused by* a treatment or independent variable, rather than by uncontrolled extraneous factors.

Interquartile range (*IQR*). A measure of variability, indicating the difference between Q_3 (the third quartile or 75th percentile) and Q_1 (the first quartile or 25th percentile); used in the construction of box plots.

Interrater reliability. A coefficient indicating agreement between raters, i.e., the extent to which the ratings of two independent raters or observers are intercorrelated.

Interval estimation. A statistical estimation approach in which the researcher uses sample data to establish a range of values that are likely, within a given level of confidence, to contain the true population parameter; the smaller the interval, the more precise the estimate.

Interval measurement. A level of measurement that involves assigning numbers to indicate both the ordering on an attribute and the distance between different amounts of the attribute.

Inverse relationship. A negative relationship between two variables; i.e., a relationship characterized by the tendency of high values on one variable to be associated with low values on the second.

Item reversal. In scoring scales, the process of reversing the direction of the scoring on certain items, often by subtracting the value of the item from 1 plus the item's maximum value.

Kaiser-Meyer-Olkin (KMO) test. A test used to assess the sampling adequacy of variables in a factor analysis, and is a means of determining the factorability of a set of variables; the closer the value of the KMO statistic is to 1, the greater the factorability.

Kendall's tau. A correlation coefficient used to indicate the magnitude of a relationship between variables measured on an ordinal scale.

Known-groups technique. A technique for assessing the construct validity of an instrument through a test of whether the instrument differentiates groups expected to differ on the construct, based on a theory or prior research evidence.

Kolmogorov-Smirnov test. A statistical test that evaluates the null hypothesis that a distribution of values in the population is normal.

Kruskal-Wallis test. A nonparametric test used to test differences between three or more independent groups, based on ranked scores.

Kurtosis. An aspect of the shape of a frequency distribution, referring to how pointed or flat its peak is.

Last observation carried forward (LOCF). An approach to imputing missing values for outcomes in a clinical trial that involves replacing missing values with a person's obtained values on the same outcome at the previous point of data collection.

Laws of probability. Established laws that stipulate the likelihood that a particular event or sequence of events will occur.

Least-squares criterion. The criterion used to estimate parameters in a model, such that the sum of the squared error terms is minimized; also called *ordinary least-squares* (OLS).

Leptokurtic distribution. A frequency distribution in which the peak is thin and pointed.

Level of measurement. A system of classifying measurements according to the nature of the measurement and the type of mathematical operations to which they are amenable; the four levels are nominal, ordinal, interval, and ratio.

Level of significance. The probability of making a Type I error, established by the researcher before the statistical analysis (e.g., the .05 level); symbolized as α, alpha.

Levene's test for equality of variances. A statistical test that tests the null hypothesis that the variances of groups being compared are equal in the population.

Likelihood index. An index used in logistic regression, indicating the probability of the observed results given the parameters estimated from the analysis; typically shown as -2 times the log of the likelihood ($-2LL$).

Likelihood ratio test. A test that can be used to evaluate the overall model in logistic regression, or to test improvement between models when predictors are added; computed by subtracting $-2LL$ for the larger model from $-2LL$ for the reduced model, resulting in a statistic distributed as a chi-square; also called a goodness-of-fit test.

Line graph. A graph used for plotting values over time, in which values are connected by a line.

Linear model. The general equation describing a straight line (that is, $Y = a + bX$).

Linear relationship. A relation between two continuous variables such that when data values are plotted in a scatter-plot, a straight line is formed.

Listwise deletion. A method of dealing with missing values in a dataset, involving the elimination of cases with missing data; also called a method of *complete case analysis*.

Loading. Coefficients summarizing the correlation between original variables and scores on linear composites (e.g., factors, canonical variate scores or discriminant scores); sometimes called *structure coefficients*.

Logistic regression. A regression procedure that uses maximum likelihood estimation for analyzing relationships between independent variables and categorical (often dichotomous) dependent variables; also called *logit analysis*.

Logit. The natural log of the odds, used as the dependent variable in logistic regression; short for logistic probability unit.

Mahalanobis distance (D^2). A statistic that is a generalized measure of the distance between groups; used in stepwise discriminant analysis as a criterion for entering predictors.

Main effect. The simple effect of an independent variable on the dependent variable, independent of other factors in the analysis.

Mann-Whitney U test. A nonparametric test of the differences between two independent groups, based on ranked scores; the nonparametric analog of the independent sample t test.

MANCOVA. See *multivariate analysis of covariance*.

MANOVA. See *multivariate analysis of variance*.

Marginal frequencies. Frequencies summarizing one of the dimensions of a crosstabs table (a row or a column), so called because they are found in the margins of the table; sometimes called *marginals*.

Marker variable. In factor analysis, a variable that is highly correlated with only one factor and that helps to define the underlying meaning of the factor.

Matrix. A rectangular arrangement of numbers with m rows (representing one dimension) and n columns (representing another dimension), resulting in an $m \times n$ configuration; examples include a correlation matrix, data matrix, and factor matrix.

Matrix algebra. A branch of mathematics that deals with rules for adding, subtracting, multiplying, and dividing matrices.

Mauchly's test. A test of the assumption of sphericity in repeated measures analyses.

Maximum likelihood estimation. An estimation approach in which the estimators are ones that estimate the parameters most likely to have generated the observed measurements.

Maximum likelihood factoring method. A method of factor analysis that uses maximum likelihood criteria in estimating parameters.

McNemar test. A nonparametric test for comparing differences in proportions when the values are derived from paired (dependent) groups.

Mean. A descriptive statistic of central tendency, computed by summing all scores and dividing by the number of participants; for samples, symbolized as M or $\overline{X}$.

Mean square. In an ANOVA context, the term used to designate the variance, often abbreviated MS; calculated by dividing a sum of squares by its respective degrees of freedom.

Mean substitution. A technique for addressing missing data problems by substituting missing values on a variable with the mean for that variable.

Measurement. The assignment of numbers to objects to designate the quantity of an attribute, according to specified rules.

Median. A descriptive statistic of central tendency, representing the exact middle score or value in a distribution of scores; the value above and below which 50% of the scores lie; symbolized as Mdn.

Meta-analysis. A method of statistically integrating effect size indexes from multiple studies addressing the same or highly similar research question; a preeminent tool in evaluating evidence for evidence-based practice.

Missing at random (MAR). Values that are missing from a dataset such that missingness is unrelated to the value of the missing data, after controlling for another variable; that is, missingness is unrelated to the value of the missing data, but *is* related to values of other variables in the dataset.

Missing completely at random (MCAR). Values that are missing from a dataset such that missingness is unrelated either to the value of the missing data, or to the value of any other variable; the subsample with missing values is a totally random subset of the original sample.

Missing not at random (MNAR). Values that are missing from a dataset such that missingness *is* related to the value of the missing data and, usually, to values of other variables as well.

Missing values. Values missing from a dataset for some participants as a result of such factors as skipped questions, refusals, withdrawals from the study, failure to complete forms, or researcher error.

Mixed design. A design in which there is both a between-subjects factor (different people in different groups) and a within-subjects factor (same people at different times or in different conditions).

Modality. A characteristic of a frequency distribution describing the number of peaks or values with high frequencies.

Mode. A descriptive statistic that indicates the score or value that occurs most frequently in a distribution of scores.

Model. A symbolic representation of concepts or variables, and interrelationships among them; in statistics and mathematics, represented by an equation.

Multicollinearity. A term that describes a correlation matrix in which two or more independent variables are highly correlated with each other.

Multifactor ANOVA. An analysis of variance used to test the relationship between two or more independent variables and a dependent variable simultaneously.

Multimodal distribution. A frequency distribution with more than one peak (high frequency).

Multinomial logistic regression. A regression procedure that uses maximum likelihood estimation to analyze relationships between independent variables and categorical dependent variables with multiple categories.

Multiple comparison procedures. Statistical tests, normally applied after preliminary results indicate overall statistically significant group differences, that compare different pairs of groups; also called *post hoc tests*.

Multiple correlation coefficient. An index that summarizes the magnitude of the relationship between two or more independent variables and a dependent variable; symbolized as *R*.

Multiple imputation (MI). The gold standard approach for dealing with missing values, involving the imputation of multiple estimates of the missing value, which are ultimately pooled and averaged in estimating parameters.

Multiple regression analysis. A statistical procedure for predicting the value of a dependent value on the basis of two or more independent variables, using least-squares estimation.

Multivariate analysis of covariance (MANCOVA). A statistical procedure used to test the significance of differences between the means of two or more groups on two or more dependent variables, after controlling for one or more covariate.

Multivariate analysis of variance (MANOVA). A statistical procedure used to test the significance of differences between the means of two or more groups on two or more dependent variables, considered simultaneously.

Multivariate normal distribution. A distribution of several variables such that each variable and all linear combinations of the variables are normally distributed; multivariate normality is assumed for many multivariate statistical tests.

Multivariate statistics. Statistical procedures for analyzing the relationships among three or more variables simultaneously.

n. The symbol used to designate the number of participants in a subgroup or in a cell of a study (e.g., "each of the four groups had an *n* of 125, for a total *N* of 500").

N. The symbol used to designate the total number of people in a study (e.g., "the total *N* was 500").

Nagelkerke R^2. One of several pseudo R^2 statistics used as an overall effect size index in logistic regression, analogous to R^2 in least-squares multiple regression, but lacking the ability to truly capture the proportion of variance explained in the outcome variable.

Negative relationship. A relationship between two variables in which there is a tendency for higher values on one variable to be associated with lower values on the other; also called an *inverse relationship*.

Negatively skewed distribution. An asymmetrical distribution of values that has a disproportionately large number of cases with high values—i.e., values falling at the upper end of the distribution; when displayed graphically, the tail points to the left.

Net effect. The effect of an independent variable on a dependent variable, after controlling for the effect of one or more covariate through multiple regression or ANCOVA.

Nominal measurement. The lowest level of measurement, involving the assignment of characteristics into categories (e.g., females, category 1; males, category 2).

Nondirectional hypothesis. A research hypothesis that does not stipulate in advance the direction and nature of the relationship between variables.

Nonparametric statistical. A general class of inferential statistical tests that does not involve rigorous assumptions about the distribution of the variables; most often used with small samples, when data are measured on the nominal or ordinal scales, or when a distribution is severely skewed.

Nonsignificant result. The result of a statistical test that indicates that the result could have occurred as a result of chance, given the researcher's level of significance; sometimes abbreviated as *NS* in research journals.

Normal distribution. A theoretical distribution that is unimodal, symmetric, and not too peaked or flat; also referred to as a *normal curve, bell-shaped curve*, or *Gaussian distribution*.

Null hypothesis (H_0). The hypothesis that states there is no relationship between the variables under study; used in connection with tests of statistical significance as the hypothesis to be rejected.

Number needed to treat (NNT). An estimate of how many people would need to receive an intervention to prevent one undesirable outcome, computed by dividing 1 by the value of the absolute risk reduction.

Oblique rotation. A rotation of factors in factor analysis such that the reference axes are allowed to move to acute or oblique angles, and hence factors are allowed to be correlated.

Odds. The ratio of two probabilities, namely the probability of an event occurring to the probability that it will not occur, calculated by dividing the number of people who experienced an event by the number for whom it did not occur.

Odds ratio (OR). The ratio of one odds to another odds, e.g., the ratio of the odds of an event in one group to the odds of an event in another group; used as a key risk index and, in logistic regression, as a measure of the effect of a predictor on the outcome, with other predictors controlled.

One-sample *t* test. The test used to evaluate the probability that the value of the sample mean equals the researcher's hypothesis about the population mean.

One-tailed test. A test of statistical significance in which only values at one extreme (tail) of a distribution are considered in determining significance; used when the researcher has predicted the direction of a relationship (i.e., posits a directional hypothesis).

One-way ANOVA. An analysis of variance used to test the relationship between a single independent variable involving three or more groups and a dependent variable.

Operational definition. The definition of a concept or variable in terms of procedures to be used to measure it.

Ordinal measurement. A level of measurement that yields an ordering of a variable along a specified dimension.

Ordinary least-squares (OLS) regression. Regression analysis that uses the least-squares criterion for estimating the parameters in the regression equation.

Orthogonal. A term used to describe variables (or factors) that are uncorrelated.

Orthogonal coding. A method of coding categorical variables in a regression analysis to make specific planned comparisons.

Orthogonal rotation. A rotation of factors in factor analysis such that the reference axes are kept at right angles, and hence the factors remain uncorrelated.

Outliers. Numerical values that are lie outside the normal range of values; by convention, a *mild outlier* is a value that lies between 1.5 and 3.0 times the interquartile range (IQR), below the first quartile (Q_1) or above the third quartile (Q_3); an extreme outlier is a value that is greater than 3.0 times the IQR, below Q_1 or above Q_3.

***p* value.** In statistical testing, the probability that the obtained results are due to chance; the probability of committing a Type I error.

Paired *t* test. A statistical test for comparing group means when people in the groups being compared are the same (e.g., before-after comparisons) or are paired (e.g., husbands and wives).

Pairwise deletion. A method of dealing with missing values in a dataset, involving the deletion of cases with missing data on a selective basis (i.e., deletion of a case only when one variable is paired with another variable that has missing data); also called a method of *available case analysis*.

Parameter. An index describing a characteristic of a population.

Parametric statistics. A class of inferential statistical tests that involves (a) assumptions about the distribution of the variables, (b) the estimation of a parameter, and usually (c) the use of interval or ratio measures.

Partial correlation. The correlation between a dependent variable (Y) and an independent variable (X_1) while controlling for the effect of a third variable (X_2); symbolized as $r_{y1 \cdot 2}$.

Partitioning variance. The process of dividing up the total variance in the dependent variable into its contributing components (e.g., between-groups variance versus within-groups variance).

Path analysis. A regression-based procedure for testing causal models, typically using nonexperimental data.

Pattern matrix. In factor analysis, the matrix that presents partial regression coefficients between variables and factors; in oblique rotation, the matrix used to interpret the meaning of the factors.

Pearson's *r*. The most widely used correlation coefficient, designating the magnitude and direction of a relationship between two variables measured on at least an interval scale; also called the *product-moment correlation*.

Percentage. The frequency of a given value, divided by the total number of observations, multiplied by 100.

Percentile. The value of a variable below which a certain percentage of observations fall (e.g., the 5th percentile is the score value below which 5% of the observations are found).

Perfect relationship. A relationship between two variables such that the values of one variable permit perfect prediction of the values of the other; indicated as 1.00 or -1.00.

Phi coefficient. An index describing the magnitude of the relationship between two dichotomous variables.

Pie chart. A graphic presentation that shows frequency distribution information in a circle, with "slices" of the pie representing the proportion for each category or score value; also known as a *circle graph*.

Pillai's trace criterion. A statistical index used in MANOVA and other multivariate tests to assess the significance of group differences.

Planned comparisons. Comparisons between group means in an ANOVA or regression analysis, for comparisons that are specified at the outset of the research.

Platykurtic distribution. A frequency distribution in which the peak is flat.

Point biserial correlation coefficient. An index of the magnitude and direction of the relationship between two variables, one of which is continuous and the other of which is dichotomous.

Point estimation. A statistical estimation procedure in which the researcher uses information from a sample to estimate a single statistic to best represent the value of the population parameter.

Pooled variance estimate. In *t* tests, the standard formula for estimating the standard error of the difference; used if the assumption of homogeneous variances is tenable or if sample sizes in the two groups are approximately equal.

Population. The entire set of individuals (or objects) having some common characteristic(s) (e.g., all AIDS patients in the United States).

Positive relationship. A relationship between two variables in which there is a tendency for high values on one variable to be associated with high values on the other.

Positively skewed distribution. An asymmetrical distribution of values that has a disproportionately large number of low values—i.e., values falling at the lower end of the distribution; when displayed graphically, the tail points to the right.

Post hoc test. A test for comparing all possible pairs of groups following a significant test of overall group differences (e.g., a significant ANOVA).

Power. The probability of correctly rejecting a false null hypothesis; power equals $1 - \beta$, the risk of a Type II error.

Power analysis. A procedure for estimating either (1) the sample size needed to minimize the risk of a Type II error; or (2) the power of a statistical test or, conversely, the likelihood of committing a Type II error.

Precision. The extent to which random errors have been reduced, usually expressed in terms of the width of the confidence interval around a parameter estimate.

Predictor variable. In correlational and regression analyses, the independent variable, used to predict the value of the dependent variable.

Principal components analysis (PCA). An analysis that is sometimes considered a type of factor analysis; PCA analyzes all variance in the observed variables, not just common factor variance.

Principal factors (PF) method. A method of factor analysis that analyzes only common factor variance, using estimates of the communality on the diagonal of the correlation matrix; sometime called *principal axis factoring*.

Probability distribution. A frequency distribution that displays all possible outcomes of some event, together with each of their probabilities; sometimes called a *probability density function* for continuous variables.

Product moment correlation coefficient (*r*). The most widely used correlation coefficient, designating the magnitude and direction of relationship between two variables measured on at least an interval scale; also referred to as *Pearson's r*.

Proportion. The frequency of a given value, divided by the total number of observations.

Protected *t* test. A post hoc test used following a significant ANOVA to test differences between all possible pairs of means; also known as *Fisher's LSD (least significant difference) test*.

Pseudo R^2. A type of statistic used to estimate the overall effect size in logistic regression, analogous to R^2 in least-squares multiple regression; the statistic should not be considered to indicate the proportion of variance explained in the outcome variable.

Qualitative data. Information that is in narrative (nonnumerical) form.

Qualitative variable. A variable measured on the nominal scale—i.e., a variable that conveys no quantitative information.

Quantitative analysis. The manipulation of numerical data through statistical procedures for the purpose of describing phenomena or assessing the magnitude and reliability of relationships among them.

Quantitative data. Information that is in a quantified (numerical) form.

Quantitative variable. A variable that conveys information about the amount of an attribute—i.e., a variable measured on the ordinal, interval, or ratio scale.

Quartile. Any of the three points (Q_1, Q_2, and Q_3) that divide a distribution into four parts, each containing one quarter of the distribution values; the first quartile (Q_1) is at the 25th percentile; the second quartile (Q_2) is at the 50th percentile, corresponding to the median; and the third quartile (Q_3) is at the 75th percentile.

***r*.** The symbol used to designate a bivariate correlation coefficient, summarizing the magnitude and direction of a relationship between two variables.

***r*-to-*z* transformation.** A logarithmic transformation of correlation coefficients to *z* scores that allows the use of the normal distribution for comparing correlation coefficients.

***R*.** The symbol used to designate the multiple correlation coefficient, indicating the magnitude (but not direction) of the relationship between the dependent variable and multiple independent variables, taken together.

R^2. The squared multiple correlation coefficient, indicating the proportion of variance in the dependent variable accounted for or explained by a group of independent variables; also called the *coefficient of determination*.

Random assignment. The assignment of participants to treatment conditions in a random manner (i.e., in a manner determined by chance alone); also known as *randomization*.

Random sample. A sample selected in such a way that each member of the population has an equal probability of being included.

Randomized block design. An experimental design involving random assignment to treatment groups within a "block" that is a nonexperimental factor (e.g., randomly assigning males and females separately to treatment conditions).

Range. A measure of variability, consisting of the difference between the highest and lowest values in a distribution.

Rank test. A type of statistical test that tests hypotheses about population group differences in terms of *locations* in a score distribution, based on their ranks.

Ratio measurement. A level of measurement with equal distances between score units, and that has a true meaningful zero point (e.g., weight in milligrams).

Raw data. The actual numerical values of collected data, prior to any transformations.

Real limits of a number. The points indicating half a measurement unit below the number (lower real limit) and half a measurement unit above the number (upper real limit).

Rectangular matrix. A matrix of data (variables × subjects) that contains no missing values for any of the variables.

Reference group. The omitted category in coding schemes for multivariate analyses, against which the effects for other categories are compared.

Regression. A statistical procedure for predicting values of a dependent variable based on the values of one or more independent variable.

Regression coefficient. The weight associated with an independent variable when predicting values of the dependent variable in regression analysis; also called a *b* weight.

Regression equation. The equation for the best fitting straight line to characterize the relationship between independent and dependent variables.

Regression imputation. An approach to imputing (estimating) a missing value by using multiple regression analysis to predict the missing value.

Relationship. A bond or association between two or more variables.

Relative frequency. The frequency of a given score value represented as a percentage (i.e., relative to other score values).

Relative risk (RR). The risk of an unfavorable event occurring given one condition, versus the risk of it occurring given another condition; computed by dividing the absolute risk for one group (e.g., an exposed group) by the absolute risk for another (e.g., the nonexposed); also called the *risk ratio*.

Relative risk reduction (RRR). The estimated proportion of baseline (untreated) risk that is reduced through exposure to the intervention, computed by dividing the absolute risk reduction (ARR) by the absolute risk for the control group.

Reliability. The degree of consistency or dependability with which an instrument measures the attribute it is designed to measure.

Reliability coefficient. A quantitative index, usually ranging in value from .00 to 1.00, that provides an estimate of how reliable or consistent an instrument is.

Repeated measures analysis of variance (RM-ANOVA). A statistical procedure for testing mean differences in a within-subjects design involving three or more conditions/observation periods or involving both within-subjects and between-subjects factors (i.e., a mixed design).

Research. Systematic inquiry that uses orderly scientific methods to answer questions or solve problems.

Research hypothesis. A researcher's prediction about variables being analyzed, typically regarding relationships between them.

Residual correlation matrix. In factor analysis, the correlation matrix that shows partial correlations between variables with the effects of factors removed.

Residual scatterplot. A scatterplot from a multivariate analysis that plots errors of prediction on one axis and predicted values of the dependent variable on the other.

Residuals. In multiple regression and other analyses, the error term or unexplained variance.

Results. The answers to research questions, obtained through an analysis of the collected data; in a quantitative study, the information obtained through statistical tests.

Robust. A characteristic of a statistical test that results in appropriate statistical decision making even when underlying assumptions have been violated.

Rotated factor matrix. A factor matrix (variables × factors) after the reference axes have been rotated in factor space.

Roy's largest root criterion (Ray's greatest characteristic root [gcr] criterion). A statistical index used in MANOVA and other multivariate tests to evaluate the significance of group differences.

Sample. A subset of a population selected to participate in a study.

Sampling distribution. A theoretical distribution of a statistic using an infinite number of samples as a basis and the values of the statistic computed from these samples as the data points in the distribution.

Sampling error. The error in the estimate of a population parameter when the estimate is based on only a portion of the population, i.e., a sample; the fluctuation of the value of a statistic from one sample from a population to another sample.

Scatterplot. A graph depicting the relationship between two continuous variables, with values of one variable on the X axis and values of the second variable on the Y axis.

Scheffé test. A post hoc test used following a significant ANOVA to test differences between all possible pairs of means; a conservative test that tends to err on the side of underestimating significance.

Scree test. One approach to deciding the appropriate number of factors in a factor analysis, which involves plotting eigenvalues against factors on a graph; discontinuities in the scree plot suggest where factoring should stop.

Selection bias. A threat to the internal validity of the study resulting from preexisting differences between the groups being compared.

Semipartial correlation. A correlation between two variables (Y and X_1) that partials out a third variable (X_2), but only from one of the variables being correlated; symbolized as $r_{y(2\cdot1)}$.

Separate variance estimate. In *t* tests, an alternative formula for estimating the standard error of the difference; used if the assumption of homogeneous variances is untenable or if sample sizes in the two groups are markedly unequal.

Significance level. The probability that an observed value or relationship could be the result of chance (i.e., the result of sampling error); significance at the .05 level indicates the probability that the observed values would be found by chance only five times out of 100.

Simultaneous multiple regression. A multiple regression analysis in which all predictor variables are entered into the equation simultaneously; sometimes called *direct* or *standard multiple regression*.

Singularity. A term that describes a correlation matrix in which two or more independent variables are perfectly correlated with each other.

Skewed distribution. A distribution of data values that is asymmetric, with the bulk of scores clustering at one end and a tail trailing off at the other end.

Slope. The rate at which a line rises across a horizontal distance; the steepness of a regression line, usually symbolized by *b* in a regression equation.

Spearman's rank-order correlation. A correlation coefficient indicating the magnitude and direction of a relationship between variables measured on the ordinal scale.

Sphericity. The assumption in repeated measures analyses that the variance of population difference scores for any two time periods is the same as the variance of population differences for any other two time periods.

Standard deviation. A descriptive statistic for measuring the degree of variability in a set of scores; an index of the average amount of deviation from the mean.

Standard error. The standard deviation of a sampling distribution (e.g., the *SD* of the sampling distribution of means is the *standard error of the mean,* abbreviated *SEM*).

Standard error of estimate. In regression analysis, the standard deviation of the errors from the regression line; used to indicate the accuracy of the predictions from regression.

Standard scores. Scores expressed in terms of standard deviations from the mean; raw scores typically are transformed to scores with a mean of zero and a standard deviation of one; sometimes called *z* scores.

Statistic. A descriptive index calculated from sample data as an estimate of a population parameter.

Statistical analysis. Mathematical methods for organizing, summarizing, and drawing conclusions about quantitative data using statistical procedures.

Statistical conclusion validity. The degree to which inferences about relationships and differences from statistical analysis of the data are accurate—i.e., free from Type I or Type II errors.

Statistical control. The use of statistical techniques to isolate or remove variance in the dependent variable that is associated with confounding variables, i.e., those extraneous to the analysis.

Statistical inference. The process of inferring attributes about the population based on information from a sample.

Statistical significance. A term indicating that the results obtained in an analysis of sample data are unlikely to have been the result of chance, at some specified level of probability.

Statistical test. An analytic procedure that allows a researcher to estimate the likelihood that obtained results from a sample reflect true population values, according to the laws of probability.

Stepdown analysis. A supplementary analysis used following a significant MANOVA to test the relative importance of the dependent variables in the analysis.

Stepwise multiple regression. A multiple regression analysis in which predictor variables are entered into the equation in steps, in the order in which the increment to *R* is greatest.

Structure coefficients. Coefficients summarizing the correlation between the original variables in the analysis and scores on linear composites (e.g., canonical variate scores or discriminant scores); also called *loadings*.

Structure matrix. The matrix that contains the correlations between variables on the one hand and linear composites (factor scores, canonical variate scores, or discriminant scores) on the other hand.

Sum of squares. The sum of squared deviation scores, often abbreviated *SS*.

Suppression. A phenomenon that sometimes occurs in multiple regression when a variable obscures (suppresses) or alters a relationship between other variables because of overlapping variability.

Symmetric distribution. A distribution of values that has two halves that are mirror images of the each other; a distribution that is not skewed.

t **distribution.** A family of theoretical probability distributions used in hypothesis testing, similar to the normal distribution in that *t* distributions are unimodal, symmetrical, and bell shaped.

t **test.** A parametric statistical test, most often used for analyzing the difference between two means (the two-sample *t* test).

Test for dependent groups. The class of statistical tests used for within-subjects (or matched-subjects) designs.

Test for independent groups. The class of statistical tests used to compare independent groups, i.e., for between-subjects designs.

Test statistic. A statistic computed to evaluate the statistical reliability of relationships between variables observed in a sample; the sampling distributions of test statistics are known for circumstances in which the null hypothesis is true.

Test-retest reliability. Assessment of the stability of an instrument by correlating the scores obtained on two separate administrations.

Tolerance. A statistical index used to detect multicollinearity among independent variables, computed by regressing each independent variable on other independent variables, and subtracting the resulting R^2 from 1.00.

True score. A hypothetical score that would be obtained if it were possible to measure a construct with no measurement error.

Tukey's honestly significant different (HSD) test. A post hoc test used following a significant ANOVA to test differences between all possible pairs of means.

Two-tailed test. A test of statistical significance in which values at both extremes (tails) of a distribution are considered in determining significance; used when the researcher has not predicted the direction of a relationship, but also the usual default in statistical testing.

Two-way ANOVA. An analysis of variance used to test the relationship between two independent variables and a dependent variable simultaneously.

Type I error. An error created by rejecting the null hypothesis when it is true (i.e., the researcher concludes that a relationship exists when in fact it does not); a false positive result.

Type II error. An error created by accepting the null hypothesis when it is false (i.e., the researcher concludes that *no* relationship exists when in fact it does); a false negative result.

Type III sum of squares. The most popular option for calculating sums of squares within the general linear model; this sum of squares is calculated by comparing the full model, to the full model without the variable of interest and so it represents the additional variability explained by adding the variable of interest.

Unimodal distribution. A distribution of values with one peak (high frequency).

Univariate statistics. Statistical procedures for analyzing a single variable at a time.

Unrotated factor matrix. A factor matrix (variables × factors) produced through factor extraction, prior to having the reference axes rotated in factor space.

Validity. A quality criterion referring to the degree to which inferences made in a study are accurate and trustworthy; in a measurement context, the degree to which an instrument measures what it is intended to measure.

Variability. The degree to which values on a variable in a set of scores are spread out or dispersed.

Variable. An attribute of a person or object that varies (i.e., takes on different values).

Variance. A measure of variability or dispersion, equal to the square of the standard deviation.

Variance–covariance matrix. A square matrix with the variances of variables on the diagonal and the covariance of pairs of variables on the off-diagonal.

Variance ratio. An approach to evaluating the homogeneity of variance assumption in many statistical tests, involving computing the ratio of variances for the groups with the highest and lowest variability; if the ratio is less than 2, homogeneity of variances can be assumed; an alternative to Levene's test.

Varimax rotation. In factor analysis, the most commonly used method of orthogonal rotation of factors following factor extraction.

Wald statistic. A statistic, distributed as a chi-square, used to evaluate the significance of individual predictors in a logistic regression equation.

Wilcoxon signed-ranks test. A nonparametric statistical test for comparing two paired groups, based on the relative ranking of values between the pairs.

Wild code. A code that is inconsistent with the coding scheme established by the researcher.

Wilks' lambda. An index used in several multivariate analyses to test the significance of group differences; indicates the proportion of variance in the dependent variable *un*accounted for by predictors.

Within-subjects test. A type of statistical test used when a single group of people is compared under different conditions or at different points in time, or when related groups of people are compared; also called a *test for dependent groups*.

X axis. The horizontal dimension of a two-dimensional graph; also known as the *abscissa*.

Y axis. The vertical dimension of a two-dimensional graph; also known as the *ordinate*.

Yates' correction. A correction to the chi-square statistic that is used when the expected frequency for any cell of a contingency table is less than 10.

z score. A standard score in a normal distribution, expressed in terms of standard deviations from the mean of zero.

Zero-order correlation. The bivariate correlation between two variables, without controlling or partialling out the effect of other variables.

APPENDIX A

Theoretical Sampling Distribution Tables

TABLE A.1 Areas of the Normal Distribution for Selected *z* Scores

Column (1):   *z* Score (or −*z*)

Column (2):   Probability of a value ⩾ *z*

               or

               Probability of a value ⩽ −*z*

Column (3):   Probability of a value ⩾ 0 and ⩽ *z*

               or

               Probability of a value ⩾ −*z* and ⩽ 0

(1) *z*	(2) ⩾ *z*	(3) ⩾ 0 and ⩽ *z*	(1) *z*	(2) ⩾ *z*	(3) ⩾ 0 and ⩽ *z*
0.00	.500	.000	1.10	.136	.364
0.05	.480	.020	1.20	.115	.385
0.10	.460	.040	1.30	.097	.403
0.15	.440	.060	1.40	.081	.419
0.20	.421	.079	1.50	.067	.433
0.25	.401	.099	1.60	.055	.445
0.30	.382	.118	1.70	.045	.455
0.35	.363	.137	1.80	.036	.464
0.40	.345	.155	1.90	.029	.471
0.45	.326	.174	1.96	.025	.474
0.50	.309	.192	2.00	.023	.477
0.55	.291	.209	2.10	.018	.482
0.60	.274	.226	2.20	.014	.486
0.65	.258	.242	2.30	.011	.489
0.70	.242	.258	2.40	.008	.492
0.75	.227	.273	2.50	.006	.494
0.80	.212	.288	2.58	.005	.495
0.85	.198	.302	2.60	.005	.495
0.90	.184	.316	2.70	.004	.496
0.95	.171	.329	2.80	.003	.497
1.00	.159	.341	2.90	.002	.498
			3.00	.001	.499

TABLE A.2 Critical Values for the *t* Distribution

df		.10	.05	.02	.01	.001
	Significance Level (α), Two-Tailed Test:	.10	.05	.02	.01	.001
	Significance Level (α), One-Tailed Test:	.05	.025	.01	.005	.0005
	Confidence Levels for *CI*s:	90%	95%	98%	99%	99.9%
1		6.31	12.71	31.82	63.66	636.62
2		2.92	4.30	6.97	9.93	31.60
3		2.35	3.18	4.54	5.84	12.94
4		2.13	2.78	3.75	4.60	8.61
5		2.02	2.57	3.37	4.03	6.86
6		1.94	2.45	3.14	3.71	5.96
7		1.90	2.37	3.00	3.45	5.41
8		1.86	2.31	2.90	3.36	5.04
9		1.83	2.26	2.82	3.25	4.78
10		1.81	2.23	2.76	3.17	4.58
11		1.80	2.20	2.72	3.11	4.44
12		1.78	2.18	2.68	3.06	4.32
13		1.77	2.16	2.65	3.01	4.22
14		1.76	2.15	2.62	2.98	4.14
15		1.75	2.13	2.60	2.95	4.07
16		1.75	2.12	2.58	2.92	4.02
17		1.74	2.11	2.57	2.90	3.97
18		1.73	2.10	2.55	2.88	3.92
19		1.73	2.09	2.54	2.86	3.88
20		1.73	2.09	2.53	2.85	3.85
21		1.72	2.08	2.52	2.83	3.82
22		1.72	2.07	2.51	2.82	3.79
23		1.71	2.07	2.50	2.81	3.77
24		1.71	2.06	2.49	2.80	3.75
25		1.71	2.06	2.49	2.79	3.73
26		1.71	2.06	2.48	2.78	3.71
27		1.71	2.05	2.47	2.77	3.69
28		1.70	2.05	2.47	2.76	3.67
29		1.70	2.05	2.46	2.76	3.66
30		1.70	2.04	2.46	2.75	3.65
40		1.68	2.02	2.42	2.70	3.55
60		1.67	2.00	2.39	2.66	3.46
120		1.66	1.98	2.36	2.62	3.73
∞		1.65	1.96	2.33	2.58	3.29

TABLE A.3 Critical Values of F: $\alpha = .05$

$\dfrac{df_B \rightarrow}{df_W \downarrow}$	1	2	3	4	5	6	8	12	24	∞
1	161.4	199.5	215.7	224.6	230.2	234.0	238.9	243.9	249.0	254.3
2	18.51	19.00	19.16	19.25	19.30	19.33	19.37	19.41	19.45	19.50
3	10.13	9.55	9.28	9.12	9.01	8.94	8.84	8.74	8.64	8.53
4	7.71	6.94	6.59	6.39	6.26	6.16	6.04	5.91	5.77	5.63
5	6.61	5.79	5.41	5.19	5.05	4.95	4.82	4.68	4.53	4.26
6	5.99	5.14	4.76	4.53	4.39	4.28	4.15	4.00	3.84	3.67
7	5.59	4.74	4.35	4.12	3.97	3.87	3.73	3.57	3.41	3.23
8	5.32	4.46	4.07	3.84	3.69	3.58	3.44	3.28	3.12	2.93
9	5.12	4.26	3.86	3.63	3.48	3.37	3.23	3.07	2.90	2.71
10	4.96	4.10	3.71	3.48	3.33	3.22	3.07	2.91	2.74	2.54
11	4.84	3.98	3.59	3.36	3.20	3.09	2.95	2.79	2.61	2.40
12	4.75	3.88	3.49	3.26	3.11	3.00	2.85	2.69	2.50	2.30
13	4.67	3.80	3.41	3.18	3.02	2.92	2.77	2.60	2.42	2.21
14	4.60	3.74	3.34	3.11	2.96	2.85	2.70	2.53	2.35	2.13
15	4.54	3.68	3.29	3.06	2.90	2.79	2.64	2.48	2.29	2.07
16	4.49	3.63	3.24	3.01	2.85	2.74	2.59	2.42	2.24	2.01
17	4.45	3.59	3.20	2.96	2.81	2.70	2.55	2.38	2.19	1.96
18	4.41	3.55	3.16	2.93	2.77	2.66	2.51	2.34	2.15	1.92
19	4.38	3.52	3.13	2.90	2.74	2.63	2.48	2.31	2.11	1.88
20	4.35	3.49	3.10	2.87	2.71	2.60	2.45	2.28	2.08	1.84
21	4.32	3.47	3.07	2.84	2.68	2.57	2.42	2.25	2.05	1.81
22	4.30	3.44	3.05	2.82	2.66	2.55	2.40	2.23	2.03	1.78
23	4.28	3.42	3.03	2.80	2.64	2.53	2.38	2.20	2.00	1.76
24	4.26	3.40	3.01	2.78	2.62	2.51	2.36	2.18	1.98	1.73
25	4.24	3.38	2.99	2.76	2.60	2.49	2.34	2.16	1.96	1.71
26	4.22	3.37	2.98	2.74	2.59	2.47	2.32	2.15	1.95	1.69
27	4.21	3.35	2.96	2.73	2.57	2.46	2.30	2.13	1.93	1.67
28	4.20	3.34	2.95	2.71	2.56	2.44	2.29	2.12	1.91	1.65
29	4.18	3.33	2.93	2.70	2.54	2.43	2.28	2.10	1.90	1.64
30	4.17	3.32	2.92	2.69	2.53	2.42	2.27	2.09	1.89	1.62
40	4.08	3.23	2.84	2.61	2.45	2.34	2.18	2.00	1.79	1.51
60	4.00	3.15	2.76	2.52	2.37	2.25	2.10	1.92	1.70	1.39
120	3.92	3.07	2.68	2.45	2.29	2.17	2.02	1.83	1.61	1.25
∞	3.84	2.99	2.60	2.37	2.21	2.09	1.94	1.75	1.52	1.00

df_B (df between) = Number of groups $- 1$
df_W (df within) = $N -$ Number of groups

(Continued)

TABLE A.3 Critical Values of F: $\alpha = .01$ *(Continued)*

$\frac{df_B \rightarrow}{df_W \downarrow}$	1	2	3	4	5	6	8	12	24	∞
1	4052	4999	5403	5625	5764	5859	5981	6106	6234	6366
2	98.49	99.00	99.17	99.25	99.30	99.33	99.36	99.42	99.46	99.50
3	34.12	30.81	29.46	28.71	28.24	27.91	27.49	27.05	26.60	26.12
4	21.20	18.00	16.69	15.98	15.52	15.21	14.80	14.37	13.93	13.46
5	16.26	13.27	12.06	11.39	10.97	10.67	10.29	9.89	9.47	9.02
6	13.74	10.92	9.78	9.15	8.75	8.47	8.10	7.72	7.31	6.88
7	12.25	9.55	8.45	7.85	7.46	7.19	6.84	6.47	6.07	5.65
8	11.26	8.65	7.59	7.01	6.63	6.37	6.03	5.67	5.28	4.86
9	10.56	8.02	6.99	6.42	6.06	5.80	5.47	5.11	4.73	4.31
10	10.04	7.56	6.55	5.99	5.64	5.39	5.06	4.71	4.33	3.91
11	9.65	7.20	6.22	5.67	5.32	5.07	4.74	4.40	4.02	3.60
12	9.33	6.93	5.95	5.41	5.06	4.82	4.50	4.16	3.78	3.36
13	9.07	6.70	5.74	5.20	4.86	4.62	4.30	3.96	3.59	3.16
14	8.86	6.51	5.56	5.03	4.69	4.46	4.14	3.80	3.43	3.00
15	8.68	6.36	5.42	4.89	4.56	4.32	4.00	3.67	3.29	2.87
16	8.53	6.23	5.29	4.77	4.44	4.20	3.89	3.55	3.18	2.75
17	8.40	6.11	5.18	4.67	4.34	4.10	3.79	3.45	3.08	2.65
18	8.28	6.01	5.09	4.58	4.25	4.01	3.71	3.37	3.00	2.57
19	8.18	5.93	5.01	4.50	4.17	3.94	3.63	3.30	2.92	2.49
20	8.10	5.85	4.94	4.43	4.10	3.87	3.56	3.23	2.86	2.42
21	8.02	5.78	4.87	4.37	4.04	3.81	3.51	3.17	2.80	2.36
22	7.94	5.72	4.82	4.31	3.99	3.76	3.45	3.12	2.75	2.31
23	7.88	5.66	4.76	4.26	3.94	3.71	3.41	3.07	2.70	2.26
24	7.82	5.61	4.72	4.22	3.90	3.67	3.36	3.03	2.66	2.21
25	7.77	5.57	4.68	4.18	3.86	3.63	3.32	2.99	2.62	2.17
26	7.72	5.53	4.64	4.14	3.82	3.59	3.29	2.96	2.58	2.13
27	7.68	5.49	4.60	4.11	3.78	3.56	3.26	2.93	2.55	2.10
28	7.64	5.45	4.57	4.07	3.75	3.53	3.23	2.90	2.52	2.06
29	7.60	5.42	4.54	4.04	3.73	3.50	3.20	2.87	2.49	2.03
30	7.56	5.39	4.51	4.02	3.70	3.47	3.17	2.84	2.47	2.01
40	7.31	5.18	4.31	3.83	3.51	3.29	2.99	2.66	2.29	1.80
60	7.08	4.98	4.13	3.65	3.34	3.12	2.82	2.50	2.12	1.60
120	6.85	4.79	3.95	3.48	3.17	2.96	2.66	2.34	1.95	1.38
∞	6.64	4.60	3.78	3.32	3.02	2.80	2.51	2.18	1.79	1.00

df_B (df between) = Number of groups − 1

df_W (df within) = N − Number of groups

TABLE A.3 Critical Values of *F:* α = .001 *(Continued)*

$df_B \rightarrow$ $df_W \downarrow$	1	2	3	4	5	6	8	12	24	∞
1	405284	500000	540379	562500	576405	585937	598144	610667	623497	636619
2	998.5	999.0	999.2	999.2	999.3	999.3	999.4	999.4	999.5	999.5
3	167.5	148.5	141.1	137.1	134.6	132.8	130.6	128.3	125.9	123.5
4	74.14	61.25	56.18	53.44	51.71	50.53	49.00	47.41	45.77	44.05
5	47.04	36.61	33.20	31.09	29.75	28.84	27.64	26.42	25.14	23.78
6	35.51	27.00	23.70	21.90	20.81	20.03	19.03	17.99	16.89	15.75
7	29.22	21.69	18.77	17.19	16.21	15.52	14.63	13.71	12.73	11.69
8	25.42	18.49	15.83	14.39	13.49	12.86	12.04	11.19	10.30	9.34
9	22.86	16.39	13.90	12.56	11.71	11.13	10.37	9.57	8.72	7.81
10	21.04	14.91	12.55	11.28	10.48	9.92	9.20	8.45	7.64	6.76
11	19.69	13.81	11.56	10.35	9.58	9.05	8.35	7.63	6.85	6.00
12	18.64	12.97	10.80	9.63	8.89	8.38	7.71	7.00	6.25	5.42
13	17.81	12.31	10.21	9.07	8.35	7.86	7.21	6.52	5.78	4.97
14	17.14	11.78	9.73	8.62	7.92	7.43	6.80	6.13	5.41	4.60
15	16.59	11.34	9.34	8.25	7.57	7.09	6.47	5.81	5.10	4.31
16	16.12	10.97	9.00	7.94	7.27	6.81	6.19	5.55	4.85	4.06
17	15.72	10.66	8.73	7.68	7.02	6.56	5.96	5.32	4.63	3.85
18	15.38	10.39	8.49	7.46	6.81	6.35	5.76	5.13	4.45	3.67
19	15.08	10.16	8.28	7.26	6.61	6.18	5.59	4.97	4.29	3.52
20	14.82	9.95	8.10	7.10	6.46	6.02	5.44	4.82	4.15	3.38
21	14.59	9.77	7.94	6.95	6.32	5.88	5.31	4.70	4.03	3.26
22	14.38	9.61	7.80	6.81	6.19	5.76	5.19	4.58	3.92	3.15
23	14.19	9.47	7.67	6.69	6.08	5.65	5.09	4.48	3.82	3.05
24	14.03	9.34	7.55	6.59	5.98	5.55	4.99	4.39	3.74	2.97
25	13.88	9.22	7.45	6.49	5.88	5.46	4.91	4.31	3.66	2.89
26	13.74	9.12	7.36	6.41	5.80	5.38	4.83	4.24	3.59	2.82
27	13.61	9.02	7.27	6.33	5.73	5.31	4.76	4.17	3.52	2.75
28	13.50	8.93	7.19	6.25	5.66	5.24	4.69	4.11	3.46	2.70
29	13.39	8.85	7.12	6.19	5.59	5.18	4.64	4.05	3.41	2.64
30	13.29	8.77	7.05	6.12	5.53	5.12	4.58	4.00	3.36	2.59
40	12.61	8.25	6.60	5.70	5.13	4.73	4.21	3.64	3.01	2.23
60	11.97	7.76	6.17	5.31	4.76	4.37	3.87	3.31	2.69	1.90
120	11.38	7.31	5.79	4.95	4.42	4.04	3.55	3.02	2.40	1.56
∞	10.83	6.91	5.42	4.62	4.10	3.74	3.27	2.74	2.13	1.00

df_B (*df* between) = Number of groups − 1

df_W (*df* within) = N − Number of groups

TABLE A.4 Critical Values of χ^2

			Level of Significance		
df	.10	.05	.02	.01	.001
1	2.71	3.84	5.41	6.63	10.83
2	4.61	5.99	7.82	9.21	13.82
3	6.25	7.82	9.84	11.34	16.27
4	7.78	9.49	11.67	13.28	18.46
5	9.24	11.07	13.39	15.09	20.52
6	10.64	12.59	15.03	16.81	22.46
7	12.02	14.07	16.62	18.48	24.32
8	13.36	15.51	18.17	20.09	26.12
9	14.68	16.92	19.68	21.67	27.88
10	15.99	18.31	21.16	23.21	29.59
11	17.28	19.68	22.62	24.72	31.26
12	18.55	21.03	24.05	26.22	32.91
13	19.81	22.36	25.47	27.69	34.53
14	21.06	23.68	26.87	29.14	36.12
15	22.31	25.00	28.26	30.58	37.70
16	23.54	26.30	29.63	32.00	39.25
17	24.77	27.59	31.00	33.41	40.79
18	25.99	28.87	32.35	34.81	42.31
19	27.20	30.14	33.69	36.19	43.82
20	28.41	31.41	35.02	37.57	45.32
21	29.62	32.67	36.34	38.93	46.80
22	30.81	33.92	37.66	40.29	48.27
23	32.01	35.17	38.97	41.64	49.73
24	33.20	36.42	40.27	42.98	51.18
25	34.38	37.65	41.57	44.31	52.62
26	35.56	38.89	42.86	45.64	54.05
27	36.74	40.11	44.14	46.96	55.48
28	37.92	41.34	45.42	48.28	56.89
29	39.09	42.56	46.69	49.59	58.30
30	40.26	43.77	47.96	50.89	59.70

TABLE A.5 Critical Values of the U Statistic (for $\alpha = .05$ Two-Tailed Test)

$n_1 \rightarrow$ $n_2 \downarrow$	1	2	3	4	5	6	7	8	9	10	11	12	13	14	15	16	17	18	19	20
1	—[a]	—	—	—	—	—	—	—	—	—	—	—	—	—	—	—	—	—	—	—
2	—	—	—	—	—	—	—	0	0	0	0	1	1	1	1	1	2	2	2	2
3	—	—	—	—	0	1	1	2	2	3	3	4	4	5	5	6	6	7	7	8
4	—	—	—	0	1	2	3	4	4	5	6	7	8	9	10	11	11	12	13	13
5	—	—	0	1	2	3	5	6	7	8	9	11	12	13	14	15	17	18	19	20
6	—	—	1	2	3	5	6	8	10	11	13	14	16	17	19	21	22	24	25	27
7	—	—	1	3	5	6	8	10	12	14	16	18	20	22	24	26	28	30	32	34
8	—	0	2	4	6	8	10	13	15	17	19	22	24	26	29	31	34	36	38	41
9	—	0	2	4	7	10	12	15	17	20	23	26	28	31	34	37	39	42	45	48
10	—	0	3	5	8	11	14	17	20	23	26	29	33	36	39	42	45	48	52	55
11	—	0	3	6	9	13	16	19	23	26	30	33	37	40	44	47	51	55	58	62
12	—	1	4	7	11	14	18	22	26	29	33	37	41	45	49	53	57	61	65	69
13	—	1	4	8	12	16	20	24	28	33	37	41	45	50	54	59	63	67	72	76
14	—	1	5	9	13	17	22	26	31	36	40	45	50	55	59	64	67	74	78	83
15	—	1	5	10	14	19	24	29	34	39	44	49	54	59	64	70	75	80	85	90
16	—	1	6	11	15	21	26	31	37	42	47	53	59	64	70	75	81	86	92	98
17	—	2	6	11	17	22	28	34	39	45	51	57	63	67	75	81	87	93	99	105
18	—	2	7	12	18	24	30	36	42	48	55	61	67	74	80	86	93	99	106	112
19	—	2	7	13	19	25	32	38	45	52	58	65	72	78	85	92	99	106	113	119
20	—	2	8	13	20	27	34	41	48	55	62	69	76	83	90	98	105	112	119	127

[a]A dash indicates that no decision is possible for the specified n.

NOTE: To be statistically significant, the calculated U must be *equal to or less than* the tabled value.

TABLE A.6 Critical Values of *r*

df 2-Tailed α: (1)	Level of Significance				
	.10 (2)	.05 (3)	.02 (4)	.01 (5)	.001 (6)
1	.988	.997	.9995	.9999	1.00
2	.900	.950	.980	.990	.999
3	.805	.878	.934	.959	.991
4	.729	.811	.882	.917	.974
5	.669	.754	.833	.874	.951
6	.622	.707	.789	.834	.925
7	.582	.666	.750	.798	.898
8	.549	.632	.716	.765	.872
9	.521	.602	.685	.735	.847
10	.497	.576	.658	.708	.823
11	.476	.553	.634	.684	.801
12	.458	.532	.612	.661	.780
13	.441	.514	.592	.641	.760
14	.426	.497	.574	.623	.742
15	.412	.482	.558	.606	.725
16	.400	.468	.542	.590	.708
17	.389	.456	.528	.575	.693
18	.378	.444	.516	.561	.679
19	.369	.433	.503	.549	.665
20	.360	.423	.492	.537	.652
25	.323	.381	.445	.487	.597
30	.296	.349	.409	.449	.554
35	.275	.325	.381	.418	.519
40	.257	.304	.358	.393	.490
45	.243	.288	.338	.372	.465
50	.231	.273	.322	.354	.443
60	.211	.250	.295	.325	.408
70	.195	.232	.274	.302	.380
80	.183	.217	.256	.283	.357
90	.173	.205	.242	.267	.338
100	.164	.195	.230	.254	.321
125	.147	.174	.206	.228	.288
150	.134	.159	.189	.208	.264
200	.116	.138	.164	.181	.235
300	.095	.113	.134	.148	.188
500	.074	.088	.104	.115	.148
1000	.052	.062	.073	.081	.104
2000	.037	.044	.056	.058	.074
df 1-Tailed α:	**.05**	**.025**	**.01**	**.005**	**.0005**

These are the critical values for testing the null hypothesis that $\rho = 0$

TABLE A.7 Transformation of r to z_r

r	z_r	r	z_r	r	z_r	r	z_r	r	z_r
.000	.000	.200	.203	.400	.424	.600	.693	.800	1.1099
.005	.005	.205	.208	.405	.430	.605	.701	.805	1.113
.010	.010	.210	.213	.410	.436	.610	.709	.810	1.127
.015	.015	.215	.218	.415	.442	.615	.717	.815	1.142
.020	.020	.220	.224	.420	.448	.620	.725	.820	1.157
.025	.025	.225	.229	.425	.454	.625	.733	.825	1.172
.030	.030	.230	.234	.430	.460	.630	.741	.830	1.188
.035	.035	.235	.239	.435	.466	.635	.750	.835	1.204
.040	.040	.240	.245	.440	.472	.640	.758	.840	1.221
.045	.045	.245	.250	.445	.478	.645	.767	.845	1.238
.050	.050	.250	.255	.450	.485	.650	.775	.850	1.256
.055	.055	.255	.261	.455	.491	.655	.784	.855	1.274
.060	.060	.260	.266	.460	.497	.660	.793	.860	1.293
.065	.065	.265	.271	.465	.504	.665	.802	.865	1.313
.070	.070	.270	.277	.470	.510	.670	.811	.870	1.333
.075	.075	.275	.282	.475	.517	.675	.820	.875	1.354
.080	.080	.280	.288	.480	.523	.680	.829	.880	1.376
.085	.085	.285	.293	.485	.530	.685	.838	.885	1.398
.090	.090	.290	.299	.490	.536	.690	.848	.890	1.422
.095	.095	.295	.304	.495	.543	.695	.858	.895	1.447
.100	.100	.300	.310	.500	.549	.700	.867	.900	1.472
.105	.105	.305	.315	.505	.556	.705	.877	.905	1.499
.110	.110	.310	.321	.510	.563	.710	.887	.910	1.528
.115	.116	.315	.326	.515	.570	.715	.897	.915	1.557
.120	.121	.320	.332	.520	.576	.720	.908	.920	1.589
.125	.126	.325	.337	.525	.583	.725	.918	.925	1.623
.130	.131	.330	.343	.530	.590	.730	.929	.930	1.658
.135	.136	.335	.348	.535	.597	.735	.940	.935	1.697
.140	.141	.340	.354	.540	.604	.740	.950	.940	1.738
.145	.146	.345	.360	.545	.611	.745	.962	.945	1.783
.150	.151	.350	.365	.550	.618	.750	.973	.950	1.832
.155	.156	.355	.371	.555	.626	.755	.984	.955	1.886
.160	.161	.360	.377	.560	.633	.760	.996	.960	1.946
.165	.167	.365	.383	.565	.640	.765	1.008	.965	2.014
.170	.172	.370	.388	.570	.648	.770	1.020	.970	2.092
.175	.177	.375	.394	.575	.655	.775	1.033	.975	2.185
.180	.182	.380	.400	.580	.662	.780	1.045	.980	2.298
.185	.187	.385	.406	.585	.670	.785	1.058	.985	2.443
.190	.192	.390	.412	.590	.678	.790	1.071	.990	2.647
.195	.198	.395	.418	.595	.685	.795	1.085	.995	2.994

TABLE A.8 Critical Values for Spearman's Rho (r_S), for $N = 5$ to 30

Test	Level of Significance			
N 2-Tailed α: (1)	.10 (2)	.05 (3)	.02 (4)	.01 (5)
5	.900	1.000	1.000	—
6	.829	.886	.943	1.000
7	.714	.786	.893	.929
8	.643	.738	.833	.881
9	.600	.683	.783	.833
10	.564	.648	.746	.794
12	.506	.591	.712	.777
14	.456	.544	.645	.715
16	.425	.506	.601	.665
18	.399	.475	.564	.625
20	.377	.450	.534	.591
22	.359	.428	.508	.562
24	.343	.409	.485	.537
25	.337	.398	.465	.510
26	.329	.392	.456	.515
28	.317	.377	.448	.496
30	.306	.363	.432	.467
N 1-Tailed α:	.05	.025	.01	.005

These are the critical values for testing the null hypothesis that $\rho_s = 0$; note that column 1 specifies the number of pairs of scores (N), not degrees of freedom. The critical values are both $+$ and $-$ for two-tailed tests.

APPENDIX B

Tables for Power Analyses

Table B.1   Power Table for d
Table B.2   Power Tables for One-Way Between-Groups ANOVA for $\alpha = .05$
Table B.3   Power Tables for One-Way Within-Groups (Repeated Measures) ANOVA for $\alpha = .05$
Table B.4   Power Tables for Chi-Square Tests as a Function of Population Values of Cramér's V ($\alpha = .05$)*

TABLE B.1 Power Table for d

Sample Size Estimates[a] to Achieve Specified Power, for Two Levels of Alpha for a Two-Tailed Test, for Various Effect Sizes (d) in a Two-Group Mean Situation

Cohen's d[b]	Power = .60		Power = .70		Power = .80		Power = .90	
	$\alpha = .10$	$\alpha = .05$	$\alpha = .10$	$\alpha = .05$	$\alpha = .10$	$\alpha = .05$	$\alpha = .10$	$\alpha = .05$
.05	2879	3915	3757	4929	4969	6304	6854	8409
.10	720	979	940	1233	1243	1576	1714	2103
.15	320	435	418	548	553	701	762	935
.20	180	245	235	309	311	394	429	526
.25	116	157	151	198	199	253	275	337
.30	80	109	105	137	139	176	191	234
.35	59	80	77	101	102	129	140	172
.40	45	62	59	78	78	99	108	132
.45	36	49	47	61	62	78	85	104
.50	29	40	38	50	50	64	69	85
.55	24	33	32	41	42	53	57	70
.60	20	28	27	35	35	44	48	59
.65	18	24	23	30	30	38	41	50
.70	15	20	20	26	26	33	35	43
.75	13	18	17	22	23	29	31	38
.80	12	16	15	20	20	25	27	33
.85	10	14	13	18	18	22	24	30
.90	9	13	12	16	16	20	22	26
1.00	8	10	10	13	13	16	18	22
1.10	6	9	8	11	11	14	15	18
1.25	5	7	7	8	8	11	11	14

[a]Sample size requirements are shown for **each group**; equal number of cases per group is assumed.

[b]The estimated effect size (d) is the estimated difference between the two population means, divided by the estimated population standard deviation, calculated with sample data as $d = (M_1 - M_2)/SD$.

TABLE B.2 Power Tables for One-Way Between-Groups ANOVA for α = .05

A. Number of Groups = 4[a]

Population Eta-Squared

POWER	.01	.03	.05	.07	.10	.15	.20	.25	.30	.40	.50	.60	.70	.80
.10	21	7	5	4	3	2	2	2	–	–	–	–	–	–
.50	144	48	28	20	14	9	7	5	4	3	2	2	2	–
.70	219	72	43	30	21	13	10	8	6	4	3	2	2	2
.80	272	90	53	37	26	17	12	9	7	5	4	3	2	2
.90	351	115	68	48	33	21	15	12	9	6	5	3	3	2
.95	426	140	83	58	40	25	18	14	11	7	5	4	3	2
.99	583	191	113	79	54	34	24	19	15	10	7	5	4	2

B. Number of Groups = 5

Population Eta-Squared

POWER	.01	.03	.05	.07	.10	.15	.20	.25	.30	.40	.50	.60	.70	.80
.10	19	7	5	3	3	2	2	2	–	–	–	–	–	–
.50	128	43	25	18	13	8	6	5	4	3	2	2	2	–
.70	193	64	38	27	18	12	9	7	6	4	3	2	2	2
.80	238	78	46	33	23	15	10	8	7	5	3	3	2	2
.90	306	101	59	42	29	18	13	10	8	6	4	3	2	2
.95	369	121	72	50	34	22	16	12	10	7	5	3	3	2
.99	501	164	97	68	46	30	21	16	13	9	6	4	3	2

C. Number of Groups = 6

Population Eta-Squared

POWER	.01	.03	.05	.07	.10	.15	.20	.25	.30	.40	.50	.60	.70	.80
.10	18	7	4	3	3	2	–	–	–	–	–	–	–	–
.50	117	39	23	17	12	8	6	5	4	3	2	2	2	–
.70	174	57	34	24	17	11	8	6	5	4	3	2	2	2
.80	213	70	42	29	20	13	9	7	6	4	3	2	2	2
.90	273	90	53	37	26	17	12	9	7	5	4	3	2	2
.95	328	108	64	45	31	20	14	11	9	6	4	3	3	2
.99	442	145	86	60	41	26	19	14	11	8	5	4	3	2

NOTE: Entries in body of table are for n, the number of participants *per group*.
[a]The power table for eta-squared for three groups is presented in the text as Table 7.5 on page 160.

TABLE B.3 Power Tables for One-Way Within-Groups (Repeated Measures) ANOVA for $\alpha = .05$

A. Number of Measurements = 3

Population Eta-Squared

POWER	.01	.03	.05	.07	.10	.15	.20	.25	.30	.40	.50	.60	.70	.80
.10	32	11	7	5	4	3	2	2	2	–	–	–	–	–
.50	247	81	48	34	23	15	11	8	7	5	3	2	2	2
.70	382	125	74	52	36	23	16	13	10	7	5	3	3	2
.80	478	157	93	65	44	28	20	15	12	8	6	4	3	2
.90	627	206	121	85	58	37	26	20	16	10	7	4	4	3
.95	765	251	148	104	70	45	32	24	19	13	9	5	4	3
.99	1060	347	204	143	97	62	44	33	26	17	12	7	6	4

B. Number of Measurements = 4

Population Eta-Squared

POWER	.01	.03	.05	.07	.10	.15	.20	.25	.30	.40	.50	.60	.70	.80
.10	27	9	6	4	3	2	2	2	2	–	–	–	–	–
.50	191	63	37	27	18	12	9	7	5	4	3	2	2	–
.70	291	96	57	40	27	18	13	10	8	5	4	3	2	2
.80	361	118	70	49	34	22	16	12	9	6	5	3	3	2
.90	469	154	91	64	44	28	20	15	12	8	6	4	3	2
.95	568	186	110	77	53	33	24	18	14	10	7	5	3	2
.99	777	254	150	105	72	45	32	25	19	13	9	6	4	3

C. Number of Measurements = 5

Population Eta-Squared

POWER	.01	.03	.05	.07	.10	.15	.20	.25	.30	.40	.50	.60	.70	.80
.10	24	8	5	4	3	2	2	2	2	–	–	–	–	–
.50	160	53	31	22	15	10	7	6	5	3	3	2	2	–
.70	241	79	47	33	23	15	11	8	7	5	3	3	2	2
.80	291	98	58	41	28	18	13	10	8	5	4	3	2	2
.90	382	126	74	52	36	23	16	13	10	7	5	4	3	2
.95	461	151	89	63	43	27	20	15	12	8	6	4	3	2
.99	626	205	121	85	58	37	26	20	16	10	7	5	4	3

NOTE: Entries in body of table are for n, the number of participants *per group*.

TABLE B.4 Power Tables for Chi-Square Tests as a Function of Population Values of Cramér's *V* (α = .05)*

A. 2 × 2 Table

Population Value of Cramér's *V* Statistic

POWER	.10	.20	.30	.40	.50	.60	.70	.80	.90
.25	165	41	18	10	7	5	3	3	2
.50	385	96	43	24	15	11	8	6	5
.60	490	122	54	31	20	14	10	8	6
.70	617	154	69	39	25	17	13	10	8
.80	785	196	87	49	31	22	16	12	10
.85	898	224	100	56	36	25	18	14	11
.90	1051	263	117	66	42	29	21	16	13
.95	1300	325	144	81	52	36	27	20	16
.99	1837	459	204	115	73	51	37	29	23

B. 2 × 3 Table

Population Value of Cramér's *V* Statistic

POWER	.10	.20	.30	.40	.50	.60	.70	.80	.90
.25	226	56	25	14	9	6	5	4	3
.50	496	124	55	31	20	14	10	8	6
.60	621	155	69	39	25	17	13	10	8
.70	770	193	86	48	31	21	16	12	10
.80	964	241	107	60	39	27	20	15	12
.85	1092	273	121	68	44	30	22	17	13
.90	1265	316	141	79	51	35	26	20	16
.95	1544	386	172	97	62	43	32	24	19
.99	2140	535	238	134	86	59	44	33	26

C. 2 × 4 Table

Population Value of Cramér's *V* Statistic

POWER	.10	.20	.30	.40	.50	.60	.70	.80	.90
.25	258	65	29	16	10	7	5	4	3
.50	576	144	64	36	23	16	12	9	7
.60	715	179	79	45	29	20	15	11	9
.70	879	220	98	55	35	24	18	14	11
.80	1090	273	121	68	44	30	22	17	13
.85	1230	308	137	77	49	34	25	19	15
.90	1417	354	157	89	57	39	29	22	17
.95	1717	429	191	107	69	48	35	27	21
.99	2352	588	261	147	94	65	48	37	29

*The entries are sample size requirements to achieve the specified power.

TABLE B.4 Power Tables for Chi-Square Tests as a Function of Population Values of Cramér's *V* (α = .05)*

D. 3 × 3 Table

Population Value of Cramér's *V* Statistic

POWER	.10	.20	.30	.40	.50	.60	.70	.80	.90
.25	154	39	17	10	6	4	3	2	2
.50	321	80	36	20	13	9	7	5	4
.60	396	99	44	25	16	11	8	6	5
.70	484	121	54	30	19	13	10	8	6
.80	536	134	60	34	21	15	11	8	7
.85	671	168	75	42	27	19	14	10	8
.90	770	193	86	48	31	21	16	12	10
.95	929	232	103	58	37	26	19	15	11
.99	1262	316	140	79	50	35	26	20	16

E. 3 × 4 Table

Population Value of Cramér's *V* Statistic

POWER	.10	.20	.30	.40	.50	.60	.70	.80	.90
.25	185	46	21	12	7	5	4	3	2
.50	375	94	42	23	15	10	8	6	5
.60	460	115	51	29	18	13	9	7	6
.70	557	139	62	35	22	15	11	9	7
.80	681	170	76	43	27	19	14	11	8
.85	763	191	85	48	31	21	16	12	9
.90	871	218	97	54	35	24	18	14	11
.95	1043	261	116	65	42	29	21	16	13
.99	1403	351	156	88	56	39	29	22	17

F. 4 × 4 Table

Population Value of Cramér's *V* Statistic

POWER	.10	.20	.30	.40	.50	.60	.70	.80	.90
.25	148	37	16	9	6	4	3	2	2
.50	294	73	33	18	12	8	6	5	4
.60	357	89	40	22	14	10	7	6	4
.70	430	107	48	27	17	12	9	7	5
.80	522	130	58	33	21	14	11	8	6
.85	582	145	65	36	23	16	12	9	7
.90	661	165	73	41	26	18	13	10	8
.95	786	197	87	49	31	22	16	12	10
.99	1046	262	116	65	42	29	21	16	13

*The entries are sample size requirements to achieve the specified power.

APPENDIX C

Answers to Exercises, Part A

CHAPTER 1

A1. a. Constant b. Variable c. Constant d. Variable

A2. a. Independent: Age; Dependent: Psychosocial adjustment

b. Independent: Handicap status; Dependent: Health self-concept

c. Independent: Self- versus nurse-administration of pain medication; Dependent: Pain rating

d. Independent: Presence versus absence of conversing visitors; Dependent: Intracranial pressure

e. Independent: Type of head covering; Dependent: Heat loss

A3. a. Discrete b. Continuous c. Discrete

d. Continuous e. Continuous

A4. a. Interval b. Ordinal c. Ratio

d. Interval (but might be considered ordinal)

e. Nominal f. Ordinal g. Nominal h. Ratio

CHAPTER 2

A1.

Number of Falls	f	%	Cum %
0	13	32.5	32.5
1	15	37.5	70.0
2	5	12.5	82.5
3	3	7.5	90.0
4	2	5.0	95.0
5	1	2.5	97.5
6	1	2.5	100.0
Total	40	100.0	

A2. a. 67.5% b. One fall c. Five and six falls

d. 82.5% e. Sample size = 40

f. There are no outliers, although it would perhaps be prudent to double check to see if the patients coded with five and six falls actually fell five/six times.

A4. The distribution is unimodal and positively skewed. The data are not normally distributed.

CHAPTER 3

A1. Mean = 30.37; median = 29.0; mode = 27. The mean is "off center," pulled slightly to the right, indicating that the distribution is positively skewed.

A2. a. 7 b. 7 c. 4 d. 5

A3. Distribution "c" has an extreme value (20) that would result in a distorted view of a "typical" value if the mean were used.

A4. Mean = 140.0; range = 60; $SD = 20.0$; variance = 400.0

A5.

Original	z Score	Transformed Standard Score
130	−0.5	450
120	−1.0	400
110	−1.5	350
150	+0.5	550
160	+1.0	600
140	0.0	500
120	−1.0	400
160	+1.0	600
170	+1.5	650
140	0.0	500

CHAPTER 4

A1.

	Experimental	Control	Total
Complied	9	5	14
	64.3% (Row)	35.7% (Row)	(100.0%)
	60.0% (Column)	33.3% (Column)	
Did not comply	6	10	16
	37.5% (Row)	62.5% (Row)	100.0%
	40.0% (Column)	66.7% (Column)	
Total	15	15	30
	100.0%	100.0%	100.0%

A2. a. The percentages shown are column percentages, i.e., within each sex group.

b. There are two infractions for which males committed fewer than 7.5% of the infractions, as determined through row percentages: working with a lapsed license (5.3% of all infractions) and providing care without a physician order (7.1%).

c. Among infractions listed in this table, male nurses were most markedly overrepresented, relative to their overall proportion among Missouri nurses, with regard to documentation errors (29.6% of all such infractions).

A3. AR_E = .30 (30.0%); AR_{NE} = .10 (10.0%); ARR = .20 (20.0%); RR = 3.0; RRR = 2.0; OR = 3.857; and NNT = 5.

A5. r = .91

CHAPTER 5

A1. The probability of drawing a spade (or a card of any particular suit): p = .25 (1 ÷ 4 suits). The probability of drawing five spades in a row: p = .0009765 ($.25^5$).

A3. The z scores for the four values = −0.5; +1.5; −2.0; +3.0

A4. The height is two *SD*s below the mean ($z = -2.00$), so $p = .023$ of randomly selecting a child whose height is lower than 50 inches tall.

A5. An *SEM* of 0.0 implies that all the sample means are equal to the population mean—there is no variability in any of the sample means as estimates of the population mean. This, in turn, implies the absence of variability of scores in the population, because under any other circumstance sampling error would result in some sample means being different from the population mean.

A6. With these values, mean = 5.0, $SD = 1.211$, and $SEM = 0.303$.

A7. The estimate for Sample B will likely be more accurate than that for Sample A. Given that the two populations have the same mean and *SD*, the *SEM* for Sample B will be smaller because the sample size is larger. Indeed, the estimated *SEM* for Sample A is 1.095 ($6.0 \div \sqrt{30}$), while that for sample B is .775 ($6.0 \div \sqrt{60}$).

A8. For the 95% *CI*, the confidence limits are 7.154 and 8.446. For the 99% *CI*, the confidence limits are wider: 6.941 and 8.659.

A9. The value of $t = 1.768$. According to Table A.2, the tabled value of *t* for $\alpha = .05$ with $df = 49$ is about 2.01. Therefore, the result is not statistically significant ($p > .05$). We cannot reject the null hypothesis that the average speed was 55 mph with a two-tailed test.

A10. The tabled value for a one-tailed test with $\alpha = .05$ and $df = 49$ is about 1.68, so the obtained result ($t = 1.768$) *is* statistically significant at the .05 level.

CHAPTER 6

A1. a. inappropriate—there are three groups, not two;

b. inappropriate—the dependent groups *t* test should be used because the parents are paired;

c. appropriate;

d. inappropriate—the DV is measured on the nominal scale;

e. inappropriate—the dependent groups *t* test should be used because it is the same people in both groups.

A2. a. appropriate, assuming the same people are used in both conversation conditions;

b. appropriate;

c. inappropriate—there are three time periods, not two;

d. inappropriate—the groups are independent (unless the data were collected longitudinally from the same people);

e. inappropriate—the DV is measured on the nominal scale.

A3. $t = 3.54$, $df = 48$, statistically significant at $\alpha = .05$

A5. $d = .91$, power is about .89, $\beta = .11$

A6. a. no;   b. yes;   c. yes;   d. yes

A7. a. about 2.02;   b. about 2.39;   c. 2.88;

d. about 1.66;   e. 2.81

A8. Power is approximately .61 and the risk of a Type II error is therefore about .39. To achieve the standard power criterion (.80), the sample should have 44 participants per group, assuming the effect size estimate is accurate.

A9. $t = 4.58$, $df = 9$, statistically significant at $\alpha = .05$ (tabled $t = 2.26$)

A10. Based on differences in sample size and variances, the separate variance estimate should be used; $t = -0.97$; with $df = 68$ this is nonsignificant at $\alpha = .05$ for a two-tailed test.

CHAPTER 7

A1. a. appropriate—one-way ANOVA;

b. appropriate—two-way (multifactor) ANOVA;

c. inappropriate—there are only two groups, an independent groups *t* test would be appropriate (although technically an *F* test *could* be used and would yield the same results);

d. inappropriate—there are only two paired groups, a dependent groups *t* test would be appropriate

e. appropriate—dependent variable is nominal level;

f. appropriate; if the same people were measured three times, RM-ANOVA; if the time-since-diagnosis groups are different people, one-way ANOVA

A2. The group means are: Nonsmokers = 21.0; Smokers = 26.0; Quitters = 35.0; the grand mean = 27.33; $SS_B = 503.33$, $SS_W = 222.00$; $df_B = 2$, $df_W = 12$; $MS_B = 251.67$, $MS_W = 18.50$; $F(2, 12) = 13.60$, significant at the .05 level.

A3. $t_{1\text{-}2} = 1.84$; $t_{1\text{-}3} = 5.15$; $t_{2\text{-}3} = 3.31$; $LSD = 5.93$. Quitters are significantly different from both nonsmokers and smokers. Smokers are not significantly different from nonsmokers.

A4. $n^2 = .69$; estimated power is greater than .99. There is a strong relationship between smoking status and somatic complaints, and the risk of a Type II error is negligible.

A6. a. not significant;   b. not significant;

c. significant;   d. significant;   e. not significant

A7. $MS_A = 74.50$; $MS_B = 37.00$; $MS_{AB} = 54.00$; $MS_W = 13.49$; $F_A = 5.52$; $F_B = 2.74$; $F_{AB} = 4.00$. With $df = 1$ and 76 for all three tests, the tabled value of *F* is 3.96. Thus, the *F* tests for sex differences (Factor A) and for the interaction (AB) are both significant, but the *F* test for differences by exercise status is not.

A9. $df_{site} = 2$; $df_{error} = 28$; $MS_{site} = 8,996.50$; $MS_{error} = 1,726.75$; the computed value of *F* for within-subjects is 5.21. With $df = 2$ and 28, the tabled value of *F* at $\alpha = .05$ is 3.34. Thus, we reject the null hypothesis that the three site means are equal.

A10. a. 9   b. 20   c. 90   d. 15   e. 319

CHAPTER 8

A1. $\chi^2 = 16.66$, $df = 2$. The tabled value of χ^2 at $\alpha = .05$ is 5.99, so the results are statistically significant. Group B's rate of obtaining a flu shot is substantially higher than expected: The value of $(O - E)^2/E$ for that cell was 7.50.

A2. Cramér's $V = .24$. If the value of V were .20, power would be between .85 and .90 (i.e., for a sample size between 273 and 316). Since V is larger than .20, power in this case exceeds .90.

A4. a. no; b. yes; c. no; d. yes

A5. a. 106; b. 159; c. 151; d. 165

A6. 1. c; 2. d; 3. b; 4. a

A7. a. Mann-Whitney U test;

    b. Repeated measures ANOVA;

    c. Cochran's Q;

    d. Chi-square test for independence;

    e. Kruskal-Wallis test;

    f. McNemar's test

CHAPTER 9

A1. a. no; b. no; c. yes; d. yes; e. no

A2. a. .578; b. .109; c. .828; d. .020

A3. a. .81; b. .36; c. .54; d. .26

A4. a. r likely would get smaller;

    b. r likely would get larger;

    c. r likely would get larger

A5. $a = 9.8$; $Y' = 9.8 - .10X$

A6. a. 4.6; b. 3.0; c. 7.5; d. 8.8

A7. Power is about .40, risk of Type II error, about .60

A8. About 200 participants

CHAPTER 10

A1. Student 19: $Y' = 3.004$, $e^2 = .009$; Student 20: $Y' = 3.397$, $e^2 = .041$

A2. a. $F(5, 114) = 25.73, p < .05$;

    b. $F(5, 24) = 5.41, p < .05$;

    c. $F(4, 59) = 5.74, p < .05$;

    d. $F(4, 59) = 2.40, p > .05$ (NS)

A3. a and c

A4. a. lowest $R^2 = .292$; b. VARA;

    c. Cannot readily be determined

A5. Male smokers = 1, female smokers = 0, male nonsmokers = 0, female nonsmokers = 0

A6. a. .04 to .40; b. .12 to .32; c. .09 to .35

A7. a. 61; b. 109; c. 141

CHAPTER 11

A1. a. Canonical analysis; b. two-way MANCOVA;

    c. mixed design RM-ANOVA; d. MANOVA;

    e. Discriminant analysis; f. ANCOVA

A3.

	Unadjusted Means	Adjusted Means
No insurance	17.96	16.63
Private insurance	24.33	25.49
Public health insurance	18.87	18.05

A4. To test for treatment effects in this RCT, we could use ANCOVA, using group as the independent variable, baseline scores as the covariate, and postintervention scores as the dependent variable. An RM-ANOVA also could be used, using group as the independent variable, and the baseline and postintervention scores as the dependent variables. Time of measurement would, in this case, be the within-subjects factor.

CHAPTER 12

A1. If the cut point were .40, 85% (rather than 80%) of the cases would be correctly classified: only one completer and two noncompleters would still be wrongly classified. Student 12, originally classified as a noncompleter when the cut point was .50, had a predicted probability of .45 and would thus now be properly classified as a completer.

A2. The equation for the logit is: $[\text{Prob}_{\text{TubalLigation}} \div \text{Prob}_{\text{NoTubalLigation}}] = -4.087 + .277X_{\text{Births}} + .074X_{\text{Age}} + .133X_{\text{Edstat1}} + .179X_{\text{Edstat2}} + .341X_{\text{Chdisabl}}$.

A4. Kanak and colleagues *could* have used the continuous variable for number of units during a hospitalization. The relationship between the logit and the predictor does appear to be fairly linear, with b coefficients declining incrementally as number of units declined—although we cannot tell if perhaps linearity ceased after five units. Their decision to use a four-category variable makes it easier to interpret the odds ratios for the effect of number of units at a glance and seems like a sensible strategy.

CHAPTER 13

A1. Item 7, absolute value = .167 (in actuality, loading was negative). This value was obtained by squaring the two loadings on item 7 shown in Figure 13.7, adding them together, subtracting the sum from the total communality of .528, then taking the square root. So, $.528 - (.491^2 + .509^2) = .0279$; the square root of $.0279 = .167$. Item 8, absolute value = .166 (this loading was also negative, although there would be no way to know this without seeing actual output).

A2. $2.955 \div 11 = 26.86$ (eigenvalue divided by number of components = % of variance)

A3. Factor I = 4.515 (.301 × 15 items); Factor II = 1.665 (.111 × 15 items); Factor III = 1.215 (.081 × 15 items)

A5. $Y = .10$; $X = .60$; test G is likely to be a quantitative aptitude test

CHAPTER 14

A1. 3.50; 1.17; 2.33; 3.33; and 2.33

A3. Using the guideline of not imputing more than 25% of missing items per case, a case with two of the seven items missing should probably not have imputed item values.

A4. 47.19; 53.94; 37.47; 46.43; and 41.05

INDEX

Note: Bolded page numbers are Glossary entries; page numbers followed by t indicate tables; page numbers followed by n indicate footnotes.

Multivariate Statistical Analyses

Name	Purpose	Measurement Level*			Number of Variables:			SPSS Commands
		IV	DV	Cov	IVs	DVs	Cov	
Multiple correlation/ regression	To test the relationship between 2+ IVs and 1 DV; to predict a DV from 2+ IVs	N,I,R	I,R	—	2+	1	—	Regression → Linear
Analysis of covariance (ANCOVA)	To test the difference between the means of 2+ groups, while controlling for 1+ covariate	N	I,R	N,I,R	1+	1	1+	General Linear Model → Univariate
Multivariate analysis of variance (MANOVA)	To test the difference between the means of 2+ groups for 2+ DVs simultaneously	N	I,R	—	1+	2+	—	General Linear Model → Multivariate
Multivariate analysis of covariance (MANCOVA)	To test the difference between the means of 2+ groups for 2+ DVs simultaneously, while controlling for 1+ covariate	N	I,R	N,I,R	1+	2+	1+	General Linear Model → Multivariate
Mixed design RM-ANOVA	To test differences between the means of 2+ independent groups (between subjects) at 2+ points in time (within subjects)	N	I, R	—	1+	1	—	General Linear Model → Repeated Measures
Canonical analysis	To test the relationship between 2 sets of variables (variables on the right, variables on the left)	N,I,R	N,I,R	—	2+	2+	—	**
Discriminant analysis	To test the relationship between 2+ IVs and 1 DV; to predict group membership; to classify cases into groups	N,I,R	N	—	2+	1	—	Classify → Discriminant
Logistic regression	To test the relationship between 2+ IVs and 1 DV; to predict the odds of an event or an outcome; to estimate relative risk	N,I,R	N	—	2+	1	—	Regression → Binary Logistic Regression
Factor analysis	To determine the dimensionality/structure of a set of variables	—	—	—	—	—	—	Data Reduction → Factor

*Measurement level of the independent variable (IV), dependent variable, (DV), and covariates (Cov):

N = nominal, I = interval, R = ratio

**SPSS requires complex syntax commands for canonical analysis